THE BONE BROTH BOOK

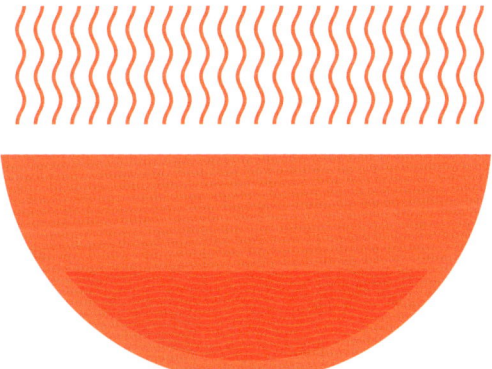

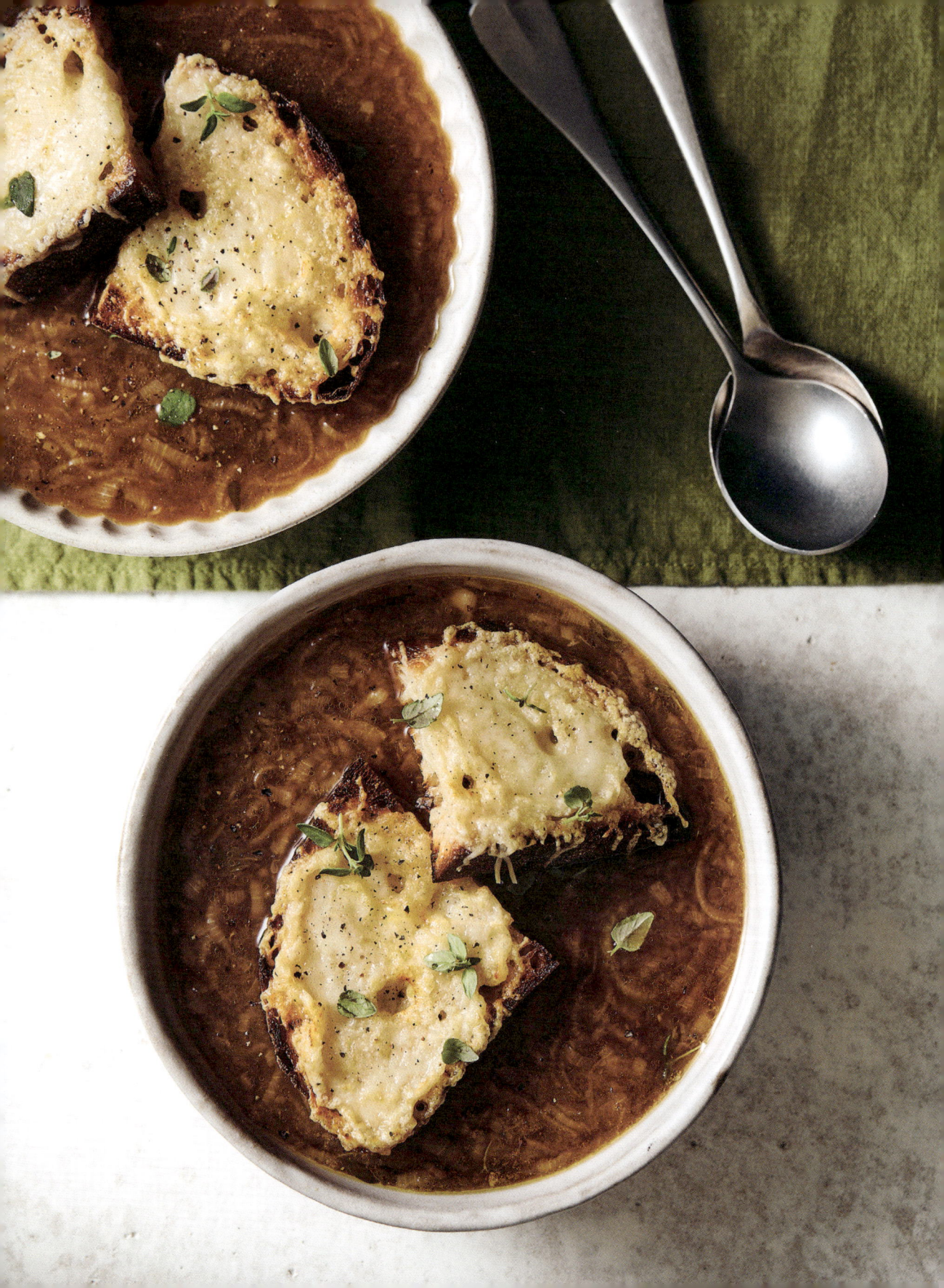

THE BONE BROTH BOOK

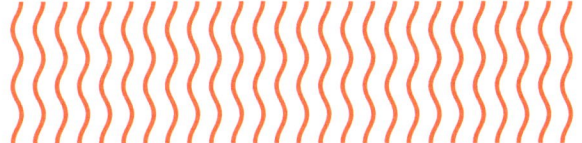

NOURISH YOURSELF NATURALLY WITH DELICIOUS, FEEL-GOOD RECIPES

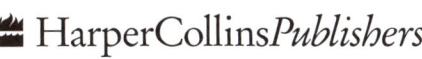   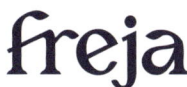

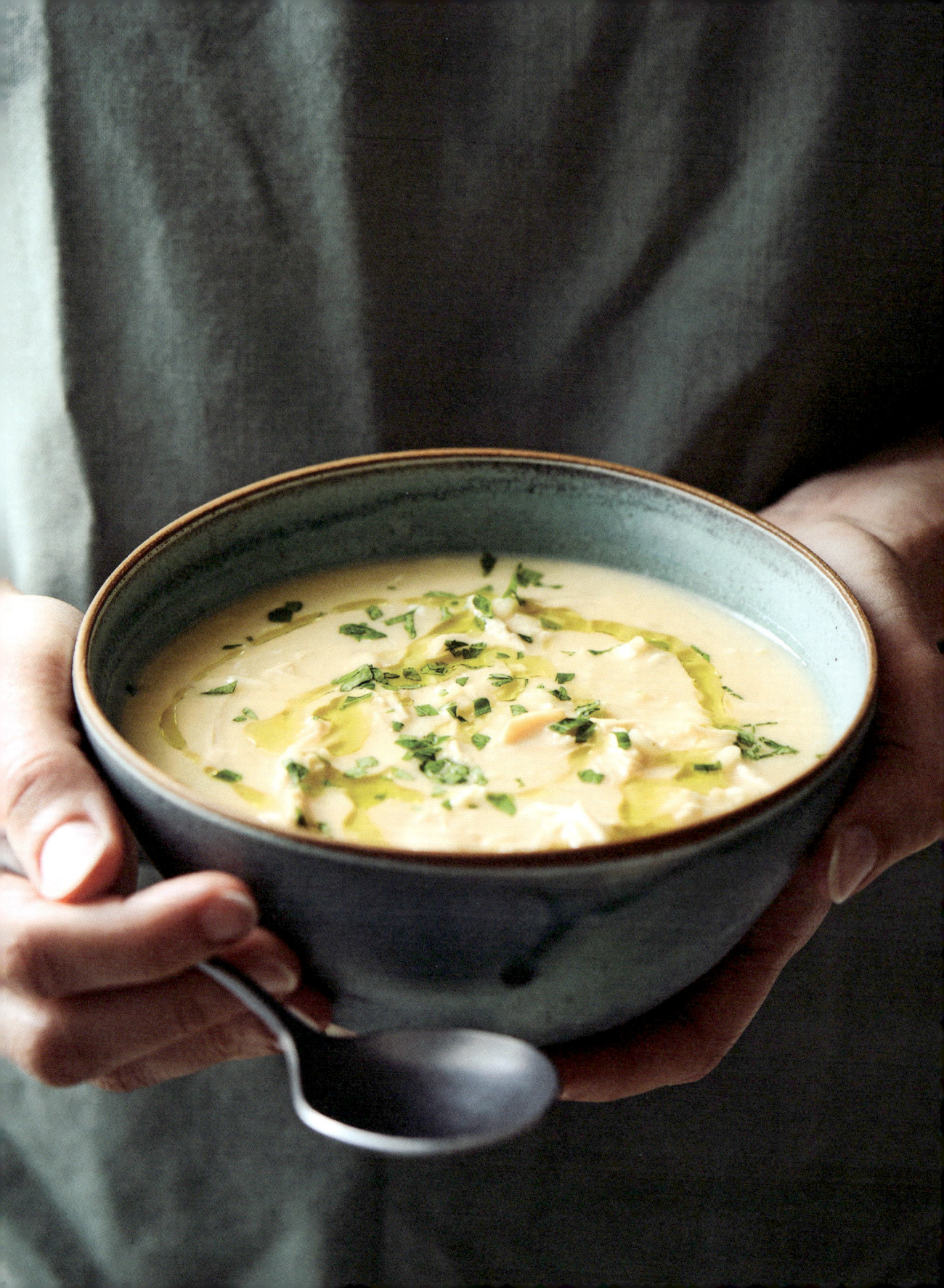

CONTENTS

Foreword	7
BONE BROTH: THE PHILOSOPHY	10
BONE BROTH: THE FOUNDATIONS	30
BONE BROTH: THE RECIPES	56
Sipping Broths	58
Brothy Soups	70
Blended Soups	88
Hearty Soups & Chowders	102
Brothy Vegetables	118
Rice, Grains & Pulses	134
Pasta & Noodles	156
Comfort Cooking	178
Bone-in Dishes	210
Broth Builder	224
References	226
Further Reading	227
Endnotes	228
Acknowledgements	229
Index	230
About Freja	238

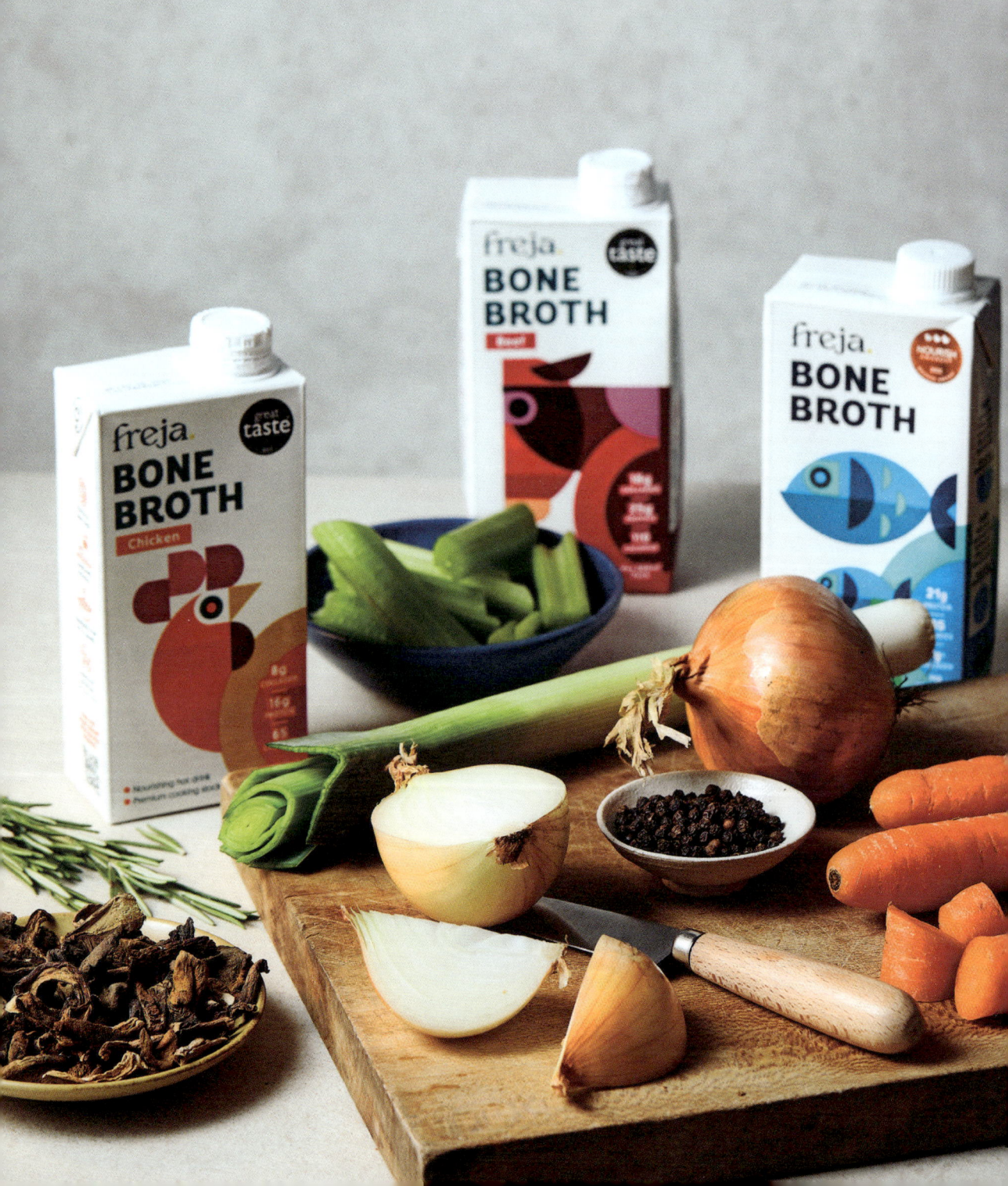

FOREWORD

There's nothing new about bone broth. Every culture has its version; every family has passed down a recipe. Broth has been both medicine and mealtime for generations. But somewhere along the way, it got lost in the noise of ultra-processed convenience and confusing nutrition advice.

When we first started selling bone broth from our kitchen table, recreating the bone-based stocks we enjoyed at home, we thought we were simply making a healthier, tastier, more natural alternative to stock cubes for those without the time, skills or access to ingredients to make it themselves.

We certainly didn't imagine we'd create a household brand or be at the forefront of a nutrition movement!

Soon after we launched Freja, we were flooded with inspiring customer reviews and messages, and we began to realise that bone broth meant so many different things to different people. For some, it was a shortcut to a childhood memory or a daily habit for gut health. For others, a postpartum nutritional essential or, in many cases, a core part of their toolkit for managing a chronic illness.

That's when we decided to give our recipe away. We didn't invent bone broth after all – it's a traditional, universal health food. And we'll always say homemade is best. Freja is just there for the days when you don't have time to simmer a stockpot for hours.

This book is an extension of that mission. Bringing together some of the ways we've come to enjoy bone broth in our own lives – on good days, tired days, slow Sundays and chaotic Wednesdays. From how to make your own from scratch to quick flavour boosts and more substantial meals, whether sipping bone broth in a mug, adding to a risotto or a five-minute noodle bowl – it's all here. From hearty Brazilian stews to classic French soups and light Keralan curries – these are all deliciously satisfying, wholesome recipes, with bone broth at their heart.

This isn't a brand book. It's not trying to sell you anything. It's a reminder of something that so often gets lost in everyday life: the power of real food, made with real ingredients, that tastes good and genuinely makes you feel better. This book is a return to common sense in a world that has made nutrition unnecessarily confusing. It's here to give you something useful. A new recipe. A new routine. Or maybe just the permission to slow down and stir up something delicious!

So, whether you're discovering bone broth for the first time or have been sipping it since childhood, we hope you find something in here that works for you.

Jess and the Freja team x

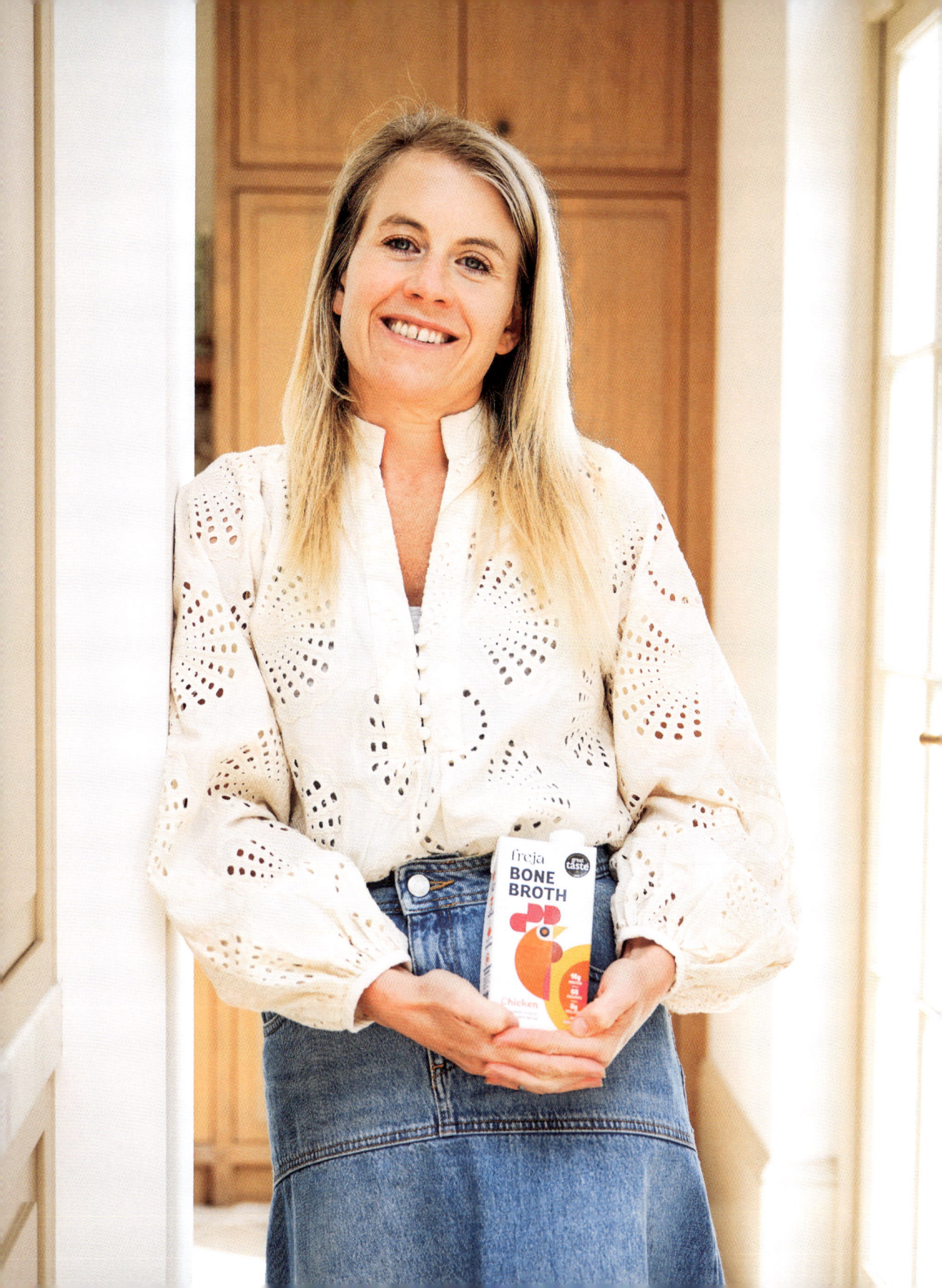

BONE BROTH: THE PHILOSOPHY

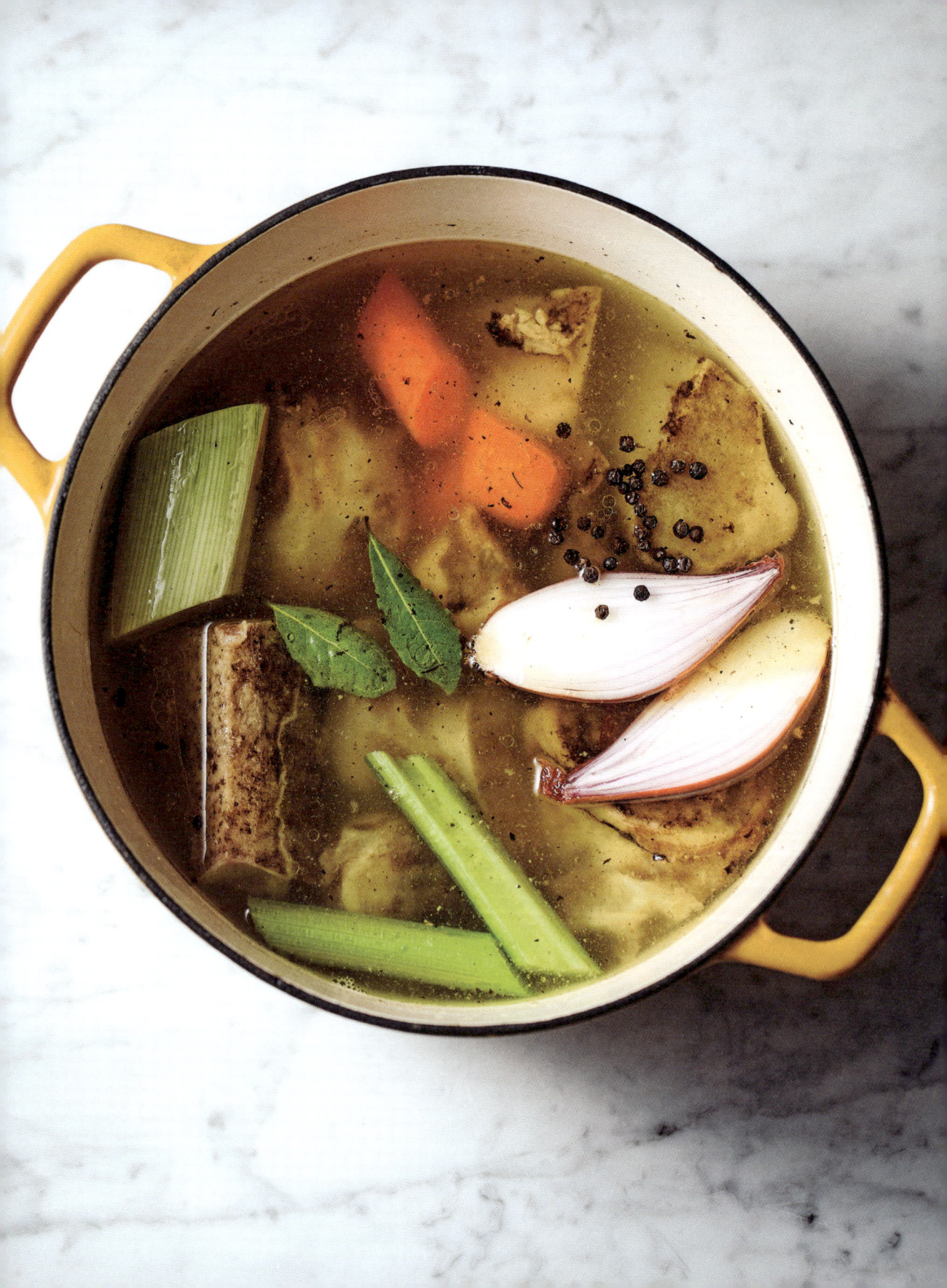

BONE BROTH 101: TIMELESS NOURISHMENT

We believe nourishing food shouldn't be hard to find, expensive to access or complicated to understand. It should be simple: rooted in tradition, yet convenient enough for modern living. We love bone broth because it embodies flavour and comfort, nourishment and nostalgia, food for both body and soul.

Bone broth is made by simmering bones for hours to extract their goodness, resulting in one of the most nutrient-dense foods you can find. That's why we often call it the *original* superfood!

What Makes Bone Broth So Special?

Bone broth has long been prized in traditional cultures, and for good reason. Slow cooking gently extracts protein, minerals, collagen, gelatine and amino acids that can be harder to find in many modern diets. These nutrients are present in forms the body can readily absorb, making bone broth an efficient way to add them to your diet. Let's take a closer look at this nutrient-rich staple.

Collagen: The Body's Glue

Collagen is the secret to a strong and flexible body, yet it's often lacking in modern diets. It accounts for around 30 per cent of the protein in the human body and is a key building block of skin, bones, joints, tendons and ligaments. Think of it as the body's glue! In fact, the word collagen comes from the Greek *kólla*, meaning 'glue', and *gen*, meaning 'producing'.

Your body produces its own collagen naturally, but production slows by roughly 1–1.5 per cent each year from early adulthood. Including bone broth in your diet can help provide collagen and its building blocks, keeping your joints healthy, your skin glowing and your gut happy.[1]

TYPES OF COLLAGEN

TYPE I: The most abundant, found in skin, bones, tendons, ligaments and organs, this is about 90 per cent of the body's collagen.

TYPE II: Builds cartilage, strengthens joints and keeps your eyes healthy.

TYPE III: Works alongside Type I to strengthen arteries and organs.

TYPE V: Supports healthy hair cell surfaces, and even the placenta during pregnancy.

Gelatine: The Jiggly Goodness

When broth is simmered slowly and steadily, collagen breaks down into gelatine. It's what gives broth its jelly-like jiggle once it has cooled, a sign it has been made the proper way. Gelatine contains the same amino acids as collagen; the protein structures are simply arranged differently.

Amino Acids: The Body's Building Blocks

ESSENTIAL AMINO ACIDS – THE ONES WE CAN'T MAKE

Essential amino acids (EAAs) are the nine building blocks of protein that our bodies can't produce, so we need to get them from our diet. They play critical roles in everything from muscle repair and immune function to hormone production. If you make broth using meaty bones rather than bare bones, you can obtain a complete amino acid profile, including the essential amino acid tryptophan, which is typically absent from processed collagen products. While bone broth isn't designed to replace complete protein foods like meat or eggs, it does contribute to your overall intake of these vital nutrients in a gentle, easy-to-digest form, making it kind on the body.

NON-ESSENTIAL AMINO ACIDS – COLLAGEN'S SIGNATURE STRENGTH

Non-essential amino acids can be produced by the body, but during times of stress, recovery, illness or pregnancy, demand often outpaces supply. Bone broth is naturally rich in certain non-essential (but incredibly important) amino acids like glycine and proline, thanks to its high collagen content. These amino acids are linked to joint health, skin elasticity, gut barrier support and the body's own collagen production. It's this unique profile that makes bone broth such a valuable addition to a varied diet.

Glycine – Small but Mighty: Glycine, the most abundant amino acid in collagen, is also the smallest, yet it plays an outsized role in the body. It supports healthy sleep, helps maintain the gut lining and aids digestion. Glycine is also involved in producing haemoglobin (the oxygen-carrying protein in red blood cells), creatine (for energy), bile salts (for fat digestion) and glutathione, often called the body's 'master antioxidant'. Its importance increases during times of stress, illness and pregnancy, when the body's demand can outpace supply.

Proline – Strong and Stable: Making up around 17 per cent of collagen, proline helps stabilise the collagen matrix, which is essential for strong, resilient tissues, from joints and skin to the gut lining. It also plays a role in wound healing and the body's own collagen production.

Glutamine – Your Gut's Best Friend: The most abundant amino acid in the bloodstream, glutamine can cross the blood-brain barrier and is a primary fuel source for intestinal cells. It supports gut barrier integrity and is especially useful for those with gut conditions such as IBS or Crohn's disease. Glutamine also teams up with glycine to produce glutathione, supporting detoxification and liver health.

PROTEOGLYCANS – YOUR JOINTS' BEST FRIEND

These water-loving molecules surround collagen in skin, cartilage and bones. One of the best known is hyaluronic acid (HA), which can hold up to one thousand times its weight in water, keeping joints cushioned and skin hydrated. Proteoglycans also contain glycosaminoglycans (GAGs) such as chondroitin and glucosamine, which are involved in maintaining cartilage and supporting gutlining health.

MIGHTY MINERALS

Bones are rich in minerals such as calcium, magnesium, iron and zinc, which support everything from nerve function and bone strength to hydration and immunity.

This is one of the reasons we see bone broth as foundational nourishment: it delivers a spectrum of nutrients that work together to support the body in countless ways. And unlike a supplement tablet or capsule, we're getting these amazing nutrients in a natural, whole-food form, making them easier for the body to absorb and generally gentler on the digestive system. It's time to bring bone broth back to the kitchen table.

Bone Broth vs Stock – What's the Difference?

As you can imagine, we get asked this a lot, and we get it: stock, broth, cubes... it can all feel a bit interchangeable. But there are some meaningful differences, especially if you're after something that does more than just taste nice.

Stock: Traditionally, stock is made by simmering meat and vegetables (sometimes with bones) for a few hours to extract flavour and create a base for soups, sauces or gravies. When done well, it's delicious and natural, although the short cooking time means it's primarily about flavour, not nutrition.

Bone broth: Bone broth, on the other hand, is simmered slowly over long periods using meaty bones as the main ingredient. This long, gentle cook extracts maximum nutrient content and gives a richer taste and a thicker, silkier texture. It draws out gelatine, protein, collagen, amino acids and minerals, turning it into something that's both comforting and nourishing.

You can generally use bone broth and stock interchangeably in recipes. We love the rich, hearty flavour and texture bone broth brings to dishes, which is far deeper and more substantial than most stock.

A word of warning: most commercially bought 'stock' is little more than water, salt and flavour enhancers, sometimes with added sugar or colourings. And don't mistake stock cubes for real stock! Stock cubes are often made from cheap industrial fats, starches and flavourings designed to imitate the taste of proper stock without offering the same benefits.

WHY COOK WITH BONE BROTH

Cooking with bone broth is a wonderful way to make meals tastier, more nourishing and more sustainable. It's versatile, helps reduce waste and connects us with traditional nose-to-tail cooking. What's not to love?

Nose-to-Tail

Our ancestors practised nose-to-tail eating, consuming all parts of the animal, including skin, cartilage, tendons and organs. Some anthropologists even believe early humans were scavengers, cracking open bones left by predators to get to the nutrient-rich marrow.

Nose-to-tail eating is everything we believe food should be: real, nourishing, respectful to the animal and better for the planet. It's how humans ate for millennia, and it's how our bodies evolved to feel our absolute best.

Why do we love this approach?

Nutrient-dense: Bones, marrow, organs, fat and skin are like the VIPs of nutrition, offering far more than muscle meat alone.

Nothing goes to waste: Turning bones into broth stretches your food further. It's budget-friendly and makes every meal count.

Respect for the animal: The practice of leaving nothing to waste honours the animal's life and the effort it took to raise it, a value understood by our hunter-gatherer ancestors as well as today's farmers.

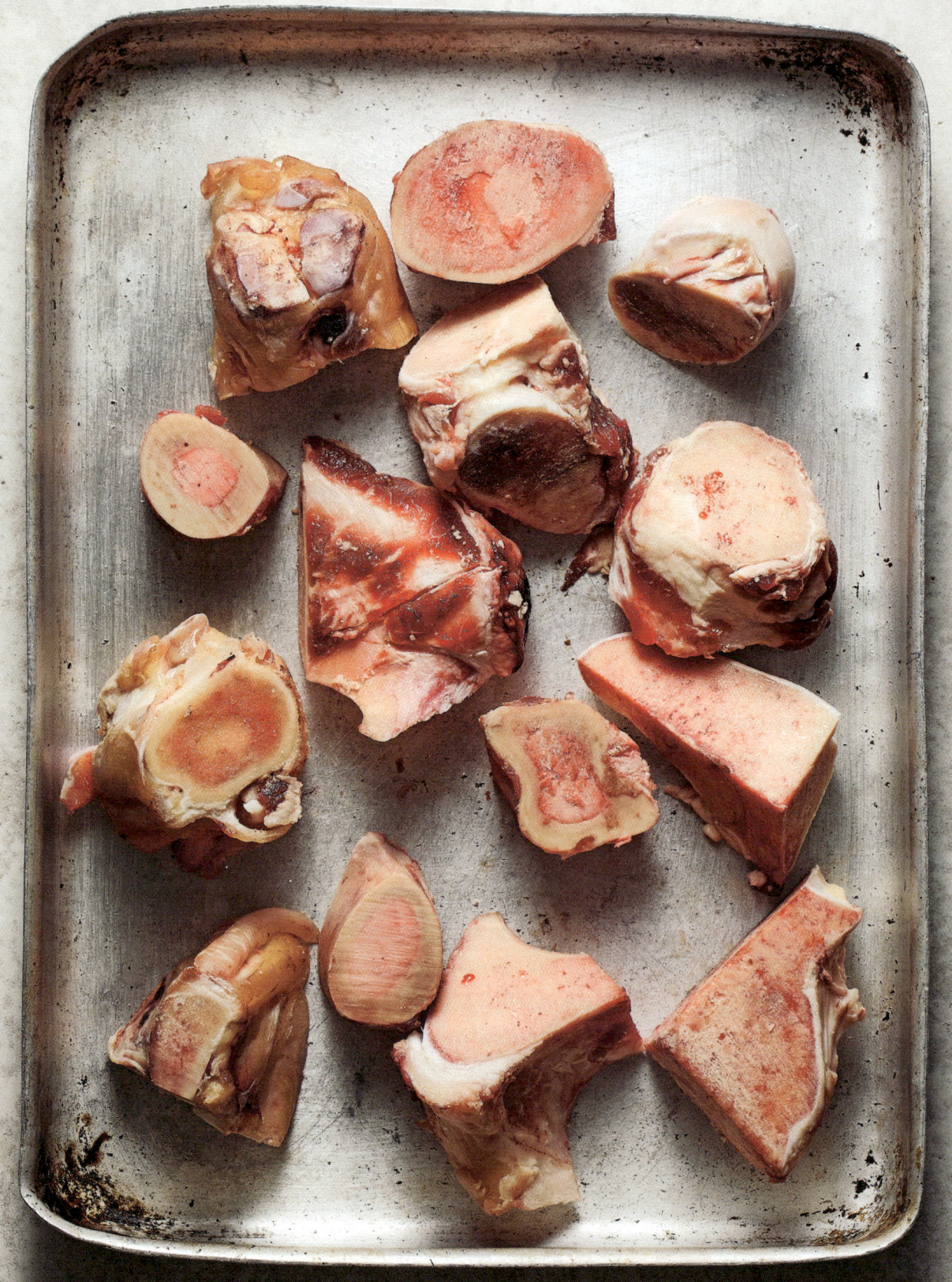

Turning Scraps into Magic

Some of our earliest memories are of childhood kitchens, filled with the rich, comforting smells coming from the simmering stockpot. Nothing was wasted; leftover bones from a roast were carefully saved and considered valuable for the next meal. Vegetable trimmings like onion skins or carrot tops, that might otherwise be discarded, were tossed into the pot, turning scraps into deep, rich flavour.

We still always try to reduce waste in our kitchen. Bone broth, in its very essence, is about minimising waste and making the most of what we already have. It's a simple way to connect us to sustainable eating.

We always look for bones from sustainably raised animals on natural diets. This isn't just better for our health, it's better for the planet. Grass-fed livestock farming is often linked with regenerative agriculture – farming methods that improve soil health and increase biodiversity. By supporting farmers who engage in these practices, we're not only ensuring that the bones we use come from healthy, well-raised animals, but we're also contributing to a farming system that replenishes, rather than depletes, our resources.

Year-Round Eating

Do you consider bone broth a traditionally wintery food? You're not alone. But we want to change that narrative – in fact it's packed with nutrients that our bodies crave all year round. It works as a base for all types of warm-weather recipes, from pastas and salad dressings to chilled soups and ramen.

And don't forget, bone broth is incredibly hydrating! Remember those mighty minerals? When present in your broth they help the body retain fluids, which is especially valuable during warmer months.

A Friend for Flexitarians

Bone broth can turn a simple veggie dish into something hearty, comforting and nourishing, without moving plants out of the spotlight. Flexitarians often tell us that bone broth is their secret weapon to extra nutrition.

Its savoury, umami flavour means a little goes a long way – you don't need a lot to get the benefits of collagen and amino acids like glycine and glutamine, which are hard to find in plant-based foods. Cooking rice, quinoa or lentils in broth instead of water boosts nutrients, adds depth of flavour, and can make plant proteins easier to digest. The long simmering process softens plant proteins, while the gelatine-rich liquid adds complementary amino acids to support the digestive system.

Just cook your rice or pasta as you would normally, but replace the water with bone broth. If there's any broth left over once the ingredient is cooked, you can add it to any accompanying sauces or save it for future dishes.

Make Bone Broth Part of Your Every Day

Looking to add more bone broth to your diet? There are so many easy, delicious ways to enjoy it. We love starting the morning with a warm mug of broth instead of coffee or sipping it at night to wind down. Try adding garlic, ginger or turmeric for a boost, or spice things up with sliced chillies and a dash of sriracha – there are countless combinations to try out.

Bone broth also makes a rich base for soups and stews, or a flavour-packed addition to sauces and gravies. Wherever a recipe calls for a stock cube, you can easily swap in bone broth for deeper flavour and extra nourishment.

Whether you're a committed nose-to-tail eater or a curious flexitarian, bone broth will support and enhance both the taste and the nutrition of your dishes. It's a simple, tasty way to connect with the cooking traditions of the past, and a sustainable choice that supports the way we want to eat today.

Sipping as a Daily Ritual

Remember Bovril? Not so long ago, sipping a warm, savoury drink like bone broth was an everyday habit for many people. Far from strange, it was a comforting tradition and a simple way to add nourishment to your day.

Bringing back this practice can be as easy as keeping a batch of broth in the fridge or freezer, ready to heat and sip whenever you need a pick-me-up. See pages 60–69 for more ideas on making sipping broth part of your routine.

THE WORLD'S ORIGINAL COMFORT FOOD

The origins of broth date back to the Stone Age, when hot stones were dropped into containers of water, meat, fat and bones to create an early form of 'stone soup'. Broth, in some form, has been a staple in many traditional cultures, and its influence remains strong today. However, many modern cultures seem to have lost the tradition of nourishing, slow-cooked broth and stock in favour of quick, convenient stock cubes and ready-made soups. These quick options may be easy, but they lack the depth, nutrition and comfort of a pot simmered low and slow. We're on a mission to bring it back.

Bone Broth Around the World

Every corner of the globe has its own love affair with bone broth. Across cultures, it has been valued for its flavour, nourishing qualities and the simple resourcefulness of using every part of an animal. In many traditions, it's even seen as medicinal – a tonic for recovery, digestion and strength.

Bone broth is the base for so many classic dishes around the world. Every culture has its own version; every family has its own recipe. Local ingredients, climate and culinary heritage have inspired endless variations on this time-honoured staple. Let's explore some of these well-loved and traditional recipes from across the globe…

ASIA: NOURISHMENT FOR BODY AND SOUL

In much of East Asia, bone broth has been a cornerstone of culinary and medicinal traditions for centuries. Known as 'long-simmered soup' or 'tonic soup', ancient Chinese traditions believed bone broth harnessed the essence of the bones and imparted their healing properties into the broth.

It is still revered today for its ability to boost energy, support digestion and promote overall wellbeing. From fragrant Vietnamese Phở to rich

Japanese Ramen, Asian bone broth recipes are as plentiful and varied as they are beloved, and many have found a permanent place on Western tables, in bustling restaurants and home kitchens alike.

EUROPEAN CULTURES

In France, broth forms the base of much classic French cooking, used in sauces, soups (e.g. consommé) and stews. Stocks made from veal, beef or chicken bones are simmered with mirepoix (carrots, celery, onions) to create rich flavours.

In Slavic cultures, bone-based soups like Russian Borscht or Polish Żurek often start with beef or pork bone broth, incorporating scraps to maximise ingredients, especially in resource-scarce times.

SCANDINAVIA: SUSTENANCE IN HARSH CLIMATES

In the cold Nordic climates, bone broth has played a vital role in traditional diets. Reindeer and fish were commonly used to create nutrient-dense and robust broths. Often infused with juniper berries, bay leaves and root vegetables, Scandinavian bone broth provided a delicious and warming base still seen in recipes today.

Finland's traditional fish soup – Lohikeitto – is made from a blend of fish bone broth, aromatic herbs like dill and hearty vegetables, and is a comforting and nourishing dish ideal for the long winter evenings.

INDIGENOUS AND NATIVE AMERICAN CULTURES

Many Indigenous groups in North America made broth from game animal bones (e.g. deer, bison), often combining them with foraged herbs or roots. The broth was used in stews or drunk for warmth and sustenance, reflecting a nose-to-tail philosophy that honoured the animal.

INDIA: SPICED AND FLAVOURFUL

Bone broth holds a special place in Indian cuisine, appearing in traditional dishes like Paya (a spicy trotter soup) and Yakhni (a fragrant mutton-based broth). These broths are richly seasoned with a blend of aromatic spices such as turmeric, cumin, cloves, caraway and ginger, creating deep, complex flavours that are both comforting and vibrant.

These broths are prized in Ayurvedic practice for their potential health benefits, including digestive support and nourishment. Bone broth also serves as a versatile base, adding richness and depth to a variety of dishes, including creamy, hearty daals, which are staples in many Indian households.

AFRICAN CULTURES

In West Africa, bone broth is used in stews and soups like Egusi or Pepper Soup, made from goat, cow or fish bones. It's a way to stretch limited resources and add nourishment to communal meals.

CENTRAL AND SOUTH AMERICA: RICH AND HEARTY

In South America, bone broth is a fundamental element of traditional cooking. In Mexico, 'caldo' refers to a variety of soups enriched with bone broth. In other South American countries like Peru, you'll find Chupe de Camarones, a shrimp and vegetable soup enriched with bone broth.

MIDDLE EAST: A NOURISHING BASE

In Middle Eastern cookery, bone broth plays an integral role, celebrated for its deep flavours and nutritional significance. A slow-cooked broth known as 'Shorba' is the key base in dishes like rice pilafs, nourishing stews and soups. In Middle Eastern households, this cherished liquid remains a symbol of hospitality and nourishment.

How We Lost the Tradition (and Why We're Bringing It Back)

In the early 1900s, the introduction of MSG (monosodium glutamate) and the stock cube to everyday cooking meant that the rich flavour of broth could be mimicked in a fraction of the time. Suddenly, convenience took priority over sustenance, and quick, easy meals like tinned soup replaced the slow-simmered stockpots in most homes. While these quick fixes were cheap and accessible, they were missing all the good stuff, stripping away the slow-cooked proteins, collagen, and minerals that gave traditional broth its depth and nutrition.

Now bone broth is making a comeback. It's the real deal, and we're all about bringing that slow-simmered goodness back to our kitchen, and to yours!

Bone broth is the basis of how we've eaten all over the world for centuries, but we're living in a world that's swapped traditional wisdom for convenience. While the nourishing stockpot simmering on the hearth has been replaced by processed soups and cubes, we are confident we can make bone broth, this incredible foundational food, a household staple again. The kitchen is the hub of the home, so let's bring the stockpot back as the hub of the modern kitchen!

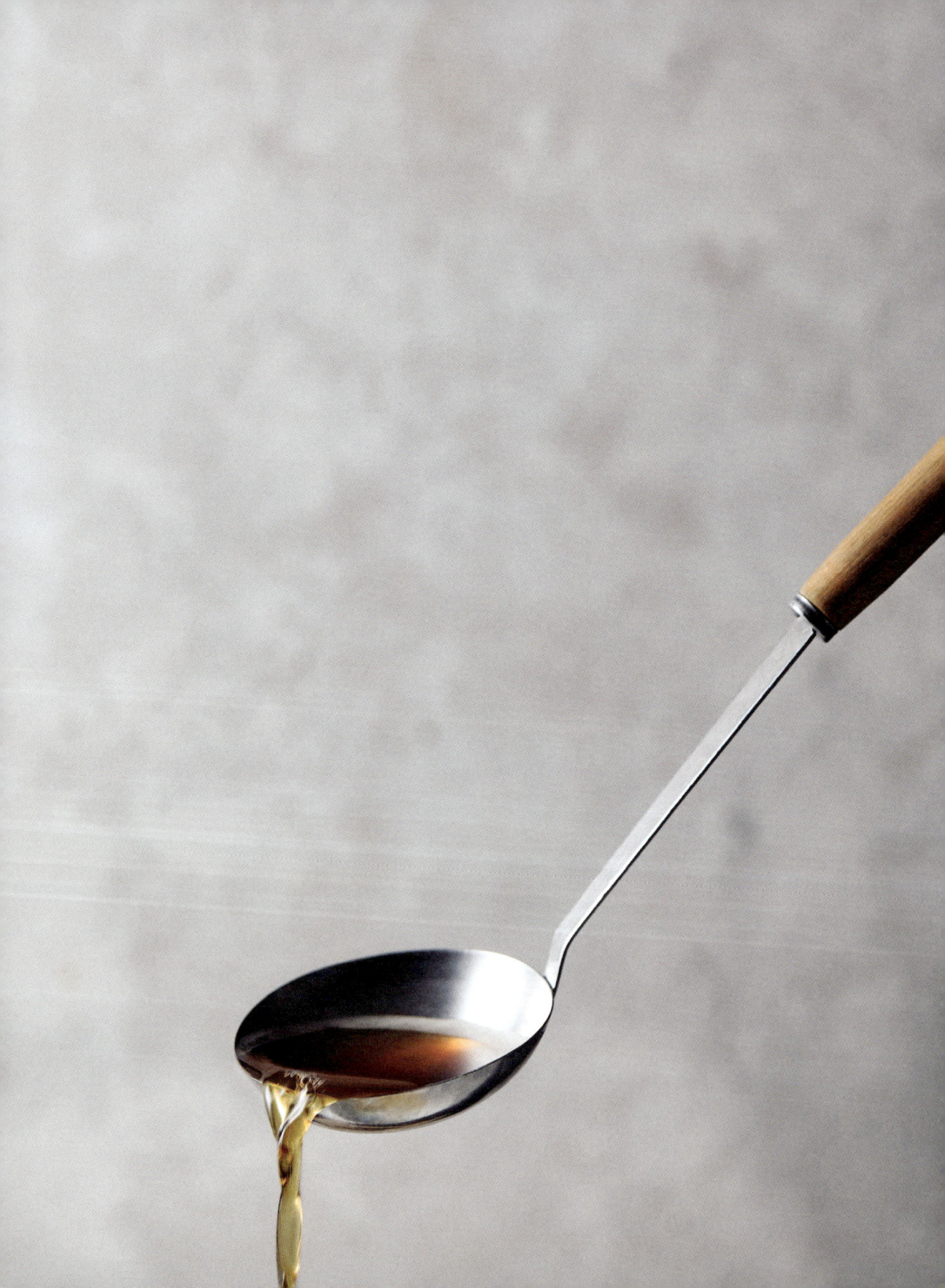

A TRADITIONAL REMEDY FOR MODERN LIFE

Good food really can act like medicine. We're always touched by the messages we receive from people telling us how bone broth has supported them, from easing digestive discomfort and soothing joint pain to helping their skin glow. For many, it feels like a gentle remedy for busy, modern lives. Since science and tradition both tell us that homemade bone broth is incredibly nourishing and healing, and we know from The Foundations chapter what components make it so, let's dive deeper into the wider range of health benefits that it can bring.

A Boost for Your Immune System

If we're feeling under the weather or need a quick pick-me-up, our go-to is a warm mug of bone broth with a pinch of ground turmeric or ginger. It's like a hug in a mug!

You may have heard of chicken soup being called 'Jewish penicillin'. Well, there's actually some truth to that. Bone broth is packed with nutrients that help your immune system stay strong. Glycine, for example, can have an anti-inflammatory and immunomodulatory effect.[2] Our grandmothers always offered broth when someone was under the weather, and it turns out they were on to something.

Glowing Skin, Strong Hair and Nails

Sipping bone broth regularly really can make your skin look brighter. This is because our skin has two layers – the outer epidermis keeps things protected, and the inner dermis is full of collagen and GAGs (glycosaminoglycans) that keep it plump and healthy. Bone broth contains collagen, gelatine and hyaluronic acid, which is known for its unique ability to retain moisture to keep your skin hydrated and happy.[3]

Collagen is just as amazing for our hair! As we age, our bodies make less collagen, and that can leave our hair thinner and weaker. Bone broth contains amino acids such as glycine and proline, plus minerals like zinc, iron and magnesium, which contribute to the production and protection of keratin, the protein that forms hair and nails.[4]

Bone Broth: The Philosophy

Ageing with Grace and Energy

We all want to get older without aches and pains, don't we? Well, bone broth can be our secret weapon. As we age, our natural collagen production declines, which can contribute to wrinkles, stiff joints and weaker bones. But broth gives us the building blocks, such as glycine, proline, glutamine, glucosamine and chondroitin, to help keep skin supple, joints flexible and bones strong.

Happy Heart and Steady Energy

Bone broth's star amino acid, glycine, can help to keep blood sugar stable. It also balances out methionine, which you get a lot of from muscle meats and eggs. Too much methionine without glycine can raise homocysteine levels, which is a risk factor for certain diseases.[5] Bone broth is a perfect addition to the modern diet to help balance things out.

Strong Bones and Flexible Joints

It turns out that drinking bone broth is good for our bones and joints, too! Collagen is a major component of bones and cartilage, after all,[6] and contains hyaluronic acid (HA), which lubricates joints, muscles and bones. Bone broth is high in protein, which contributes to the maintenance of normal muscles and bones, and also contains minerals that are important for skeletal health, including calcium, magnesium and phosphorus.

A Healthy Gut

Broth's reputation for supporting digestive health goes back thousands of years. Amino acids such as glutamine and glycine help maintain the integrity of the gut lining, reducing the risk of unwanted particles passing into the bloodstream and causing inflammation, sometimes known as 'leaky gut'. Glutamine is the primary fuel source for the cells lining the intestines, while glycine supports stomach acid and bile production, aiding food breakdown and reducing inflammation.[7]

You may notice improved digestion if you sip bone broth before meals. Glycine boosts stomach acid and bile, which helps break down food and keeps things moving smoothly.[8] We've even heard from people who say bone broth has helped with issues like colitis and Crohn's. While more research is needed, centuries of culinary tradition – and countless personal accounts – point to its effectiveness in treating this type of illness.

Better Mood and Deeper Sleep

We all know just how important sleep is for our health. Well, bone broth contains nutrients that have been shown to help us achieve a better night's sleep! Glycine acts as an inhibitory neurotransmitter, sending calming signals to your brain, easing anxiety and helping you fall asleep more quickly.[9] It also works alongside tryptophan to aid serotonin (the 'happy chemical') and melatonin (the sleep hormone) production, both of which are key to good mood and restful nights. Magnesium, naturally present in broth, is also key – acting like nature's chill pill, relaxing muscles and calming nerves for a good night's rest.

That's why including a warm cup of broth in the evening is much more than just a comforting drink – it may help your body overcome barriers to a healthy night's sleep!

A Friend for Weight Management

Bone broth can be a helpful tool if you're looking to maintain a healthy weight or support gradual weight loss. It's naturally high in protein but very low in calories, which helps keep you feeling fuller for longer. This satiety effect can lead to fewer between-meal cravings and make it easier to avoid high-sugar or ultra-processed snacks.

Gelatine, one of bone broth's hallmark nutrients, plays an important role here. It slows gastric emptying (meaning food stays in your stomach longer) and supports healthy digestion, which can help your body absorb nutrients more efficiently and improve your metabolism. When digestion is working well, energy levels are more stable, making it easier to stick to balanced eating patterns.

Because it's both light and nourishing, bone broth can also be used as a daily meal-time accompaniment. Many people enjoy a small cup before lunch or dinner; the warmth and protein help take the edge off hunger, so you're less likely to overeat. It's also a satisfying alternative to late-night snacking as it's gentle on the stomach and low in calories, yet still comforting and full of flavour.

Incorporating broth into your daily and weekly cooking can further support healthy eating goals. Swapping it for oil or cream in soups, stews, risottos or sauces can boost protein without adding unnecessary fats, while still delivering that deep, savoury flavour. It's a small change with a big impact over time.

Nourishment for Pregnancy and Beyond

Nutrient-dense foods to support your body during this transformative stage of life are essential, and we believe bone broth should be at the top of the list! It has been used by expecting and new mothers for centuries for a variety of reasons, from providing easy nourishment during morning sickness to helping with postpartum healing. It's gentle on the stomach and packed with protein and electrolytes to keep you hydrated and energised, even when other foods seem unappealing.

Glycine is especially important during pregnancy for foetal growth and maternal tissue support. Your body needs it for your baby's growth, and it can help keep your skin supple, joints happy and blood pressure steady. A fun fact: the uterus at the end of pregnancy contains 800 per cent more collagen than in a non-pregnant state![10]

As pregnancy progresses, your need for fluids and electrolytes increases. Staying well hydrated supports circulation and can help ease common symptoms like cramps, headaches, fatigue and brain fog. Bone broth is a natural source of electrolytes, making it a simple way to support hydration during this time.

Hydration remains just as important after birth, especially while breastfeeding, as dehydration can affect milk supply. Bone broth can be a nourishing addition to your diet, helping to replenish fluids and electrolytes while supporting lactation.

It's also rich in the amino acid glycine, which supports tissue repair and recovery. It's no wonder many traditional cultures emphasise collagen-rich meals during pregnancy and postpartum.

Keeping Strong and Healthy During Menopause

Menopause and perimenopause often bring changes in muscle mass, joint comfort and weight distribution. Your body might start losing muscle mass and strength in a process called sarcopenia. This can affect how you feel day-to-day and, in some cases, lead to physical challenges. The good news is that eating the right nutrients can help keep your muscles strong and healthy.

Protein is your muscles' best friend. Research shows that getting enough protein in your diet can help slow down muscle loss. Aim for around 25–30g (1oz) of protein at each meal.[11]

For a little protein boost, bone broth can be a great addition to your meals. For example, a 100ml (3½fl oz) serving of chicken bone broth should have on average 2–3g of protein, while beef bone broth can pack up to 4g per 100ml (3½fl oz). For a standard mug (about 250ml/9fl oz), that means you're getting roughly 5–10g of protein per serving.

While bone broth alone probably won't hit your full protein needs, it's a tasty way to add extra nutrients to your day, or even your usual cooking.

Menopause can also bring on symptoms like hot flushes. Women with higher body mass are more likely to have hot flushes, so maintaining a healthy weight by incorporating bone broth into your daily diet can be an effective way to manage these symptoms.[12] Research in *The Journal of Nutrition* suggests that the gelatine in bone can help curb your appetite, so bone broth might leave you feeling fuller for longer.[13]

In partnership with an NHS menopause and digestive health clinic, Freja Bone Broth was trialled by a group of peri- and post-menopausal women and ulcerative colitis patients. After adding bone broth to their diet daily for just 6 weeks, 94 per cent of participants self-reported in the survey visible improvements in the quality of their skin, hair or nails; 90 per cent self-reported in the survey improved joint comfort; 85 per cent found it easier to manage digestion and everyday energy; and 75 per cent reported a reduction in their overall menopause symptoms.[14]

Bone broth is one of the most enduring and nutrient-dense foods, which has helped people flourish across cultures and generations. Despite its rise in popularity in the health space, it's certainly not just a passing fad. There's something special about the way its ingredients work together, creating a powerful kind of medicine that's bigger than just the sum of its parts.

BONE BROTH: THE FOUNDATIONS

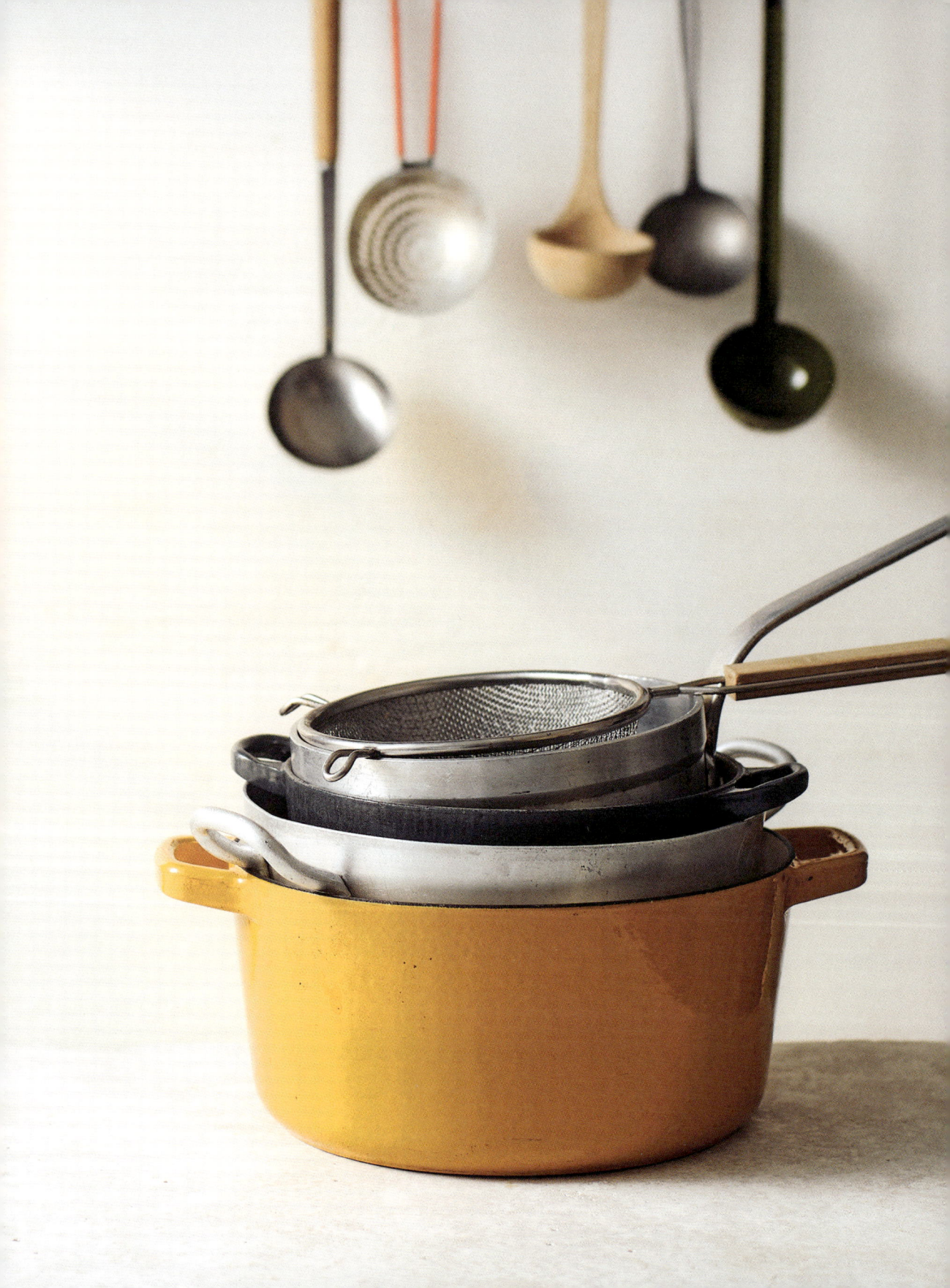

HOW TO MAKE BONE BROTH AT HOME

Now that we've explored the many benefits of bone broth, let's get in the kitchen and try it for ourselves. Bone broth is not only delicious but also incredibly versatile – the perfect base for soups, stews, sauces, curries and so much more. Whether you choose beef, chicken or fish, the method is simple: start with good ingredients, give them time and let the heat work its magic. It's easier than you may think!

In this chapter, we'll cover everything you need to know to master the basics of bone broth: what to use, how to prepare it and how to troubleshoot any hiccups along the way. You'll see how basic tools and simple techniques can turn humble ingredients into something rich and nourishing with never-ending possibilities. Let's get started!

What You'll Need

You don't need a fancy kitchen or top-notch equipment to make bone broth – just good-quality ingredients, a few simple tools and patience! Here's what you'll want to have on hand.

EQUIPMENT

Stockpot: A tall, narrow pot (height greater than the diameter) is ideal, as it minimises evaporation during a long simmer. A large saucepan works too, just make sure there's enough room to fully cover the bones with water.

Pressure cooker: If you're short on time, a pressure cooker really can be a game-changer. The collagen in the bones is converted to gelatine in the broth much more quickly in the pressurised environment. Flavour is also extracted from vegetables in about a third of the time it takes to make veg stock on the hob.

Slow cooker: If you prefer not to stand over a stockpot – whether because of time or patience – this might be perfect for you. You can just walk away and let the cooker work its magic. The broth might have a bit less gelatine, but it'll still be packed with flavour and nutrients.

Skimmer: This handy tool makes it easy to scoop off any impurities that rise to the top while cooking. It's worth having one, but if you don't, a small hand sieve would also work well.

Strainer: A fine-mesh sieve is perfect for catching all the little bits when you strain your broth.

INGREDIENTS – THE BUILDING BLOCKS OF FLAVOUR

Bones: The flavour comes from the meat on the bones, so meaty cuts like short ribs or beef shin, or leftover roast chicken carcasses will give you a richer, heartier broth. You also want to use the bones that are the richest in collagen and nutrients to ensure a gelatine-rich broth. If you're making beef bone broth, include knuckles and marrow bones. For chicken, buy a whole bird from the butcher and include the wings, neck and the feet if possible. Further ingredients are discussed on pages 42–47.

Pork Bone Broth

You won't find pork bone broth in this book, not because it isn't delicious, but because it's not a staple in most British kitchens. Our focus is on simple, practical broths you can make with ingredients you're likely to have at home, or can easily pick up from your butcher or fishmonger. These are the versatile bases that show up across many cuisines and will feel familiar to everyday cooks. That said, pork broth has a rich tradition, especially in Japanese cooking, where it forms the base of iconic ramen styles like tonkotsu. Creating a truly authentic ramen broth is best learnt from those who have dedicated themselves to the craft. If you'd like to explore it further, we recommend the following:

Ramen Forever – Tim Anderson
Japanese Soul Cooking – Tadashi Ono and Harris Salat
Ramen: Japanese Noodles and Small Dishes – Tove Nilsson

These will take you deeper into the techniques and traditions of pork and Ramen broths than we could hope to cover, while we focus on bringing you everyday broths for the home cook.

CHICKEN BUTCHER CUTS

CUT	WHY CHOOSE IT?	FLAVOUR PROFILE	GELATINE CONTENT	NOTES
WHOLE CHICKEN	BALANCED MEAT AND BONE	LIGHT, SAVOURY	MODERATE	GIVES BROTH PLUS COOKED MEAT
WINGS	SKIN, CARTILAGE, SMALL BONES	RICH, SLIGHTLY FATTY	HIGH	ESSENTIAL FOR A GEL JIGGLE
LEGS (DRUMSTICKS/ THIGHS)	MEAT AND CONNECTIVE TISSUE	FULL CHICKEN FLAVOUR	HIGH	ECONOMICAL CHOICE
FEET	CARTILAGE-RICH	NEUTRAL CHICKEN FLAVOUR	VERY HIGH	BOOSTS GEL, BLANCH FIRST
BACKS AND CARCASSES	BONE AND CARTILAGE	SAVOURY	HIGH	OFTEN LEFT OVER FROM ROASTS

BEEF BUTCHER CUTS

CUT	WHY CHOOSE IT?	FLAVOUR PROFILE	GELATINE CONTENT	NOTES
MARROW BONES	RICH IN MARROW AND MINERALS	DEEP, FATTY RICHNESS	LOW (ADD CARTILAGE BONES TOO)	BEST ROASTED FOR DEPTH
KNUCKLE (SHIN END)	LOTS OF CONNECTIVE TISSUE	SAVOURY, BEEFY	VERY HIGH	GELATINE POWERHOUSE
OXTAIL	MEAT, BONE AND CARTILAGE	INTENSELY BEEFY	HIGH	ADDS BOTH FLAVOUR AND TEXTURE
BEEF SHIN (BONE-IN)	MUSCLE AND BONE	MEATY, SAVOURY	MODERATE-HIGH	ADDS BODY AND DEPTH
NECK BONES	MEAT AND CARTILAGE	SAVOURY, BALANCED	HIGH	OFTEN INEXPENSIVE
SHORT RIBS (ON BONE)	RICH MEAT AND BONE	DEEP BEEFINESS	MODERATE	GREAT FOR FLAVOUR BASE

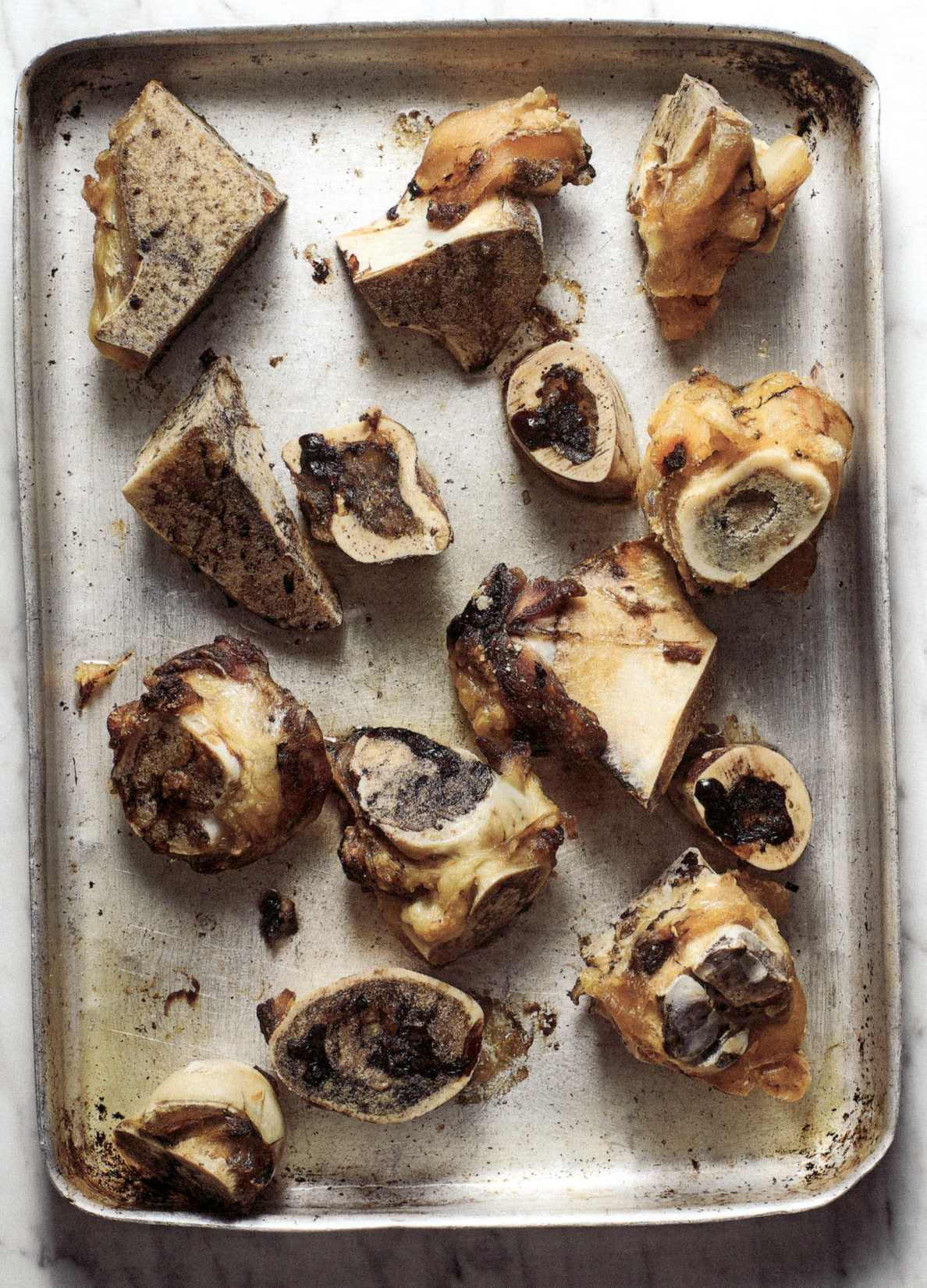

FISH AND SHELLFISH FISHMONGER PIECES

FISH/SHELLFISH PART	WHY CHOOSE IT?	FLAVOUR PROFILE	GELATINE CONTENT	NOTES
FISH HEADS (SALMON, COD, TURBOT, HALIBUT)	COLLAGEN IN CHEEKS, EYES AND SKIN	DEEP, SAVOURY, RICH	VERY HIGH	ALWAYS REMOVE GILLS (BITTER) AND RINSE WELL
FISH FRAMES/ SKELETONS	BONES AND SCRAPS OF MEAT	LIGHT, CLEAN	HIGH	IDEAL FOR CLEAR CONSOMMÉ-STYLE BROTHS
FISH COLLARS	MEAT, SKIN AND BONE	RICH, FATTY	MODERATE	ESPECIALLY FROM OILY FISH, LIKE SALMON
PRAWN/SHRIMP SHELLS	SWEET, AROMATIC	LIGHT SEAFOOD	LOW	HEADS ADD DEPTH – INCLUDE THEM IF AVAILABLE
LOBSTER SHELLS	INTENSE, SWEET, LUXURIOUS	BISQUE-LIKE	LOW	AVOID OVERCOOKING – CAN GO BITTER
CRAB SHELLS	SAVOURY, NUTTY	RICH SEAFOOD	LOW	FENNEL, TOMATO AND SAFFRON WORK WELL
LANGOUSTINE SHELLS	DELICATE, REFINED	LIGHT SEAFOOD	LOW	PERFECT FOR RISOTTOS AND SAUCES

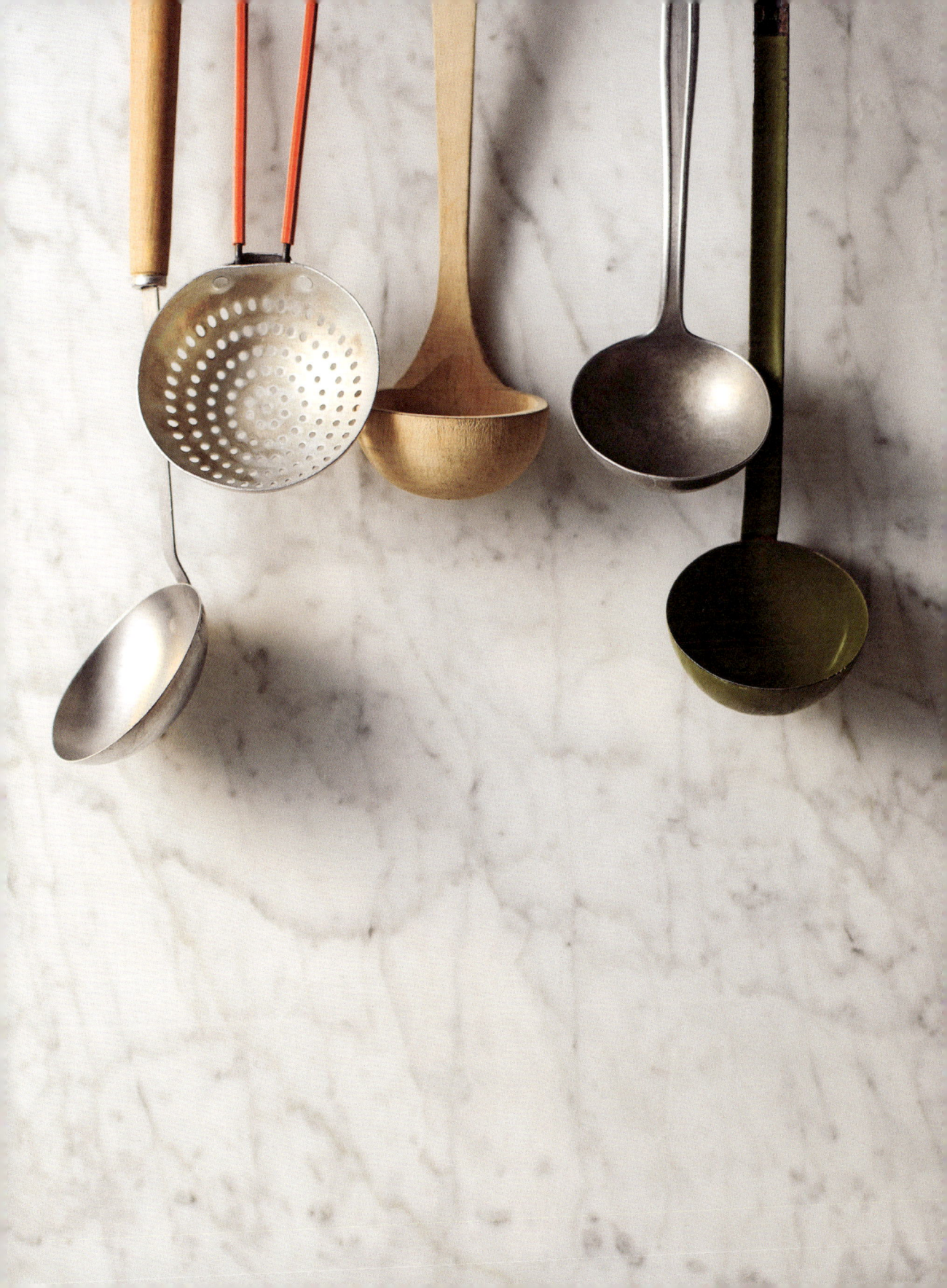

TO ROAST OR NOT TO ROAST?

Whether you roast your bones before simmering or drop them straight into the pot can dramatically change the flavour, colour and overall character of your broth. Roasting triggers the Maillard reaction, creating those deep, caramelised, savoury notes that make a broth taste richer and more complex. It also transforms the colour, giving chicken broth a warm golden hue and beef broth a darker, heartier tone. If you roast your bones alongside vegetables and herbs, the heat helps their flavours develop early, adding depth from the very first stage.

Skipping roasting has its advantages too. It produces a cleaner, more delicate flavour, which is especially important for lighter broths like Japanese-style chicken or fish stocks. It can also give you a clearer gelatine set, with a bright, almost translucent finish. And, of course, it's quicker; going straight into the pot can save you half an hour or more without sacrificing the nourishing qualities of your broth.

In our household, we always make bone broth after a roast chicken (in fact, this is the most commonly made broth in the UK), but we use unroasted bones in some of our Freja broths for a lighter, cleaner taste. It's entirely up to personal preference and we'd encourage you to experiment!

PRACTICAL TIPS
* Don't over-roast shellfish – bitterness creeps in quickly.
* Combine techniques – e.g. roast half your chicken bones for depth, leave half raw for freshness.
* If in doubt, roast beef and shellfish but skip roasting white fish unless you want a stronger flavour.

A Healthy Animal Makes Healthy Bones!

Bones from grass-fed and pasture-raised animals are the way to go. They're richer in collagen, omega-3 fatty acids, antioxidants and certain vitamins.[15] Healthy and happy animals produce nutrient-dense bones with a richer flavour and more gelatine than poorly raised alternatives.

WHEN TO ROAST VS WHEN TO SKIP

PROTEIN TYPE	ROAST FOR	SKIP ROASTING FOR	NOTES
BEEF	DEEP, HEARTY FLAVOUR FOR SOUPS, STEWS, GRAVIES	LIGHTER CONSOMMÉS	ROAST AT 200°C (180°C FAN)/400°F/GAS 6 FOR 30–40 MINUTES
CHICKEN	RICH GOLDEN BROTH, ROAST CHICKEN FLAVOUR	DELICATE BROTHS OR ASIAN-STYLE SOUPS	ROAST AT 200°C (180°C FAN)/400°F/GAS 6 FOR 25–30 MINUTES
FISH	STRONG, ROBUST SEAFOOD SOUPS (MEDITERRANEAN, BISQUE)	CLEAN, LIGHT JAPANESE-STYLE STOCKS (DASHI-STYLE)	ROAST AT 200°C (180°C FAN)/400°F/GAS 6 FOR 10–15 MINUTES IF USING OILY FISH
SHELLFISH (PRAWNS, CRAB, LOBSTER, LANGOUSTINES)	SWEET, INTENSE BISQUES AND SEAFOOD STEWS	VERY DELICATE SHELLFISH CONSOMMÉS	ROAST AT 200°C (180°C FAN)/400°F/GAS 6 FOR 10–20 MINUTES DEPENDING ON SIZE OF SHELLS

AROMATICS – YOUR FLAVOUR BOOSTERS

Bone broth is a blank canvas, and aromatics (vegetables, spices and herbs) are the way to build a unique flavour that suits your own tastebuds or your desire to experiment! Onions, carrots, parsnips, garlic, leeks and fennel all work beautifully. When we make beef broth, we love to add root veggies like parsnips, which add a touch of sweetness. If you have any slightly wilted veg or scraps, such as onion or potato peelings, carrot tops or leek ends, toss them in – they're perfect for enhancing a broth. For fish broth, we include fennel as it brings a subtle anise flavour. Fresh herbs like parsley, thyme, rosemary and bay leaves are also fantastic, especially for chicken broth. Spices, used sparingly, can deliver extra warmth, depth and global influences.

Flavour balance tip: Aromatics should enhance, not dominate. Aim for vegetables to be 20–25 per cent of bone weight. Add spices by the teaspoon unless aiming for a spice-forward broth (e.g. phở).

Seasoning: Hold off on adding salt until the end to avoid an overly salty broth. Peppercorns add a nice kick though! Use high-quality unrefined sea salt if you can.

Water: Filtered water is best since it's free of impurities like chlorine, which can concentrate during the long simmer, affecting the flavour and counteracting all those amazing health benefits.

Skimming: Ideally, your veg and herbs are added after the initial skimming process, as veg can rise to the surface and make the broth hard to skim.

See our aromatics table on pages 44–47 for a simple but absolutely non-exhaustive list of ingredients you can choose to add to your broth during cooking.

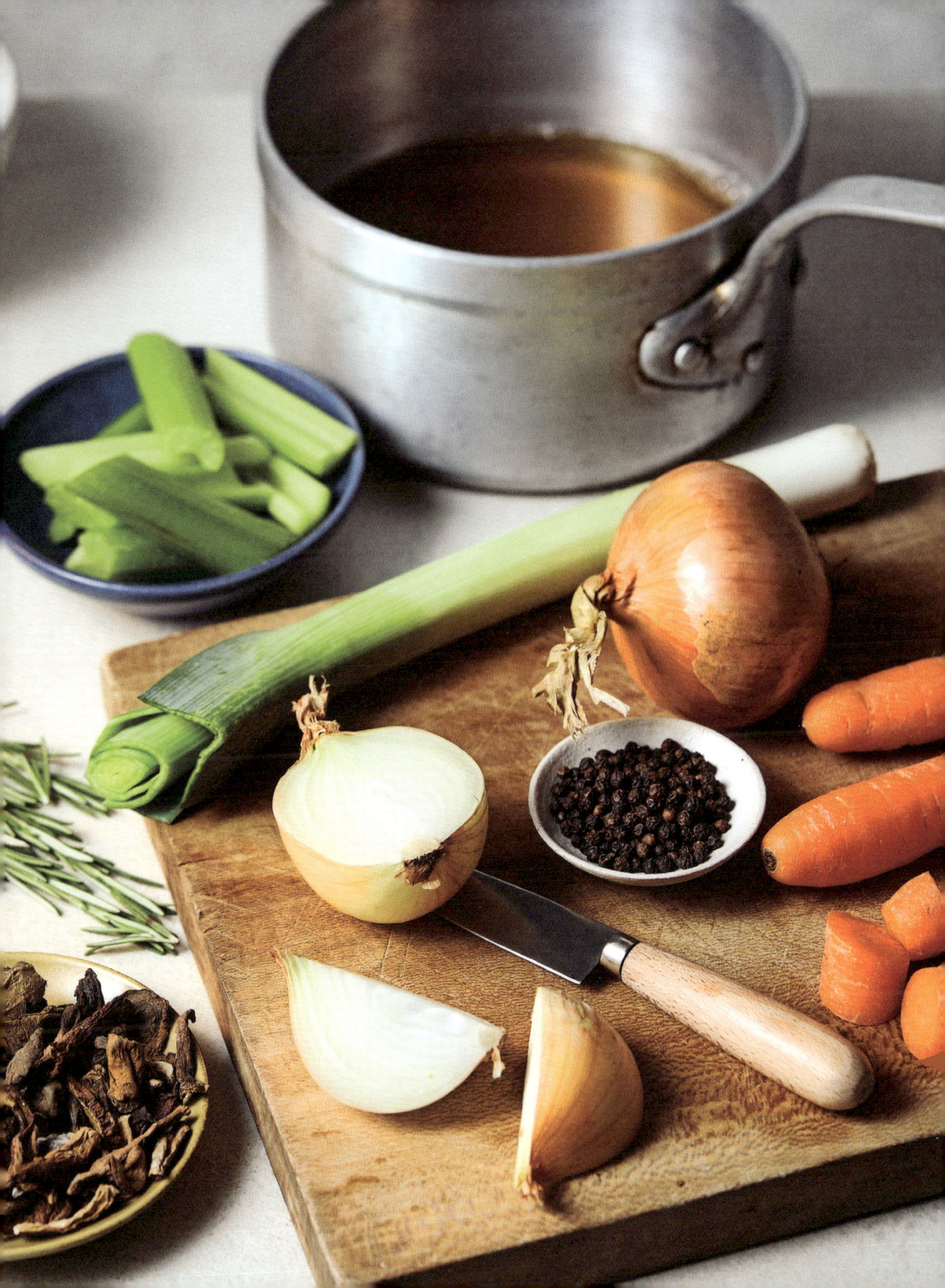

AROMATICS

AROMATIC	FLAVOUR NOTES	GLOBAL INSPIRATION	WHEN TO ADD	HOW MUCH	TIPS
ONION (BROWN, WHITE, RED)	SWEET, EARTHY BASE	FRENCH, INDIAN, MEXICAN	EARLY, AFTER FIRST SKIM	1–2 MEDIUM, QUARTERED	LEAVE SKINS ON FOR GOLDEN COLOUR
LEEK	MILD, SWEET ONION FLAVOUR	FRENCH, JAPANESE	EARLY, AFTER FIRST SKIM	1–2, CHOPPED INTO LARGE CHUNKS	USE ONLY WHITE/LIGHT GREEN PART FOR DELICATE BROTHS
GARLIC	SAVOURY, AROMATIC	MEDITERRANEAN, CHINESE, MIDDLE EASTERN	MIDWAY	3–6 CLOVES, LIGHTLY CRUSHED	TOO MUCH CAN OVERPOWER IN LONG COOKS
CARROT	SWEETNESS, BALANCE	FRENCH, EASTERN EUROPEAN	EARLY, AFTER FIRST SKIM	2–3 MEDIUM, CUT INTO LARGE CHUNKS	AVOID OVERCOOKING TO PREVENT CLOUDY BROTH
PARSNIP	SWEET, EARTHY DEPTH	BRITISH, EASTERN EUROPEAN	EARLY	1 LARGE	GREAT FOR BEEF BROTH RICHNESS
CELERY	HERBAL, SAVOURY	FRENCH, ITALIAN, AMERICAN	EARLY	2–3 STALKS	USE LEAVES SPARINGLY – STRONG FLAVOUR

AROMATIC	FLAVOUR NOTES	GLOBAL INSPIRATION	WHEN TO ADD	HOW MUCH	TIPS
FENNEL BULB	SWEET, ANISEED	MEDITERRANEAN, JAPANESE (FISH)	EARLY	½–1 BULB	EXCELLENT FOR FISH/SHELLFISH
BAY LEAF	SUBTLE HERBAL NOTE	EUROPEAN, CARIBBEAN	EARLY	2–3 LEAVES	REMOVE AFTER COOKING – BITTER IF LEFT TOO LONG
PARSLEY STEMS	FRESH, GREEN	FRENCH, MIDDLE EASTERN	EARLY	SMALL HANDFUL	STEMS HOLD MORE FLAVOUR THAN LEAVES
THYME	WOODY, SAVOURY	FRENCH, BRITISH	EARLY	3–4 SPRIGS	HARDY HERB – SURVIVES LONG SIMMERS
ROSEMARY	PINEY, RESINOUS	MEDITERRANEAN	EARLY	1–2 SMALL SPRIGS	USE SPARINGLY – STRONG FLAVOUR
GINGER	WARM, SPICY	CHINESE, VIETNAMESE	MIDWAY	3–5 SLICES	GREAT FOR CHICKEN/FISH, DIGESTION BENEFITS

AROMATICS

AROMATIC	FLAVOUR NOTES	GLOBAL INSPIRATION	WHEN TO ADD	HOW MUCH	TIPS
TURMERIC (FRESH)	EARTHY, VIBRANT COLOUR	INDIAN, INDONESIAN	MIDWAY	5–6 SLICES	STAINS – USE GLOVES
LIME LEAVES	CITRUSY, FLORAL	THAI, INDONESIAN	LAST 30–60 MINUTES	2–3 LEAVES	BEST FOR LIGHT CHICKEN AND FISH BROTHS
STAR ANISE	SWEET LIQUORICE	CHINESE, VIETNAMESE	MIDWAY	1–2 WHOLE	COMPLEMENTS BEEF AND DUCK BROTHS
CINNAMON STICK	WARM, SWEET SPICE	MIDDLE EASTERN, MEXICAN	MIDWAY	1 STICK	ESPECIALLY GOOD IN RED MEAT BROTHS
CLOVES	WARM, PUNGENT	INDIAN, CARIBBEAN	EARLY (STUDDED INTO ONION)	3–4	STRONG – USE SPARINGLY
CORIANDER SEEDS	CITRUSY, WARM	INDIAN, MEXICAN	EARLY	1 TBSP	CRUSH LIGHTLY BEFORE ADDING

AROMATIC	FLAVOUR NOTES	GLOBAL INSPIRATION	WHEN TO ADD	HOW MUCH	TIPS
PEPPERCORNS (BLACK, WHITE)	SPICY HEAT	GLOBAL	EARLY	1–2 TSP	BLACK = STRONGER, WHITE = SUBTLE
TOMATO (FRESH, PASTE)	UMAMI, COLOUR	ITALIAN, SPANISH	EARLY	1–2 TBSP PASTE OR 1 LARGE TOMATO	BEST IN BEEF OR CHICKEN BROTHS
DRIED MUSHROOMS (SHIITAKE, PORCINI)	UMAMI DEPTH	JAPANESE, ITALIAN	EARLY	3–5 MUSHROOMS	REHYDRATE AND ADD SOAKING LIQUID
SEAWEED (KOMBU)	MINERAL UMAMI	JAPANESE	LAST 30 MINUTES	1–2 STRIPS	REMOVE BEFORE BOILING TO AVOID BITTERNESS

METHOD FOR BONE BROTH

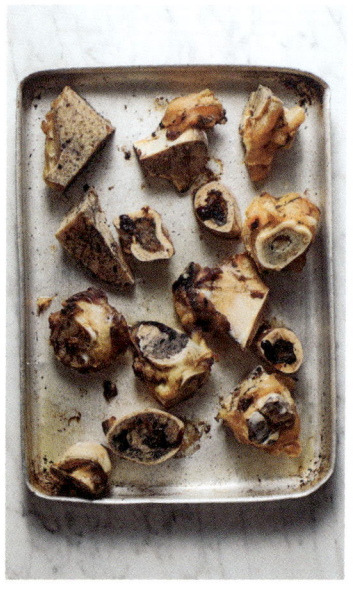
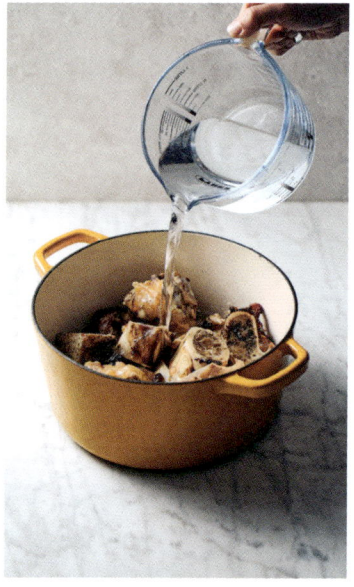
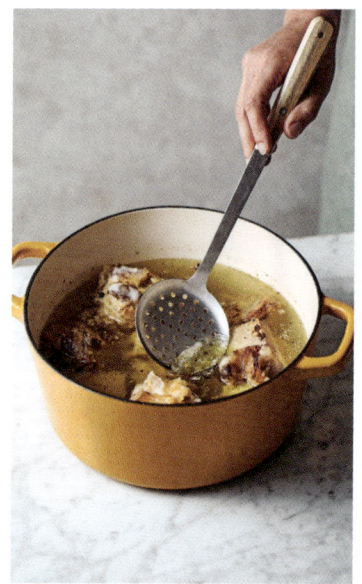

1

Start by giving your bones a quick rinse under cold water. This washes away any surface impurities that can cloud the broth later. If you're going for that deep, rich flavour, now's the time to roast them (see pages 40–41), otherwise, they can go straight into the pot.

2

Add your bones to a large stockpot, slow cooker or pressure cooker, and cover them with cold, filtered water – just enough to fully submerge them. Bringing the temperature up slowly is key. Keep the lid off at this stage; it helps you keep an eye on the surface and encourages a cleaner, clearer broth.

3

As the water begins to warm, you'll notice a pale foam, or 'scum', rising to the surface. Skim this off gently with a skimmer or spoon. It's a small step, but it makes a big difference to the clarity and taste of your final broth.

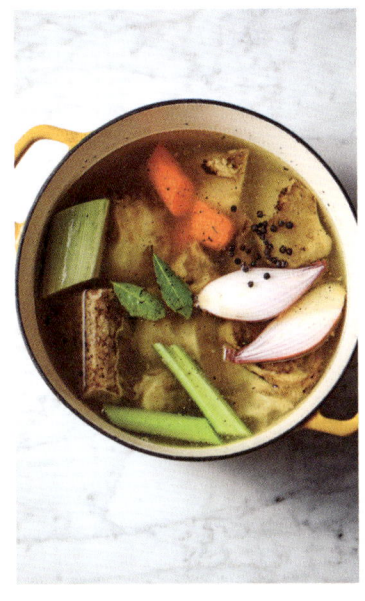 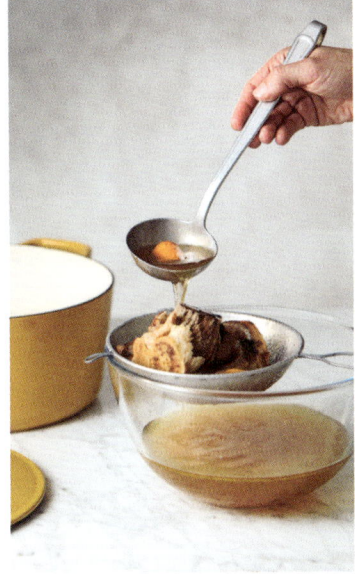 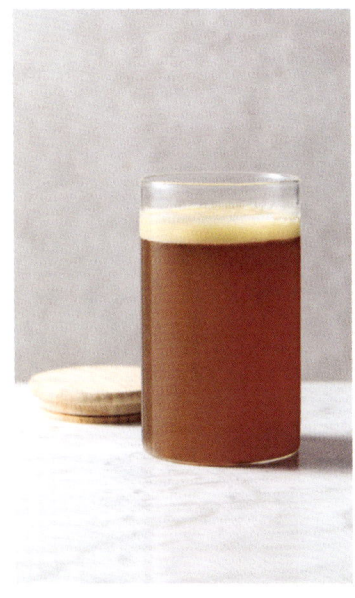

4

Once you've done your initial skim, it's time to build flavour. Add your aromatics in stages so they add the best flavour. Sturdy vegetables and robust spices go in first as they can handle the long simmer. Medium-bodied herbs and spices, like ginger slices or cinnamon sticks, join halfway through. Save your most delicate additions, the leafy herbs, seaweed, citrus leaves, etc., for the last hour, so their brightness comes through without turning bitter.

5

Now comes the slow, patient part. Keep your broth at a gentle simmer, never a rolling boil, so you preserve both clarity and gelatine. As a guide: chicken bones need 6–12 hours but can go for longer; beef needs 12–24 hours minimum; and fish or shellfish will reward you after 6–8 hours. When it's ready, lift out the solids, let the broth rest briefly, then strain through a fine mesh sieve for a clear result.

6

Cool the broth completely in the fridge. As it chills, the fat will rise and set into a firm layer, easy to lift off and save for cooking. Beneath it, you'll hopefully find that beautiful, wobbly gel that means you've coaxed every last bit of goodness from your ingredients.

STORAGE

In our kitchen, the freezer is never without a good supply of light chicken bone broth, rich roast beef broth and delicate fish broth. Having them on hand means a nourishing base is always just minutes away.

In the fridge: Chicken and beef broth will happily keep for up to a week because the natural gelatine acts as a gentle preservative. Fish broth is best enjoyed within 2 days, when its flavour is at its freshest. And remember, if your broth ever smells off, trust your senses – don't risk it!

In the freezer: For longer storage, the freezer is your best friend. Pour cooled broth into freezer-safe glass jars, leaving enough space at the top for expansion as it freezes. Ice cube trays are another brilliant option. Once frozen, pop the cubes into reusable bags for easy portioning. You can even simmer your broth down into a rich concentrate before freezing in cubes; just top up with hot water when you're ready to use. Properly stored, your frozen broth will stay delicious for up to 6 months.

So, are you ready to fill your kitchen with the comforting aroma of your first batch of bone broth?

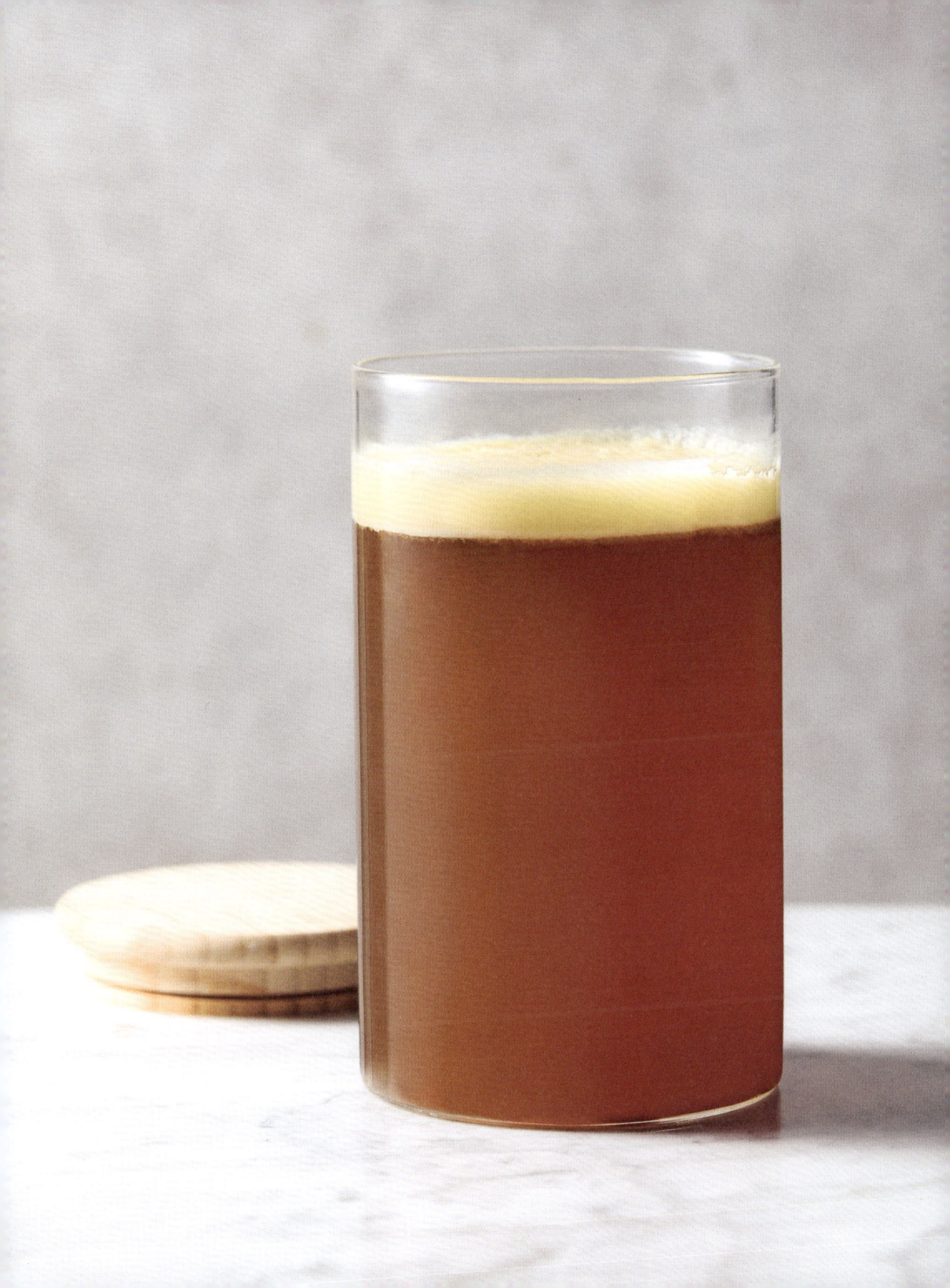

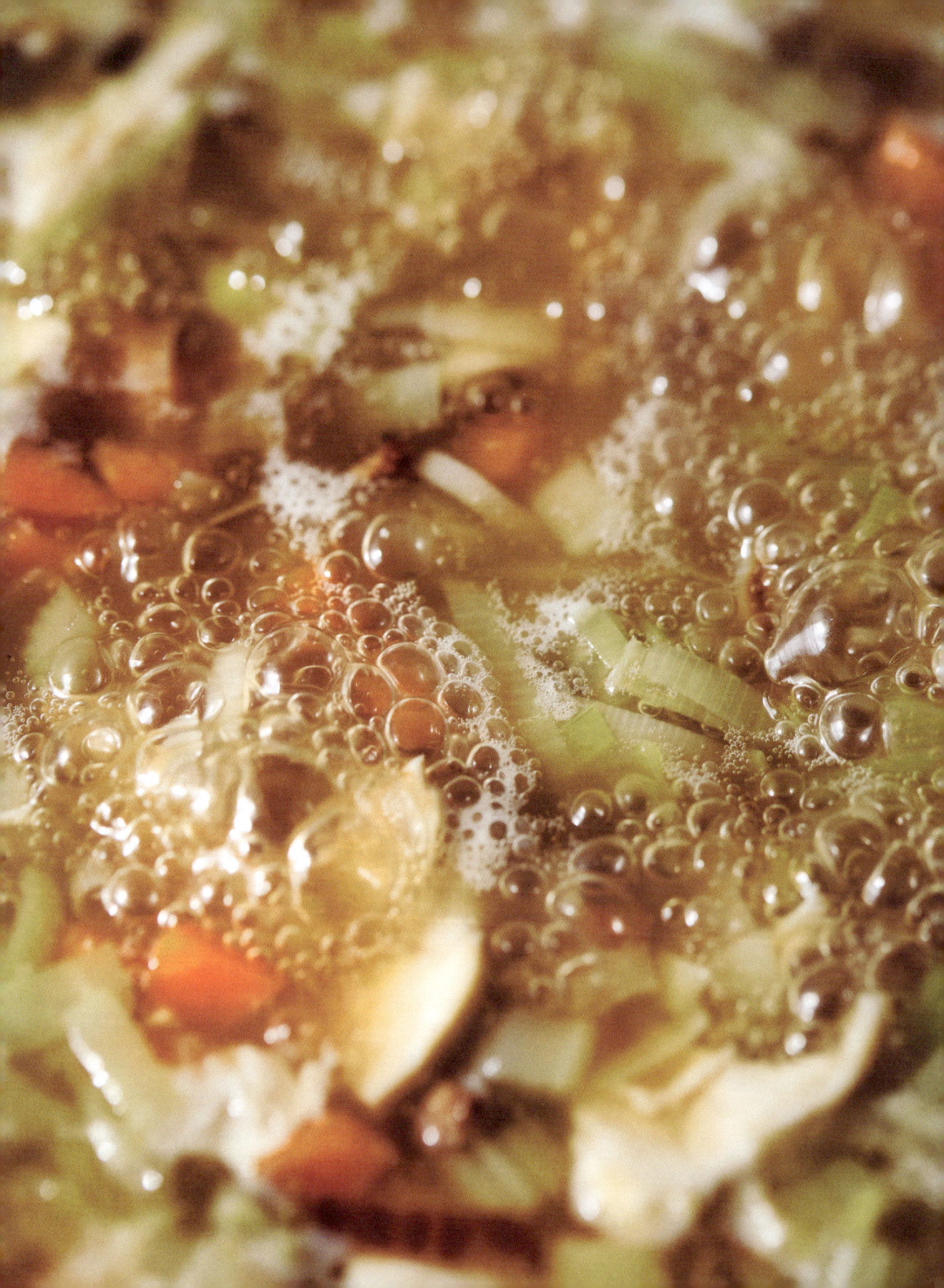

BROTH-BUSTING: FIXING COMMON BONE BROTH PROBLEMS

Even the most seasoned broth-makers run into the occasional hiccup. Sometimes your broth looks a little murky, other times it refuses to set into that glorious, wobbly gel. Don't worry as both are more common than you think, and both are easily fixed.

My Broth is Cloudy!

Bone broth can turn cloudy for a few reasons. Here are some of the things to watch out for.

Boiling too hard: A cloudy broth is usually the result of a little too much excitement in the pot. A rolling boil can whisk impurities into the liquid, emulsifying them so they stay suspended rather than rising to the surface. A gentle, steady simmer is the secret, with the lid off or slightly ajar, so everything stays calm and clear.

Not skimming the surface: Skipping the skimming step is another culprit. As the broth simmers, foam (sometimes called 'scum') will appear on the surface. This is simply proteins and other natural compounds being released from the bones. Left unchecked, they'll mix back into the liquid, slightly muddying the flavour as well as the look.

Impurities in the bones: The bones themselves can play a role, too. Industrially raised animals sometimes produce more impurities than pasture-raised or grass-fed ones. A quick rinse in cold water, or a short roast in the oven before simmering, can help keep things cleaner.

Overcooking the veg: Vegetables have their part to play. If you simmer them too long they start to break down, releasing fine particles that drift through the broth.

Not letting the broth sit after cooking: After you've finished cooking, give your broth 10 minutes to rest before straining, so any last bits can settle at the bottom. Ladle off the clear liquid, leaving that cloudy layer behind.

If you do end up with a cloudy broth, it's still perfectly good to drink and cloudiness won't affect the nutrient content in any way – the only thing affected is appearance. But if you want it crystal clear, whisk a couple of egg whites into the cooled broth, then gently reheat and simmer for about an hour. The egg whites will gather up the particles, ready to be strained away, leaving you with a beautifully clear result.

My Broth Doesn't Jiggle!

A perfectly gelled broth is one of life's little kitchen triumphs. It means your bones have given up plenty of collagen, which has set into gelatine. But if yours stays liquid in the fridge, don't despair. It's still nutritious and flavour-packed, and it will still contain plenty of collagen, just in a form that hasn't set firmly. Less gelatine doesn't necessarily mean less collagen; the collagen may simply have broken down into smaller peptides that stay liquid when chilled. They're still there, still beneficial, and still worth every sip.

It often comes down to the bones. For chicken, wings, legs, and especially feet are full of tendons and cartilage – the real gelatine powerhouses. Using a whole chicken will give you broth plus tender meat for other dishes. For beef, ask your butcher for knuckles, short ribs, shin or oxtail. Fish bones are naturally high in cartilage and usually set easily.

The quality of the bones matters too. Pasture-raised animals generally produce bones with more collagen, which means better gelling.

Then there's the bone-to-water ratio. You want just enough water to cover the bones. Any more and you dilute the gelatine. As a guide, use around 4 litres (136fl oz) water for 1.5kg (3lb 5oz) chicken bones, and the same volume for about 3kg (6lb 12oz) beef bones.

Temperature is another factor. A hard boil can break collagen down into shorter strands that won't gel. Keep your broth at a low, gentle simmer throughout.

Finally, time matters. Cut it short and you won't extract enough collagen; let it go too long, and the collagen strands can break apart. For chicken, aim for 6–12 hours; beef, 12–24 hours; fish, 6–8 hours.

Even without a wobble, your broth will still be rich in goodness. But if you follow these tips, your next batch is far more likely to have that satisfying jelly-like set when cooled.

How to Choose Ready-Made Broth

Sometimes life's too busy for simmering pots and careful skimming, and that's okay. If you're reaching for a ready-made bone broth, the good news is there are some excellent options out there. The trick is knowing what to look for so you're getting something as close as possible to the real, homemade deal.

Start with the ingredients list. The best broths are refreshingly simple: meaty bones, water, vegetables (think onions, carrots, parsnips, fennel) and herbs like thyme, bay leaf and parsley. If you see a string of additives, artificial flavours and preservatives, you're not looking at a homemade-style bone broth.

Quality sourcing matters. Bones from grass-fed or pasture-raised animals are naturally richer in collagen, omega-3s and minerals, and they're free from hormones and antibiotics. Look for brands that work with independent farms and are transparent about their supply chain – it makes a difference both for your health and the planet.

Check the nutrition. A proper bone broth will proudly list its protein and collagen content. And it should gel when chilled – a sure sign of a healthy dose of gelatine. If it's thin and watery straight from the fridge, it's likely lighter on the good stuff.

Check their website – if a broth has hundreds of glowing reviews praising its flavour, that's usually a good sign you've found a keeper!

BONE BROTH: THE RECIPES

SIPPING BROTHS

There's something deliciously comforting about wrapping your hands around a warm mug of broth. It's simple, soothing and, more often than not, exactly what your body needs. These sipping broths are designed to be just that – easy, nourishing pick-me-ups for any time of day.

Whether you're fighting off a cold, winding down for the evening or just in need of a savoury reset between meals, these recipes are fast, flavourful and restorative. No fancy kit required, just a few good ingredients that warm you from the inside out.

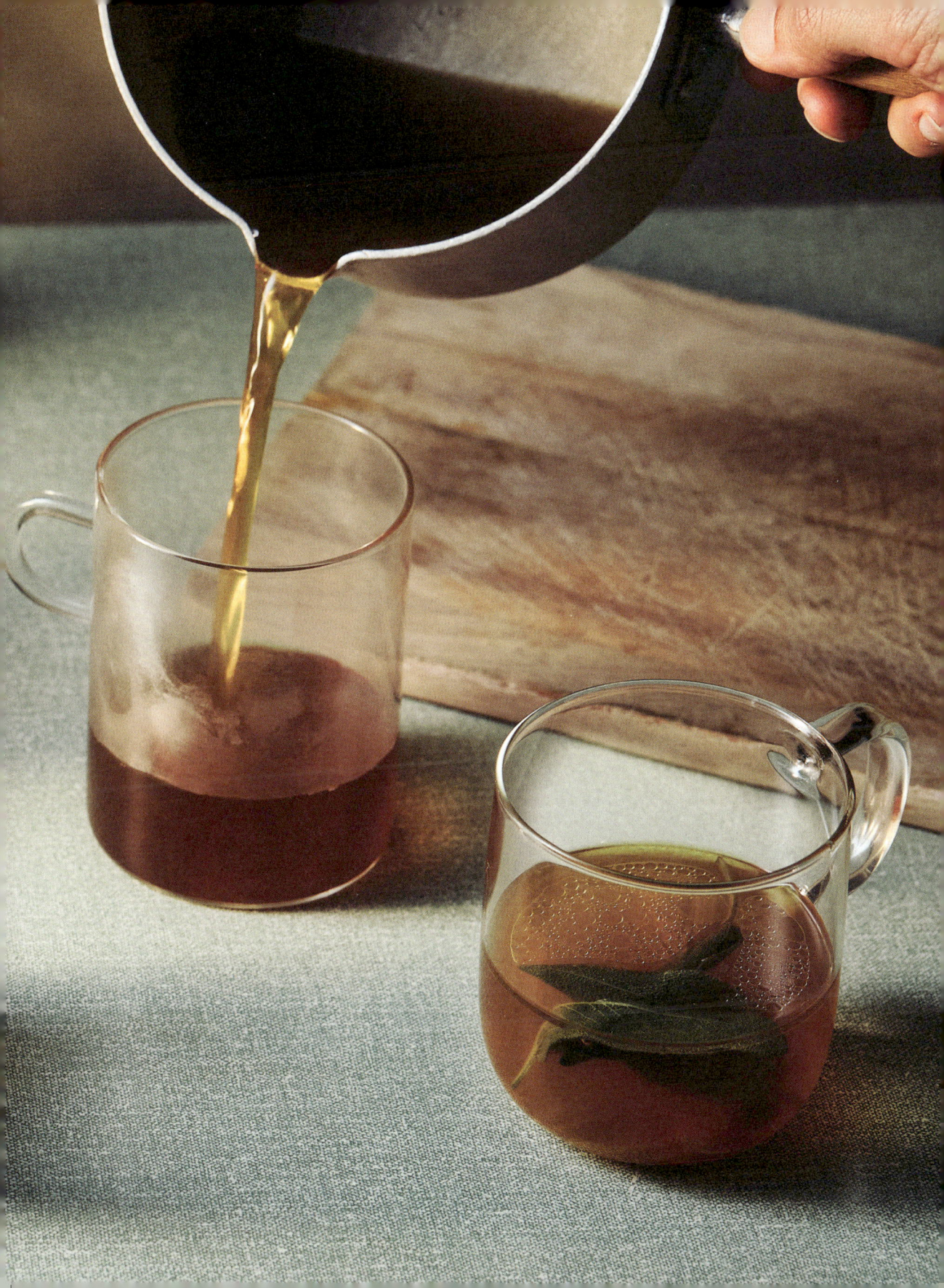

GET-WELL-SOON CHICKEN BROTH

There's a reason chicken broth has long been the go-to remedy for colds, flus and general under-the-weatheriness. It's gentle, nourishing and easy on the gut – just what you need when you're not feeling your best. This is comfort in a cup. A hug in a mug. Light yet savoury, soothing and full of flavour.

SERVES 1
PREP TIME: 5 MINUTES

250ml (9fl oz) chicken bone broth

Simply pour your chicken bone broth into a small saucepan, warm gently until steaming (but not boiling) and sip slowly from your favourite mug.

TO SERVE
Add a slice of fresh ginger, a squeeze of lemon or a pinch of sea salt if you like – but honestly, it's perfect just as it is.

PROPER BEEF TEA

This old-school staple is as British as it gets. Traditionally known as 'beef tea', it's essentially just hot beef broth sipped straight from the mug. Rich, savoury and full-bodied, this is a broth with backbone. Drink it mid-morning for a savoury pick-me-up or in the evening as a warming wind-down.

SERVES 1
PREP TIME: 5 MINUTES

250ml (9fl oz) beef bone broth

To serve, pour beef bone broth into a small saucepan and gently heat until piping hot. Tip into a mug and sip slowly.

TO SERVE
The deep, beefy flavour speaks for itself, but for an extra kick, stir in a few drops of Worcestershire sauce or a grind of black pepper.

IMMUNE-BOOSTING TONIC

This golden broth is full of gently warming ingredients like ginger and turmeric. This particular blend of spices is a play on 'golden milk', traditionally consumed in Indian cultures for its anti-inflammatory properties, but here we've added it to broth instead of milk for extra depth of flavour. It's naturally soothing and restorative, especially when you feel run-down or need a gentle reset.

SERVES 1
PREP TIME: 2 MINUTES
COOK TIME: 5–7 MINUTES

250ml (9fl oz) chicken bone broth
1 thumb-sized piece of fresh ginger, thinly sliced or grated
¼ teaspoon ground turmeric
1 teaspoon honey
1 tablespoon lemon juice

1. Pour the bone broth into a small saucepan.

2. Add the ginger and turmeric and bring to a gentle simmer.

3. Let it simmer gently and infuse for 5–7 minutes, then strain into a mug.

4. Stir in the honey and lemon juice until fully dissolved.

TO SERVE
Sip slowly while hot. Feel it warm you from the inside out.

PROVENÇAL GARLIC & SAGE BROTH

This savoury, herb-scented broth is inspired by a traditional French hangover cure. It's rich in garlic, calming in flavour and surprisingly reviving, no matter whether you've overdone it or not.

SERVES: 1
PREP TIME: 2 MINUTES
COOK TIME: 6–8 MINUTES

1 teaspoon olive oil
2 garlic cloves, thinly sliced
250ml (9fl oz) chicken bone broth
3 sage leaves
1 small strip of lemon zest
Sea salt

1. Gently warm the olive oil in a small saucepan.

2. Add the sliced garlic and cook for 1–2 minutes until soft but not browned.

3. Pour in the chicken bone broth and add the sage leaves and lemon zest.

4. Simmer gently for 5–6 minutes, then strain into a mug and season with salt to taste.

TO SERVE
Best sipped slowly in peace and quiet.

Sipping Broths

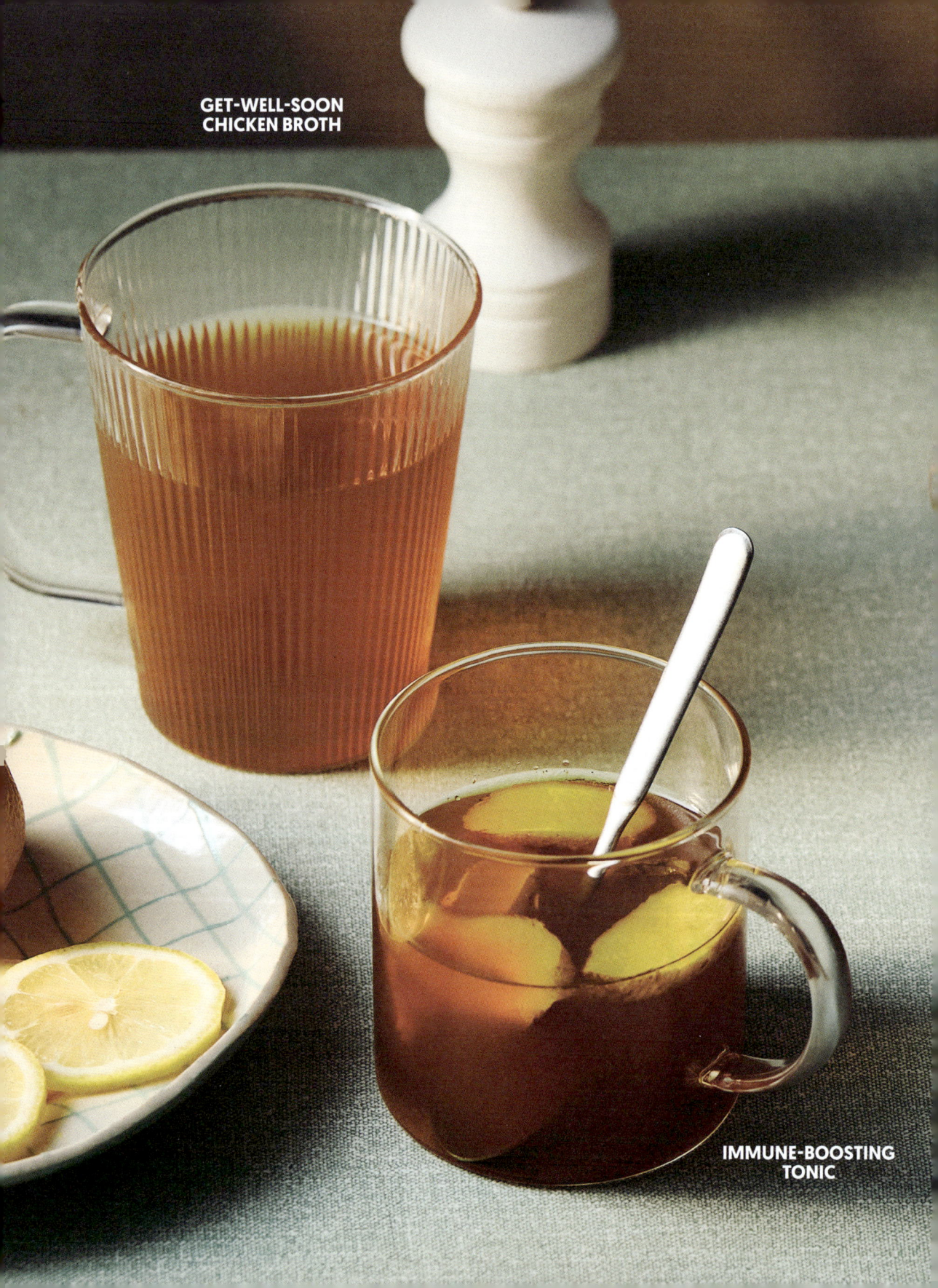

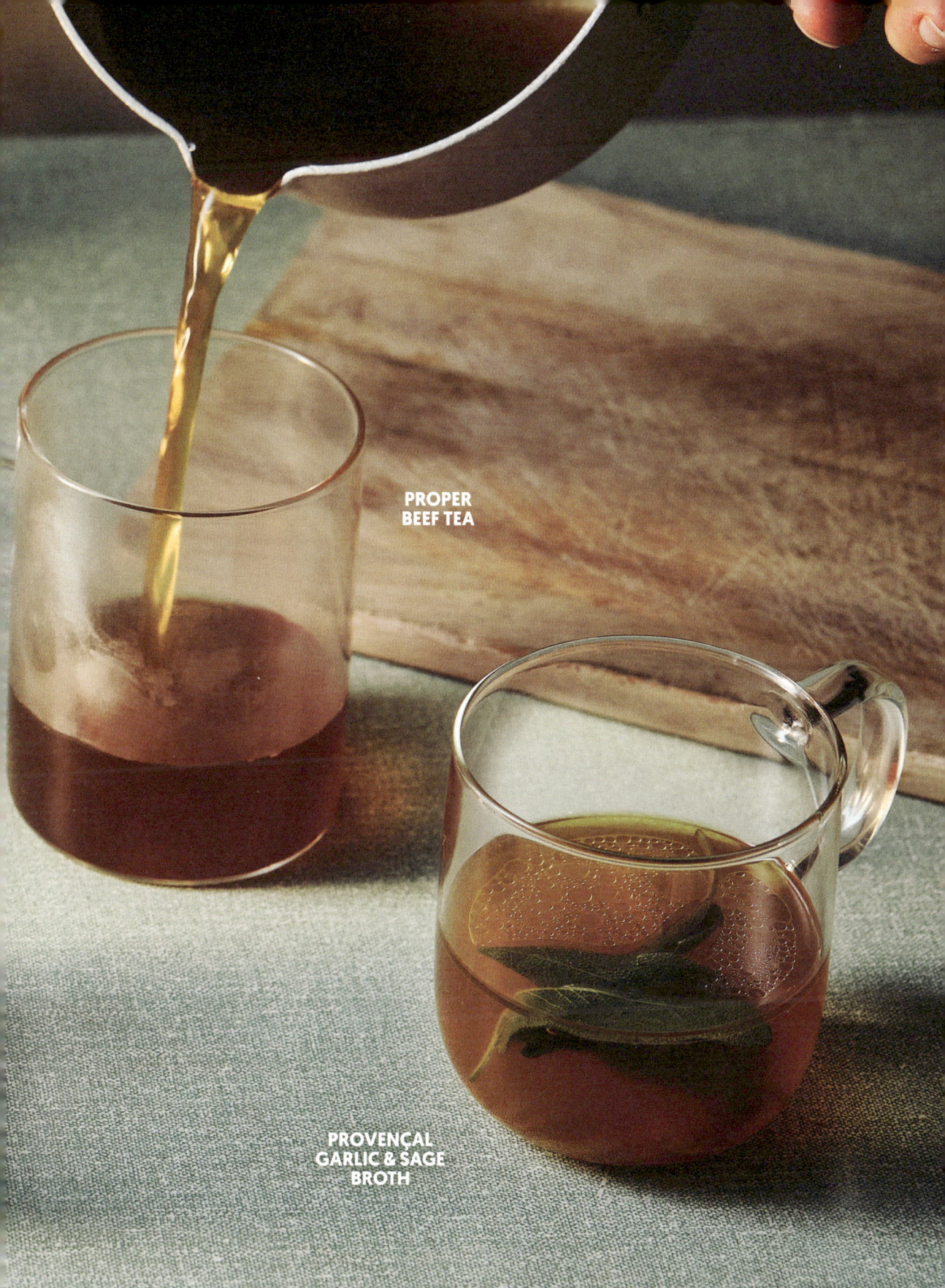

PROPER BEEF TEA

PROVENÇAL GARLIC & SAGE BROTH

HOT BROTH TODDY

A richly comforting take on the classic hot toddy, this version swaps hot water for broth to add additional nutrition and a deeper, more savoury flavour. It's soothing yet also punchy and guaranteed to give you a boost.

SERVES 1
PREP TIME: 2 MINUTES
COOK TIME: 3–5 MINUTES

250ml (9fl oz) chicken bone broth
1 tablespoon lemon juice
1 teaspoon honey
25ml (¾fl oz) whisky (optional)

1. Warm the bone broth in a small saucepan until steaming.

2. Stir in the lemon juice and honey until fully dissolved.

3. Add the whisky, if using, and heat gently for 1 minute more.

TO SERVE
Pour into a mug and clear your schedule – this one might relax you so much you need a snooze after.

PROTEIN POWER-UP
(EGG DROP BROTH)

Fancy a light, silky twist on breakfast? This has you covered. Soft ribbons of egg stirred straight into hot broth. It's simple, nourishing and packed with protein. What a way to start the day!

SERVES 1
PREP TIME: 1 MINUTE
COOK TIME: 2–3 MINUTES

250ml (9fl oz) chicken bone broth
1 egg
Pinch of sea salt

1. Bring the broth to a gentle simmer in a small saucepan.

2. Beat the egg in a small bowl.

3. Stir the broth to create a whirlpool, then slowly drizzle in the egg while stirring.

4. Let it cook for 30 seconds, then season lightly with salt.

TO SERVE
Pour into a mug or bowl and enjoy warm.

UMAMI MARMITE TEA

Love it or hate it, this is a savoury, salty-smooth drink with serious depth. It's as satisfying as it is simple, delivering big flavour for minimal effort. Ideal for mid-morning or as a lighter alternative to a snack.

SERVES 1
PREP TIME: 1 MINUTE
COOK TIME: 2–3 MINUTES

250ml (9fl oz) beef bone broth
½ teaspoon Marmite

1. Warm the beef bone broth in a small saucepan until piping hot.

2. Stir in the Marmite until fully dissolved.

TO SERVE
Pour into a mug and enjoy as is.

MISO BONE BROTH

Two ingredients, one super-satisfying cup. This savoury, umami-rich broth is quick, comforting and makes a brilliant mid-morning reset.

SERVES 1
PREP TIME: 1 MINUTE
COOK TIME: 2–3 MINUTES

250ml (9fl oz) chicken bone broth
1 teaspoon white miso paste

1. Warm the broth gently in a small saucepan until just below boiling point.

2. Remove from the heat and whisk in the miso paste until fully dissolved.

TO SERVE
Pour into a mug and enjoy hot. Simple. Swap chicken for beef bone broth for a deeper flavour.

SPICED CHAI BONE BROTH

Earthy, creamy and gently spiced, this sipping broth takes inspiration from traditional masala chai, but keeps things pared back and balances the aromatics with a savoury undertone. It's a wonderfully soothing way to start the day, especially on colder mornings.

SERVES 1
PREP TIME: 2 MINUTES
COOK TIME: 5–7 MINUTES

250ml (9fl oz) chicken bone broth
2 slices of fresh ginger
1 cinnamon stick
2 cardamom pods, lightly crushed
2 black peppercorns
1 black tea bag or 1 teaspoon loose-leaf black tea
50ml (1¾fl oz) whole milk

1. Pour the bone broth into a small saucepan.

2. Add the ginger, cinnamon, cardamom, peppercorns and black tea.

3. Bring to a gentle simmer and let the broth infuse for 5–7 minutes.

4. Remove the ginger, cinnamon, cardamom pods, peppercorns and tea bag (use a tea strainer if you use loose-leaf tea). Gently stir in the milk.

TO SERVE
Pour into a mug and sip slowly. Feel free to add honey or maple syrup for a sweeter finish.

BULLETPROOF COFFEE BONE BROTH

A broth-meets-caffeine blend that brings together coffee, broth and healthy fats. It's savoury, creamy and energising – the ultimate morning pick-me-up.

SERVES 1
PREP TIME: 2 MINUTES
COOK TIME: 2–3 MINUTES

125ml (4fl oz) strong black coffee or espresso
125ml (4fl oz) beef bone broth
1 teaspoon unsalted butter

1. Warm the coffee and broth together in a small saucepan until steaming.

2. Add the butter and blend with a hand blender until smooth and frothy.

TO SERVE
Pour into your mug of choice and drink while warm.

BONE BROTH HOT CHOCOLATE

Using beef broth as the base gives this hot chocolate a savoury depth, as does the dark chocolate, but this is balanced beautifully with the subtle sweet creaminess of full-fat milk. Comforting, rich and just a little indulgent, it's an unexpected combination, but once you try it, you'll be coming back for more. Trust us.

SERVES 1
PREP TIME: 2 MINUTES
COOK TIME: 3–5 MINUTES

250ml (9fl oz) beef bone broth
2 teaspoons unsweetened cocoa powder
1 square (10g/¼oz) dark chocolate (70% cocoa solids)
100ml (3½fl oz) whole milk

1. Warm the bone broth in a small saucepan over low heat.

2. Whisk in the cocoa powder until smooth.

3. Add the chocolate and stir until melted.

4. Pour in the milk and heat gently while stirring for 1–2 minutes more, until steaming and fully blended.

TO SERVE
Tip into a mug and get cosy.

BLOODY BULLSHOT

A bold, savoury spin on a Bloody Mary. Beef broth replaces most of the tomato juice for a rich, peppery pick-me-up that works just as well first thing as it does late at night. It's tangy, beefy and packs a proper punch.

SERVES 1
PREP TIME: 2 MINUTES
COOK TIME: 2–3 MINUTES

250ml (9fl oz) beef bone broth
50ml (1¾fl oz) tomato juice
½ teaspoon Worcestershire sauce
½ teaspoon lemon juice
A few drops of Tabasco
Pinch of celery salt
50ml (1¾fl oz) vodka (optional)
Freshly ground black pepper

1. Combine the beef broth and tomato juice in a small saucepan.

2. Warm gently until steaming but not boiling.

3. Stir in the Worcestershire sauce, lemon juice, Tabasco, celery salt and black pepper.

4. Add vodka, if using, and stir to combine.

TO SERVE
Pour into a heatproof glass, a thermos or mug and sip hot.

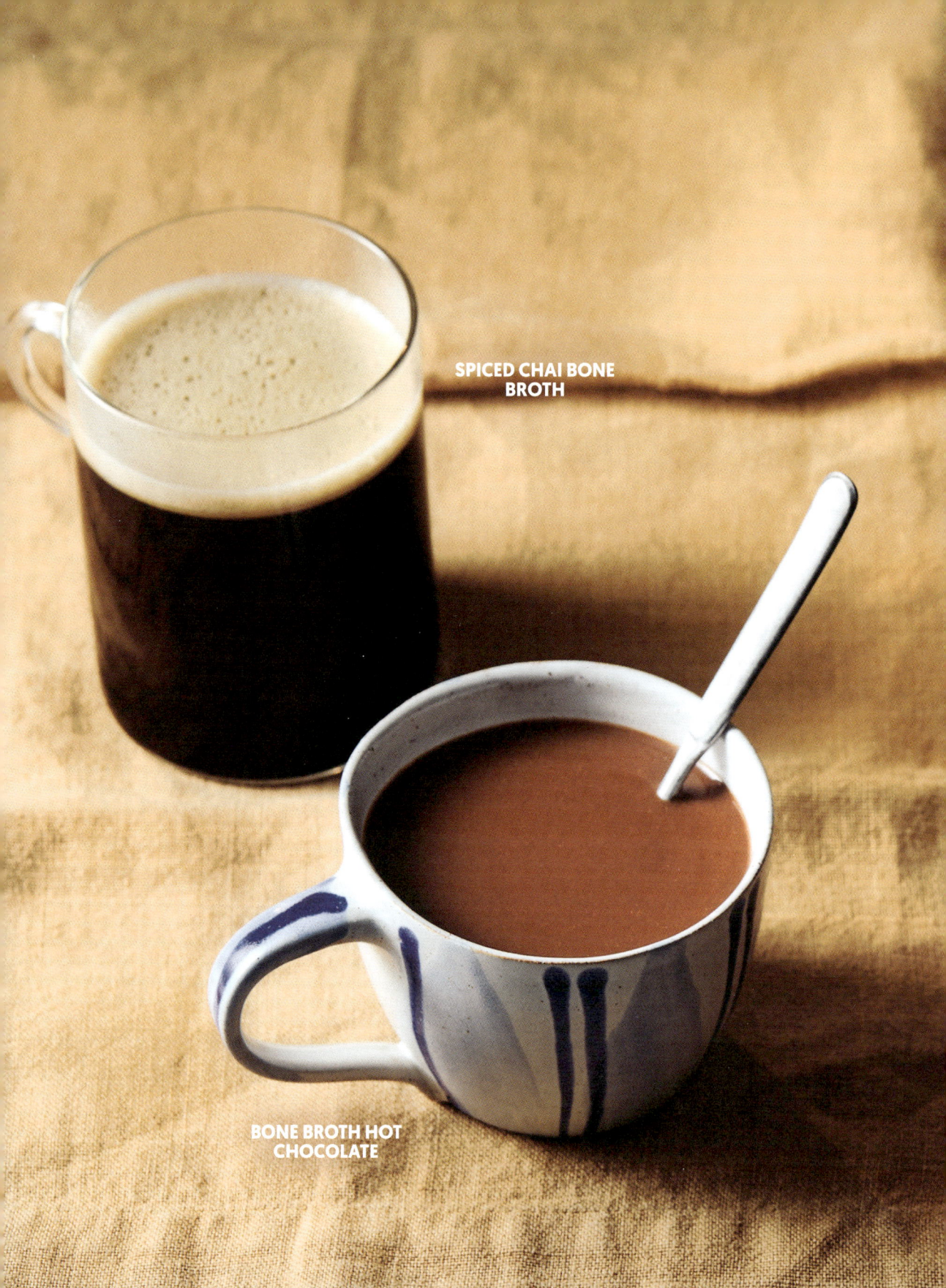

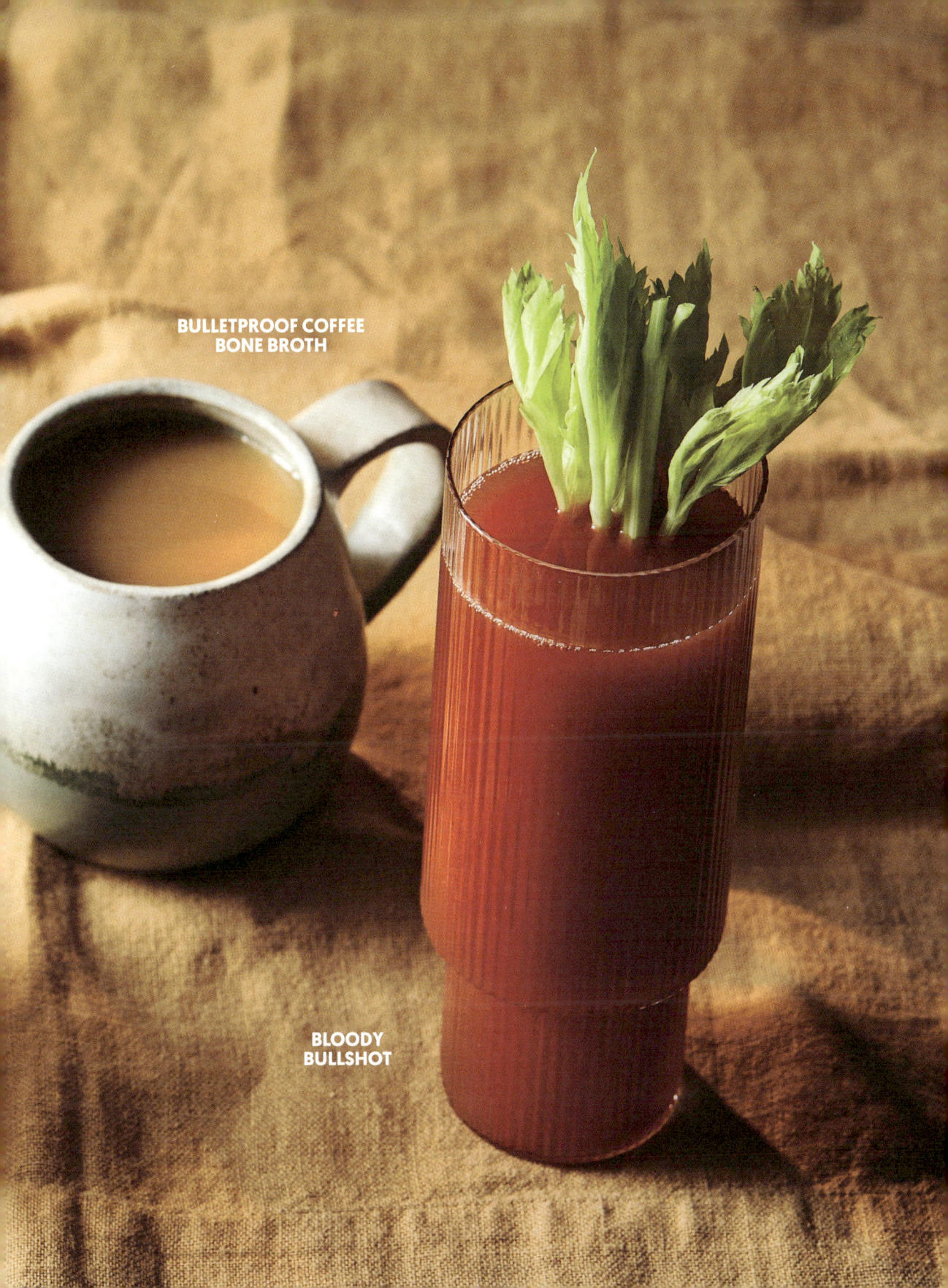

BROTHY SOUPS

Not every soup needs to be thick or creamy to be satisfying. The brothy soups in this chapter are naturally thinner than their blended cousins, but still rich with flavour. The lighter broth creates a robust, umami-rich base, ready to be finished with an endless variety of seasonings, textures and toppings.

Some, like Korean Miyeok-Guk – often served for postpartum healing – are rooted in culture and tradition, while others are modern twists on familiar favourites. What they all share is a focus on letting the broth take centre stage.

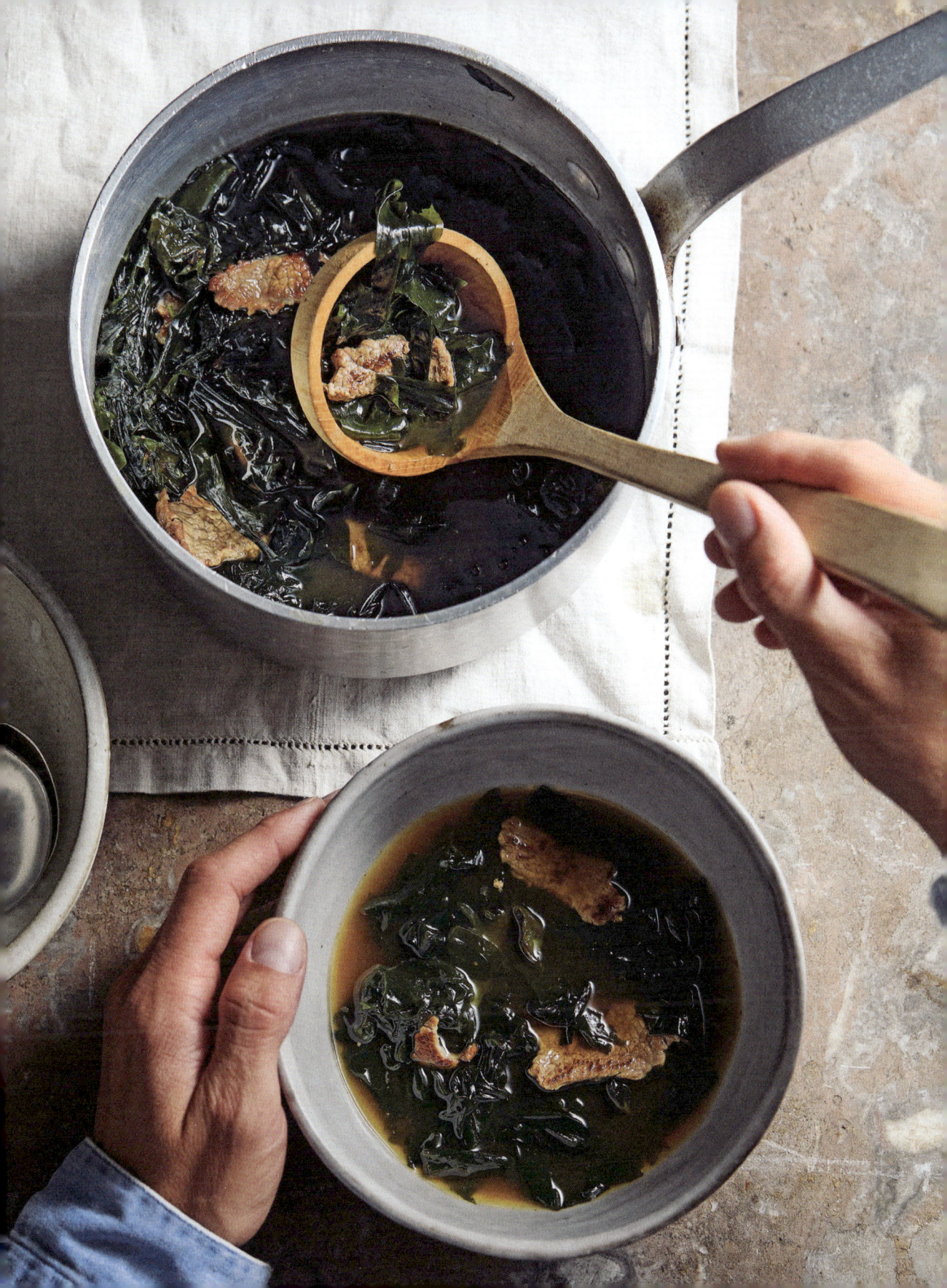

HOT & SOUR PRAWN TOM YUM

This fiery, fragrant Thai soup gets its kick from the lemongrass, lime and chilli. A splash of fish sauce and a squeeze of lime juice create the classic hot-sour balance. Using bone broth is an ideal way to deepen the flavour, add extra nutrition and create a glossier texture.

SERVES 4
PREP TIME: 15 MINUTES
COOK TIME: 15 MINUTES

1 litre (35fl oz) fish bone broth
3 stalks of lemongrass, bruised and halved
6 lime leaves, torn
4cm (1½ inch) piece of galangal, sliced
3 red chillies, halved lengthways (adjust to taste)
250g (9oz) oyster or shiitake mushrooms, torn or sliced
2 small tomatoes, cut into wedges
1 small red onion or 2 shallots, thinly sliced
400g (14oz) raw prawns, peeled and deveined
2 tablespoons fish sauce, plus more to taste
Juice of 2–3 limes
2 teaspoons palm sugar or brown sugar

TO SERVE
Handful of coriander leaves
Thai chilli oil or extra sliced chilli (optional)

HEAT THE BONE BROTH
Put the bone broth and 500ml (17fl oz) water in a large saucepan and bring to a gentle simmer.

ADD THE AROMATICS TO THE BONE BROTH
Add the lemongrass, lime leaves, galangal and chillies. Simmer for 5–7 minutes to infuse the broth.

INCORPORATE THE VEG
Stir in the mushrooms, tomatoes and onion. Simmer for another 3–4 minutes until just softened.

COOK THE PRAWNS
Add the prawns and cook until pink and just cooked through – around 2–3 minutes.

FINISH OFF THE SOUP
Stir in the fish sauce, lime juice and sugar. Taste and adjust the balance – it should be bright, hot and savoury.

PREPARE FOR SERVING
Remove the aromatics (lemongrass, galangal and lime leaves). Leave the chillies in or remove for less heat.

TO SERVE
Serve hot, scattered with fresh coriander and optional chilli oil or sliced fresh chilli. Great paired with a bowl of steaming sticky rice.

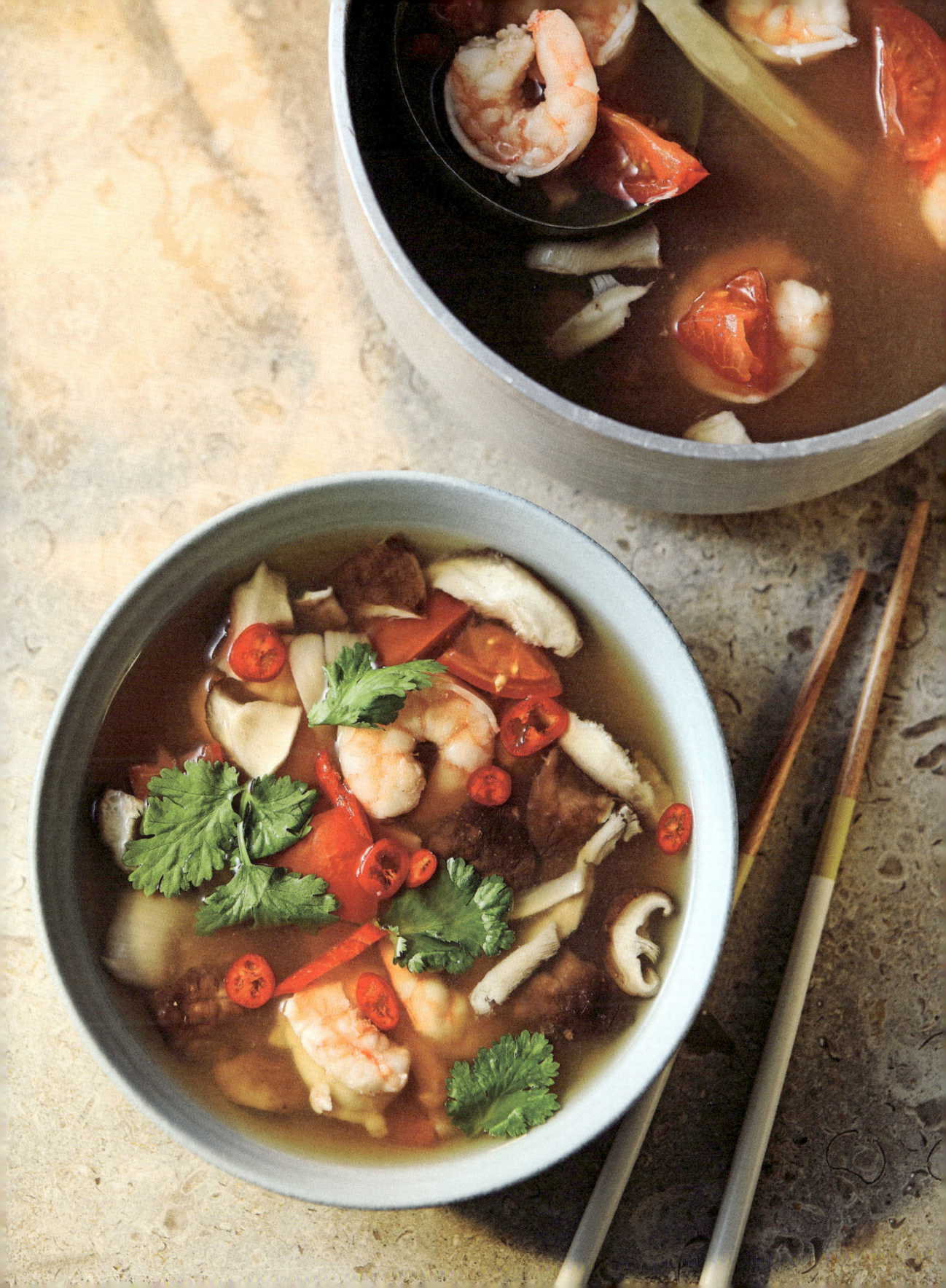

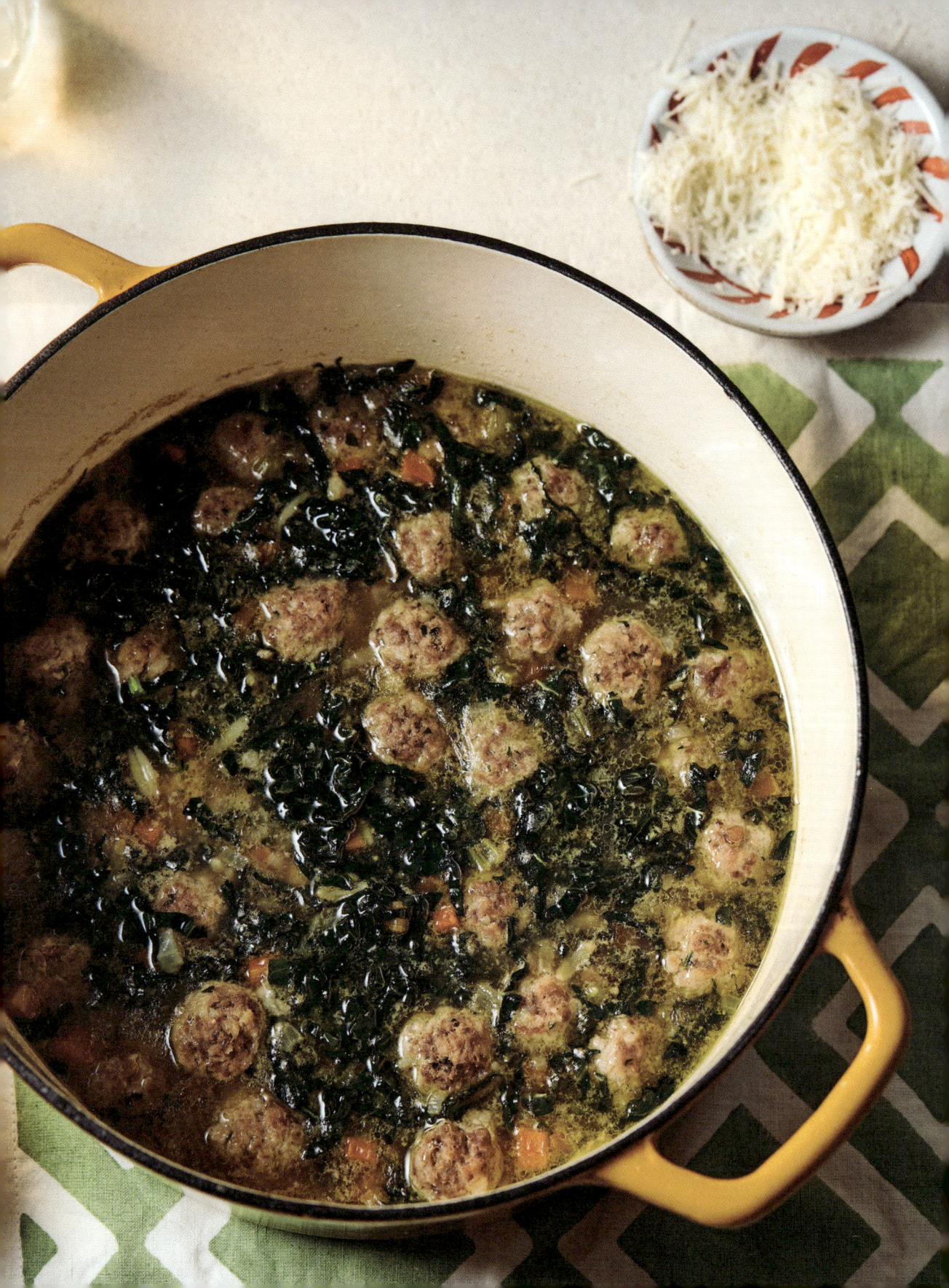

ITALIAN WEDDING SOUP

A rustic Italian classic where the 'wedding' refers to the perfect marriage of flavours: savoury broth, delicate meatballs, bitter greens and comforting pasta. Using bone broth elevates the umami richness of the soup, turning this everyday dish into something worth raising a toast to.

SERVES 4
PREP TIME: 25 MINUTES
COOK TIME: 25 MINUTES

FOR THE MEATBALLS
250g (9oz) pork mince
250g (9oz) beef mince
1 garlic clove, finely grated
30g (1oz) Parmesan cheese, finely grated
30g (1oz) breadcrumbs
1 egg
1 tablespoon chopped flat-leaf parsley
Sea salt and freshly ground black pepper

FOR THE SOUP
1 tablespoon olive oil
1 small onion, finely chopped
1 carrot, diced
1 celery stick, diced
1 litre (35fl oz) chicken bone broth
60g (2¼oz) small pasta (acini di pepe, orzo or stelline)
100g (3½oz) spinach or cavolo nero, chopped

TO SERVE
Extra Parmesan cheese

MAKE THE MEATBALLS
In a bowl, mix the pork, beef, garlic, Parmesan, breadcrumbs, egg, parsley and a good pinch of salt and pepper. Roll into small meatballs, around the size of a cherry. Chill while you prepare the soup.

COOK YOUR SOFRITO
Warm the olive oil in a large pan over medium heat. Add the onion, carrot and celery. Cook for 5–7 minutes until softened but not coloured.

COOK YOUR MEATBALLS
Pour in the bone broth and bring to a gentle simmer. Drop in the meatballs and cook for 8–10 minutes until just cooked.

COOK THE PASTA
Add the pasta and simmer for a further 8–10 minutes until al dente.

ADD THE GREENS
Stir in the greens and cook for 1–2 minutes until wilted. Taste and adjust the seasoning. Add a splash of boiling water if it looks a little thick.

TO SERVE
Ladle into bowls, evenly distributing the meatballs, and serve with lashings of extra Parmesan.

CHINESE CHICKEN & SWEETCORN SOUP

A real crowd pleaser, this light, comforting Chinese soup is made with chicken bone broth, tender shredded chicken and sweetcorn. It is finished with a classic egg ribbon and lightly thickened for a silky texture – just enough to make it richer without losing that clean, brothy feel.

SERVES 4
PREP TIME: 10 MINUTES
COOK TIME: 15 MINUTES

- 1 tablespoon sunflower oil
- 2 spring onions, finely sliced (reserve some green tops for garnish)
- 1 garlic clove, finely grated
- 1 small piece of fresh ginger (about 10g/¼oz), peeled and grated
- 1 litre (35fl oz) chicken bone broth
- 300g (10½oz) cooked chicken, shredded
- 200g (7oz) tinned or frozen sweetcorn
- 1 tablespoon cornflour mixed with 2 tablespoons cold water
- 2 eggs, beaten
- 1 teaspoon light soy sauce
- ½ teaspoon sesame oil
- Sea salt and ground white pepper

TO SERVE
Crispy chilli oil (optional)

COOK THE BASE
Heat the oil in a saucepan over medium heat. Add the spring onion whites, garlic and ginger. Fry for 1–2 minutes until fragrant but not coloured.

SIMMER THE BONE BROTH
Pour in the chicken bone broth and bring to a gentle simmer.

MIX THROUGH THE CHICKEN AND SWEETCORN
Add the shredded chicken and sweetcorn. Simmer for about 5–7 minutes until everything is warmed through.

LIGHTLY THICKEN
Stir in the cornflour slurry and let it bubble for 1–2 minutes – just enough to give the broth a little body while keeping it light.

CREATE THE EGG RIBBONS
Slowly drizzle in the beaten eggs while gently stirring to form soft ribbons through the soup. Season with soy sauce, sesame oil, salt and white pepper.

TO SERVE
Serve hot, garnished with the reserved spring onion tops. Add a spoonful of crispy chilli oil if you like it spicy.

LIVERPUDLIAN BEEF SCOUSE BROTH

A dish so beloved, Liverpudlians proudly take their nickname from it. This is a warming, chunky beef and vegetable broth with all the comforting flavours of a traditional Scouse, just lighter and more brothy.
A delicious, hearty bowlful that doesn't weigh you down.

SERVES 4
PREP TIME: 15 MINUTES
COOK TIME: 1 HOUR 20 MINUTES

1 tablespoon olive oil
400g (14oz) stewing beef, cut into large chunks
1 large onion, roughly chopped
2 garlic cloves, crushed
3 carrots, peeled and cut into large pieces
2 celery sticks, chopped
1 bay leaf
1 litre (35fl oz) beef bone broth
1 teaspoon dried thyme
1 teaspoon Marmite (for extra umami)
3 large potatoes, peeled and cut into chunks
Sea salt and freshly ground black pepper

TO SERVE
Chopped flat-leaf parsley
Crusty bread

BROWN THE BEEF
Heat the olive oil in a large saucepan over medium heat. Add the beef chunks and brown on all sides for 6–8 minutes. Remove and set aside.

SOFTEN THE ONION
Add the onion and garlic to the same pan. Cook for 5 minutes until softened and fragrant.

ADD THE VEG AND LIQUID
Return the beef to the pot along with the carrot, celery and bay leaf. Pour in the beef bone broth and 500ml (17fl oz) water. Bring to a gentle simmer.

SIMMER AWAY
Add the dried thyme and Marmite and season lightly with salt and pepper. Cover partially and cook gently for 45 minutes.

COOK THE POTATOES
Add the potatoes and simmer for a further 20–25 minutes until all the vegetables are tender but still hold their shape.

SEASON
Adjust the seasoning with salt and pepper to taste. Remove the bay leaf.

TO SERVE
Ladle into bowls, sprinkle with the chopped parsley and serve with crusty bread (non-negotiable!).

AVGOLEMONO
(GREEK EGG & LEMON CHICKEN SOUP)

This is the kind of soup that feels like it's doing you good with every spoonful. A Greek classic, it's gently thickened with egg and lifted with lemon, giving it a silky texture and a bright, clean flavour. One of our family favourites.

SERVES 4
PREP TIME: 5 MINUTES
COOK TIME: 15 MINUTES

1 litre (35fl oz) chicken bone broth
100g (3½oz) long-grain rice
300g (10½oz) cooked chicken, shredded
2 eggs
Juice of 1 large lemon (about 40ml/1¼fl oz)
Sea salt and ground white pepper

TO SERVE
Drizzle of extra virgin olive oil
Finely chopped dill or parsley

SIMMER THE BONE BROTH
Bring the chicken bone broth and 200ml (7fl oz) water to a gentle simmer in a large saucepan.

COOK THE RICE
Add the rice and cook for 8–10 minutes until just tender.

ADD THE CHICKEN
Stir in the shredded chicken and warm through for 2–3 minutes.

MAKE YOUR EGG-LEMON MIX
In a small bowl, whisk together the eggs and lemon juice until smooth.

TEMPER THE EGG
Slowly ladle in a few spoonfuls of hot broth to temper the egg mixture, whisking constantly.

THICKEN THE SOUP
Pour the tempered mixture back into the pan off the heat, stirring gently for 1–2 minutes to thicken the soup without it curdling.

SEASON
Season with salt and white pepper to taste.

TO SERVE
Ladle into bowls and finish with a drizzle of olive oil and a scattering of chopped dill or parsley.

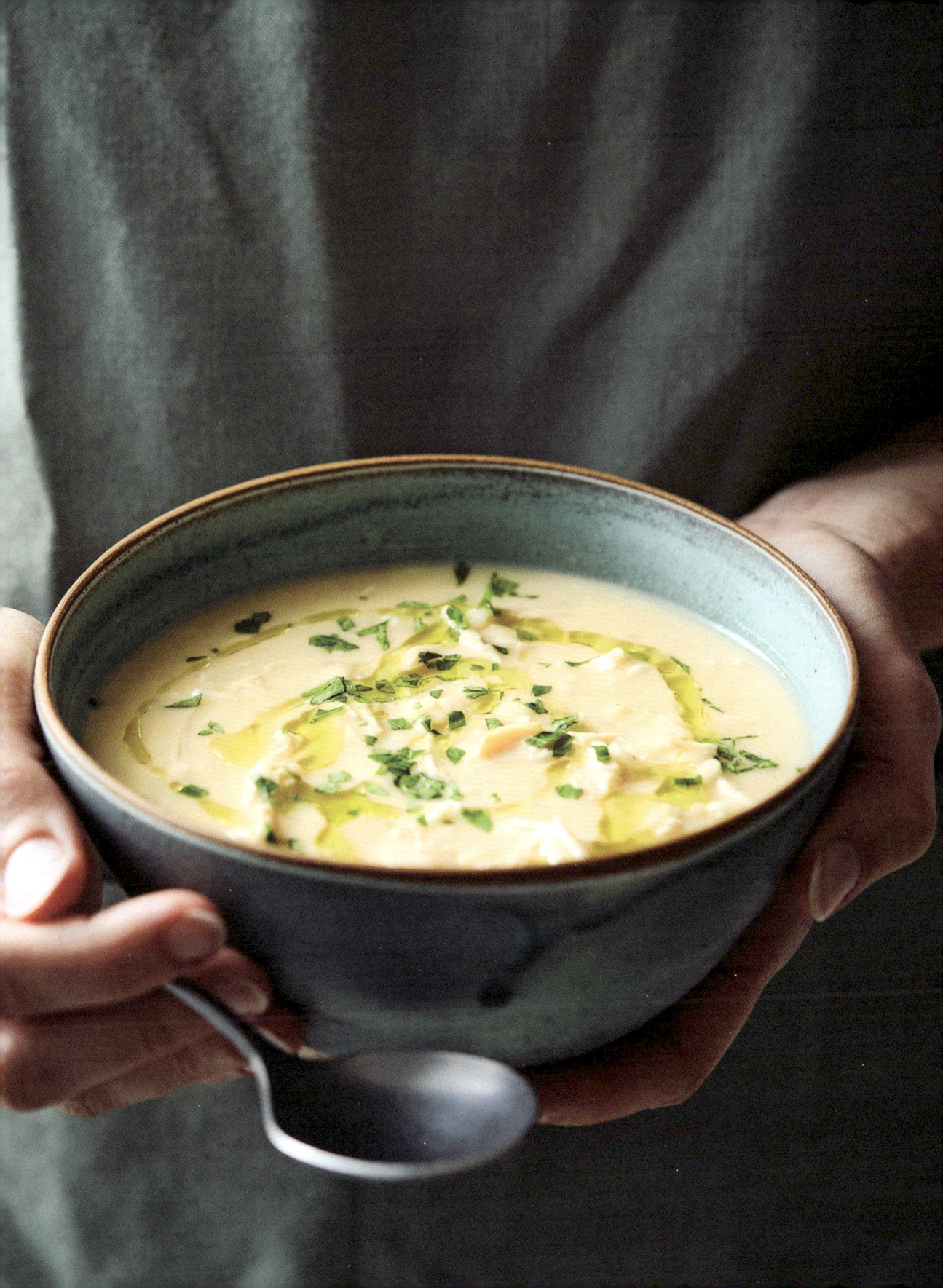

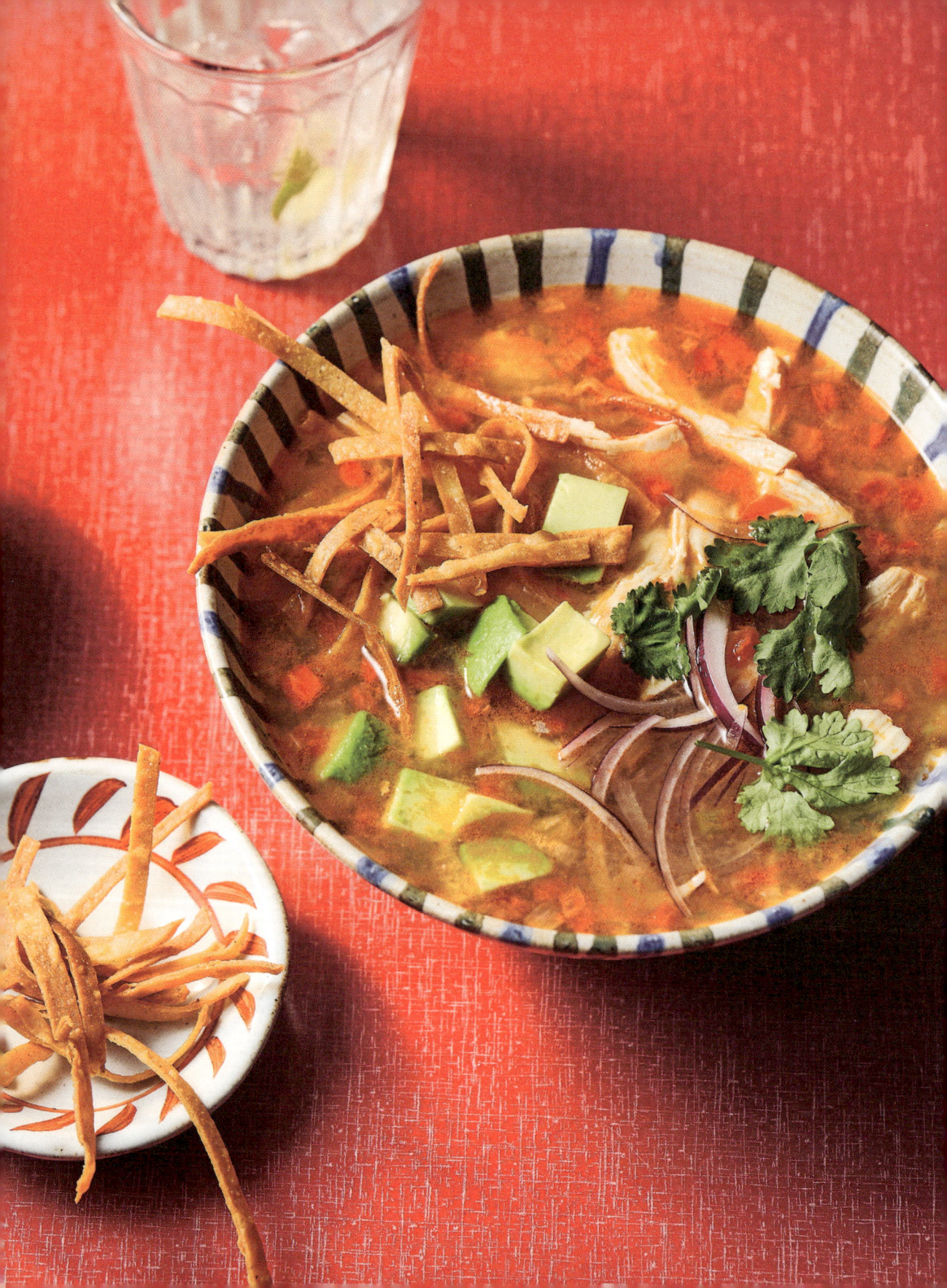

SOPA DE LIMA
(MEXICAN LIME & CHICKEN SOUP)

Fresh with lime, rich with bone broth and layered with warming herbs and spice, this bright Mexican soup from Yucatán can be hot or mild, depending on how brave you're feeling. Crunchy tortillas and fresh garnishes add contrast to the light, zesty broth, packing it with flavour.

SERVES 4
PREP TIME: 10 MINUTES
COOK TIME: 25 MINUTES

1 tablespoon sunflower oil
1 small white onion, finely chopped
1 garlic clove, finely grated
1 green chilli, deseeded and chopped (optional)
1 tomato, finely chopped
1 litre (35fl oz) chicken bone broth
1 bay leaf
½ teaspoon ground cumin
300g (10½oz) cooked chicken, shredded
Juice of 2 limes (about 40ml/ 1¼fl oz)
Sea salt

TO SERVE

Neutral oil (vegetable or sunflower), for frying
4 corn tortillas, sliced into thin strips
1 avocado, diced
½ red onion, finely sliced
Coriander leaves
Extra lime wedges

SOFTEN THE ONION
Heat the tablespoon of oil in a large saucepan over medium heat. Add the onion and cook for 3–4 minutes until soft.

MAKE YOUR TOMATO BASE
Stir in the garlic, green chilli and tomato. Cook for 3–4 minutes until the tomato breaks down.

ADD THE BONE BROTH
Add the chicken bone broth, 200ml (7fl oz) boiled water, bay leaf and cumin. Bring to a simmer.

ADD THE CHICKEN
Add the shredded chicken and cook for 5–7 minutes until warmed through.

FRESHEN UP THE SOUP WITH LIME
Stir in the lime juice and season with salt to taste. Remove the bay leaf.

MAKE CRISPY TORTILLA STRIPS
For the tortillas, heat a layer of oil in a frying pan and fry the strips in batches for 1–2 minutes until crisp. Drain on kitchen paper.

TO SERVE
Ladle the soup into wide, deep bowls. Top with avocado, red onion, coriander and crispy tortilla strips. Serve with the extra lime wedges.

CHEAT'S BOUILLABAISSE
(CLASSIC FRENCH FISH SOUP)

Bring the warmth of Marseille to your table in under an hour with this rustic, aromatic fish stew. Traditionally, bouillabaisse takes time, built on layers of fish stock, saffron and slow-cooked flavour. This version is a shortcut, but a good one. Using ready-made bone broth in place of hours-long fish stock gives you the same deep richness, without the wait. It's bold, briny and perfect with a hunk of crusty bread for dipping.

SERVES 4
PREP TIME: 15 MINUTES
COOK TIME: 35 MINUTES

2 tablespoons olive oil
1 small fennel bulb, finely sliced
1 leek, white part only, sliced
1 celery stick, chopped
3 garlic cloves, finely sliced
1 tablespoon tomato purée
Large pinch of saffron threads
1 teaspoon smoked paprika
150ml (5fl oz) dry white wine
1 litre (35fl oz) fish bone broth
1 x 400g tin chopped tomatoes
1 bay leaf
300g (10½oz) firm white fish (like cod or hake), cut into chunks
200g (7oz) raw prawns, peeled and deveined
250g (9oz) mussels, cleaned
Zest of ½ orange
Drizzle of extra virgin olive oil (optional)
Sea salt and freshly ground black pepper

GARLIC AIOLI
50g (1¾oz) mayonnaise
1 garlic clove, grated
Juice of 1 lemon wedge
Pinch of salt

TO SERVE
Toasted sourdough or baguette
Chopped flat-leaf parsley

SOFTEN THE VEG
Heat the olive oil in a large saucepan over medium heat. Add the fennel, leek and celery and cook for 6–8 minutes until soft and translucent.

ADD THE SPICES
Stir in the garlic, tomato purée, saffron and paprika. Cook for 1–2 minutes until fragrant.

DEGLAZE WITH WINE
Pour in the wine and let it bubble for 2–3 minutes to reduce the liquid slightly.

ADD THE BONE BROTH
Add the bone broth, tomatoes and bay leaf. Simmer gently for 15 minutes.

ADD THE FISH
Season with salt and pepper, then add the white fish. Simmer for 4–5 minutes.

ADD THE SHELLFISH
Add the prawns and mussels and cook for a further 3–4 minutes until just cooked through and the mussel shells have opened. Discard any that don't.

MAKE THE GARLIC AIOLI
Mix the mayonnaise with the grated garlic, lemon juice and a pinch of salt. Mix well until combined.

FINISH THE SOUP
Finish with the orange zest and a swirl of extra virgin olive oil, if you like.

TO SERVE
Ladle into bowls and serve with the toasted bread, aioli and a scattering of parsley.

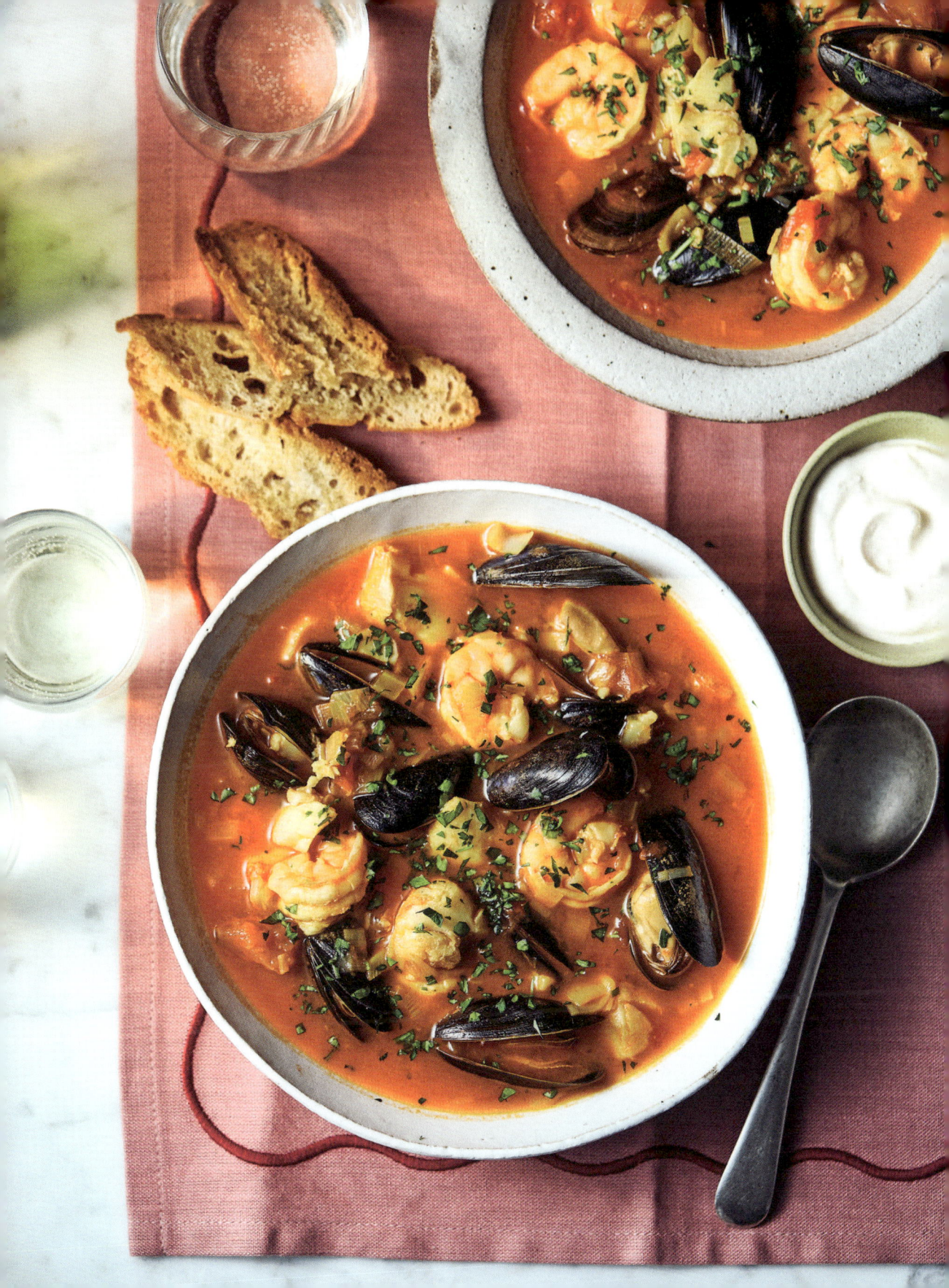

YUKGAEJANG
(KOREAN SPICY BEEF SOUP)

A deeply warming Korean soup made with tender shredded beef, vegetables and a spicy, umami-rich bone broth. It's hearty without being heavy, made for the days you need something flavour-packed and nourishing.

SERVES 4
PREP TIME: 20 MINUTES
COOK TIME: 1 HOUR 30 MINUTES

400g (14oz) beef brisket or stewing beef
1 small onion, halved
3 garlic cloves, smashed
1 thumb-sized piece of fresh ginger, sliced
1 litre (35fl oz) beef bone broth
1 tablespoon sesame oil
2 tablespoons gochugaru (Korean red chilli flakes)
1 tablespoon soy sauce
1 tablespoon fish sauce
150g (5½oz) beansprouts
Handful of oyster mushrooms, torn
½ leek, halved and sliced lengthways
Sea salt

TO SERVE
Chopped spring onion
Sesame seeds
Steamed rice

SIMMER THE BEEF
Place the beef, onion, garlic and ginger into a large saucepan with the bone broth and 500ml (17fl oz) water. Bring to the boil, then quickly reduce to a simmer for 1 hour 15 minutes, skimming occasionally.

PULL THE BEEF
Remove the beef and shred into long strips with a fork. Strain and reserve the broth.

COOK THE GOCHUGARU
Heat the sesame oil in a clean large saucepan over medium heat. Add the gochugaru and stir for 30 seconds to bloom.

ADD THE BONE BROTH BACK
Pour in the reserved broth, then add the soy sauce and fish sauce. Simmer for 10 minutes.

RETURN THE BEEF AND VEG
Add the shredded beef, beansprouts, mushrooms and leek. Simmer gently for 8–10 minutes.

SEASON
Taste and season with salt as needed.

TO SERVE
Ladle into bowls and top with the chopped spring onion and sesame seeds. Serve with rice on the side.

RUSTIC CABBAGE & SMOKED SAUSAGE BROTH

This kind of broth has long roots in rural French cooking – where frugality meets flavour, and nothing goes to waste. Smoked sausage, tender cabbage and silky bone broth come together in a bowl that's simple, hearty and deeply satisfying. It's a cold-weather staple built on comfort, not fuss.

SERVES 4
PREP TIME: 10 MINUTES
COOK TIME: 40 MINUTES

1 tablespoon olive oil
1 onion, finely chopped
1 carrot, diced
1 celery stick, diced
2 garlic cloves, finely sliced
1 teaspoon caraway seeds (optional)
250g (9oz) smoked sausage (like kielbasa), sliced into coins
½ white cabbage, cored and shredded
1 litre (35fl oz) chicken bone broth
1 bay leaf
1 tablespoon cider vinegar or white wine vinegar
Sea salt and freshly ground black pepper

TO SERVE
Chopped dill or flat-leaf parsley
Crusty bread

SOFTEN THE VEG
Warm the olive oil in a heavy-based soup pot over medium heat. Add the onion, carrot and celery, cooking for 6–8 minutes until softened but not coloured.

GET THE AROMAS GOING
Stir in the garlic and caraway seeds, if using, and cook for about 1–2 minutes until fragrant.

SIZZLE THE SMOKED SAUSAGE
Add the smoked sausage and let it sizzle for 3–4 minutes until starting to caramelise at the edges.

ADD THE CABBAGE
Tip in the cabbage and stir through to coat in the fat. Cook for 2–3 minutes until just wilting.

ADD THE BONE BROTH
Pour in the bone broth and 300ml (10½fl oz) water. Add the bay leaf and bring to a simmer.

BUBBLE AWAY
Cover and cook for 25–30 minutes until the cabbage is silky and the broth deeply flavoured.

SEASON
Season the broth generously with salt and black pepper. Stir in the vinegar just before serving.

TO SERVE
Ladle into bowls, top with chopped dill or parsley and serve with crusty bread on the side.

MIYEOK-GUK
(KOREAN SEAWEED SOUP)

Traditionally eaten on birthdays and after childbirth, Miyeok-Guk is a soup rooted in ritual and made with care. It's packed with mineral-rich seaweed, tender beef and a clear, savoury bone broth. Nourishing and restorative, it's deeply familiar in Korean households – served to mark milestones, aid recovery or simply offer everyday comfort.

SERVES 4
PREP TIME: 10 MINUTES, PLUS SOAKING
COOK TIME: 30 MINUTES

15g (½oz) dried miyeok (wakame seaweed)
Drizzle of sunflower oil
150g (5½oz) beef brisket or stewing beef, thinly sliced
1 garlic clove, minced
1 litre (35fl oz) beef bone broth
1 tablespoon soy sauce
1 teaspoon sesame oil
1 teaspoon fish sauce (optional)
Sea salt

TO SERVE
Steamed rice
Extra sesame oil or toasted sesame seeds (optional)

SOAK THE SEAWEED
Soak the dried miyeok (seaweed) in 500ml (17fl oz) cold water for 15–20 minutes until fully rehydrated and soft. Drain, rinse well, then cut into bite-size lengths.

BROWN THE BEEF
Heat the sunflower oil in a heavy-based soup pot over medium heat. Add the beef and sauté for 3–4 minutes until browned all over.

ADD THE SEAWEED AND GARLIC
Add the drained seaweed and garlic to the pan and cook, stirring, for 2–3 minutes to coat and deepen the flavour.

SIMMER THE BONE BROTH
Pour in the bone broth and bring to a gentle boil. Skim any foam, then reduce to a simmer for 25–30 minutes.

SEASON
Season with soy sauce, sesame oil and fish sauce, if using. Taste and add salt as needed.

TO SERVE
Serve simply with steamed rice on the side and a drizzle of sesame oil or sprinkling of toasted sesame seeds, if using.

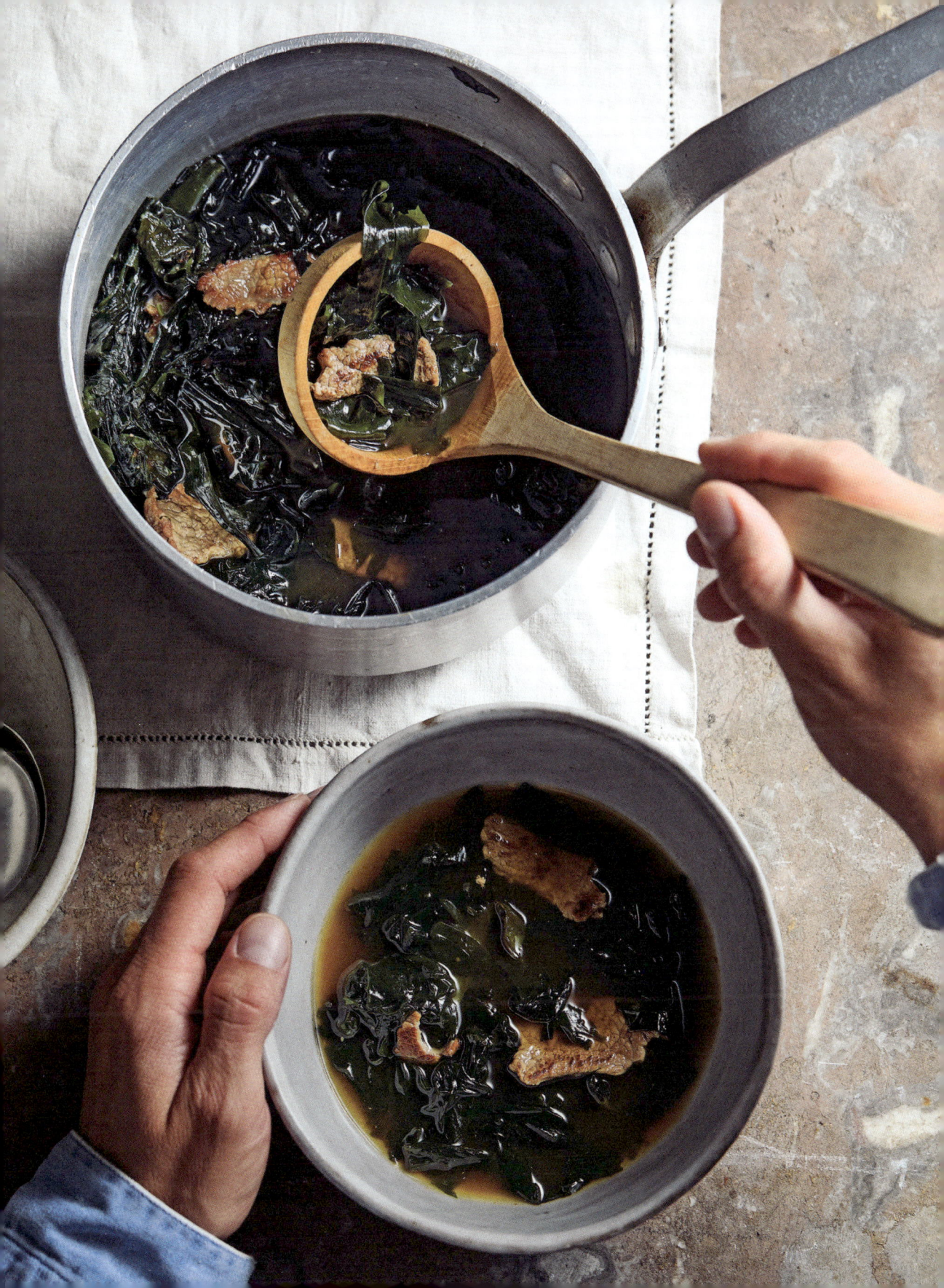

BLENDED SOUPS

We're firm believers that there's a soup for every season, whether it's a light and fresh Gazpacho to transport you to the Spanish sunshine or a Classic Cream of Mushroom to throw you back to the joy of childhood winters.

With bone broth as the base for these blended soups, you get a deeper flavour and a smoother finish, plus all the benefits of extra nourishment. Most of these recipes can be made in one pot and blitzed straight in the pan, ready in under an hour. Ideal for lunch, dinner or anything in between.

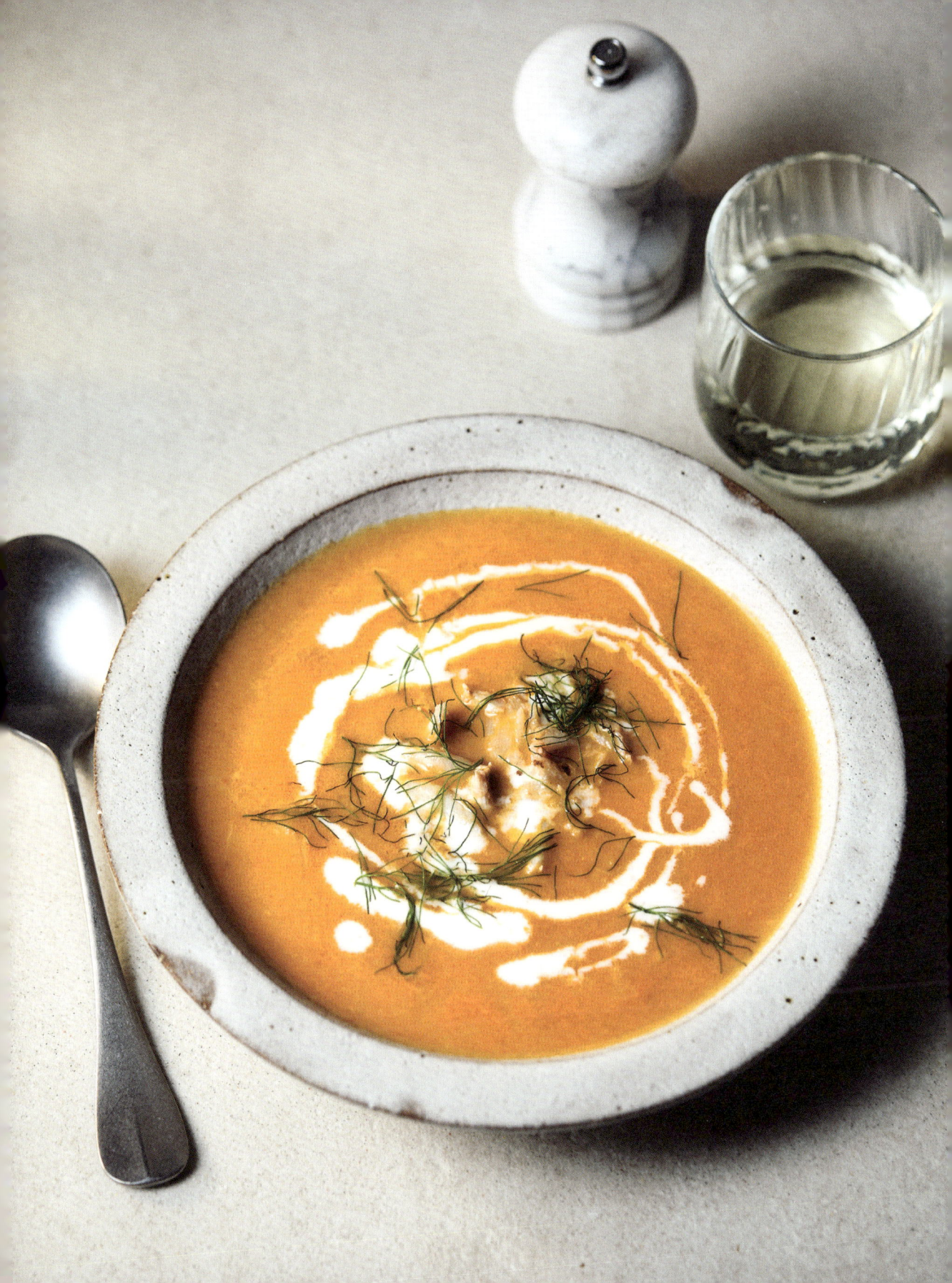

EGGS FLORENTINE SOUP

This is everything you love about Eggs Florentine – spinach, savoury depth and a runny yolk – reimagined as a silky, comforting soup. It's hearty but not heavy, built on proper bone broth and finished with a poached egg that makes it feel like more than just lunch. Great for using up frozen spinach and a brilliant way to turn a few humble ingredients into something more.

SERVES 4
PREP TIME: 15 MINUTES
COOK TIME: 40 MINUTES

- 1 tablespoon butter
- 1 tablespoon olive oil
- 1 onion, finely chopped
- 2 garlic cloves, finely chopped
- ½ teaspoon fine sea salt
- Pinch of ground nutmeg
- 1 potato, peeled and chopped
- 750ml (26fl oz) beef bone broth
- 250g (9oz) frozen spinach or 300g (10½oz) fresh spinach
- Small handful of flat-leaf parsley or tarragon (optional, for brightness)
- 30g (1oz) hard cheese (Cheddar, Comté or Parmesan), chopped or grated
- Small knob of cold butter
- Lemon juice, to taste
- Freshly ground black pepper

TO SERVE
- 4 eggs
- Crème fraîche

START WITH A SLOW SWEAT
In a large saucepan, melt the butter with the olive oil over low heat. Add the onion, garlic and salt. Cook gently for about 10–15 minutes until completely soft and sweet, stirring now and then to prevent browning.

ADD SPICE AND SIMMER
Stir in the nutmeg, then add the chopped potato and pour in the bone broth. Bring to a gentle simmer and cook for about 15–20 minutes, or until the potato is soft enough to mash with a spoon.

ADD SPINACH AND HERBS
Stir in the spinach (frozen or fresh) and cook until wilted and heated through. Add the fresh herbs if using.

BLEND UNTIL SMOOTH
Use a hand blender to blitz the soup in the pan until completely smooth and velvety. For an ultra-smooth texture, pass it through a fine-mesh sieve.

ENRICH AND BALANCE
Add the grated cheese and a small knob of cold butter. Stir or blend again briefly to melt and emulsify. Add the lemon juice to brighten and black pepper to finish.

POACH THE EGGS
Bring a saucepan of water to a gentle simmer. Crack each egg into a small cup, swirl the water and gently slide in the egg. Poach for 3–4 minutes until the white is set but the yolk is still runny. Remove with a slotted spoon and drain on kitchen paper.

TO SERVE
Ladle the hot soup into bowls and gently top each one with a poached egg. Finish with a spoonful of crème fraîche and a crack of black pepper.

BAKED POTATO SOUP WITH SOUR CREAM & CHIVES

This creamy, comforting soup transforms baked potatoes into hearty, velvety bowls of goodness, thickened with their natural starchiness and boosted with bone broth. Top with sour cream and crisp toppings and you're on to a guaranteed weeknight winner.

SERVES 4
PREP TIME: 10 MINUTES
COOK TIME: 1 HOUR 10 MINUTES

4 large floury potatoes (about 900g/2lb), whole and unpeeled
1 tablespoon olive oil
1 onion, finely chopped
2 garlic cloves, crushed
500ml (17fl oz) chicken bone broth
300ml (10½fl oz) whole milk
100g (3½oz) sour cream
80g (2¾oz) grated mature Cheddar cheese
1 tablespoon finely chopped chives
Sea salt and freshly ground black pepper

TO SERVE
Extra sour cream
Extra finely chopped chives
Crispy bacon bits (optional)
Fried shallots (optional)

ROAST THE POTATOES
Preheat the oven to 200°C (180°C fan)/400°F/gas 6. Prick the potatoes and bake directly on the oven shelf for 1 hour, or until tender with crisp skins.

COOL AND SCOOP
Let the potatoes cool slightly, then cut in half and scoop out the flesh into a bowl. Set aside.

SOFTEN THE ONIONS
In a large saucepan, heat the olive oil and cook the onion for 6–8 minutes until soft. Stir in the garlic and cook for a further 1–2 minutes.

MAKE THE SOUP BASE
Add the baked potato flesh, bone broth and milk. Bring to a simmer, breaking up the potatoes with a spoon.

BLITZ THE SOUP
Simmer gently for 10–12 minutes, stirring often. Blitz the soup with a hand blender until it's creamy with a bit of texture.

FINISH THE SOUP
Stir in the sour cream, grated cheese and chives. Season generously with salt and pepper. Heat through gently but don't let it boil.

TO SERVE
Ladle into bowls and top with a spoonful of sour cream, extra chives and crispy bacon bits and fried shallots if you're feeling fancy.

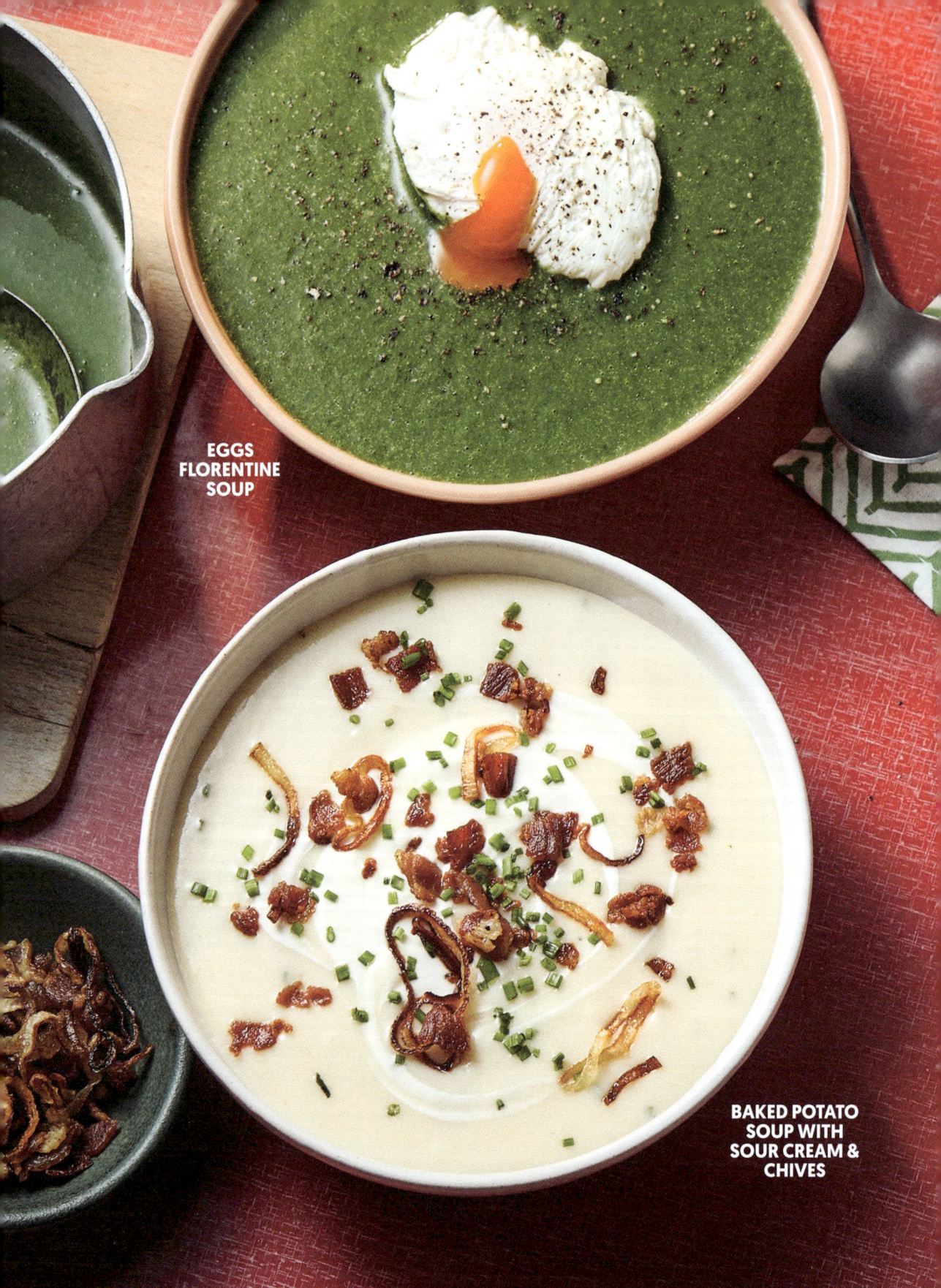

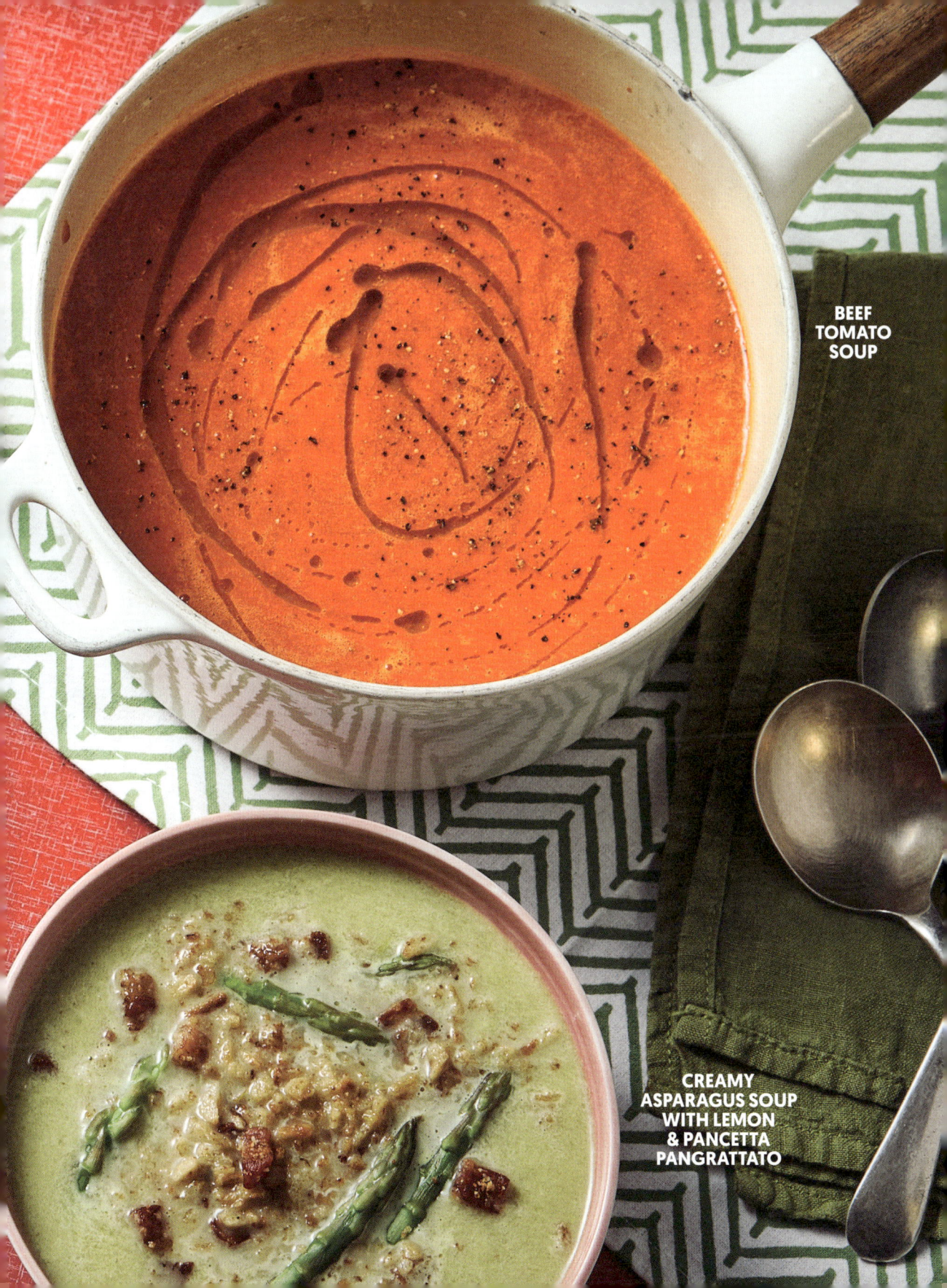

BEEF TOMATO SOUP

CREAMY ASPARAGUS SOUP WITH LEMON & PANCETTA PANGRATTATO

BEEF TOMATO SOUP

This is a proper cold-weather soup, the kind you want with a melting cheese toastie or just on its own in a big mug. Roasting the tomatoes brings out their sweetness, and using beef bone broth instead of water or stock adds a deeper, more rounded flavour with extra nutrition. It's a great one to batch cook, and it gets better after a day in the fridge.

SERVES 4
PREP TIME: 15 MINUTES
COOK TIME: 55 MINUTES

1kg (2lb 4oz) ripe beef tomatoes or large vine tomatoes, halved
1 red onion, cut into wedges
3 garlic cloves, unpeeled
3 thyme sprigs
2 tablespoons olive oil
1 tablespoon balsamic vinegar
½ teaspoon sugar
1 tablespoon unsalted butter
1 tablespoon tomato purée
750ml (26fl oz) beef bone broth
1 teaspoon Worcestershire sauce
Sea salt and freshly ground black pepper

TO SERVE
Crème fraîche
Drizzle of extra virgin olive oil

ROAST THE TOMATOES
Preheat your oven to 210°C (190°C fan)/400°F/gas 6–7. Place the halved tomatoes, cut-side up, on a large roasting tray. Add the red onion, garlic cloves and thyme sprigs. Drizzle with the olive oil and balsamic vinegar, then season well with salt, pepper and a little sugar. Roast for 40–45 minutes until soft and starting to brown at the edges.

MAKE THE SOUP BASE
When the veg are done, squeeze the garlic from their skins and discard the thyme stems. Blend the tomatoes, onion and garlic together to a smooth purée. Add a bit of broth to loosen if needed.

BUILD THE FLAVOUR
In a large saucepan, melt the butter over medium heat. Add the tomato purée and cook for 1–2 minutes until it darkens slightly and smells sweet. Pour in the blended tomato mixture, beef bone broth and Worcestershire sauce. Bring to a simmer and cook gently for 10–15 minutes.

STRAIN (OPTIONAL)
For a silky finish, blend again and pass through a fine-mesh sieve into a clean pan. Discard any pulp.

SEASON
Taste and adjust the seasoning.

TO SERVE
Serve hot in warm bowls or mugs. Top with a spoon of crème fraîche or a drizzle of olive oil as preferred. Ideal with a cheese toastie on the side.

CREAMY ASPARAGUS SOUP WITH LEMON & PANCETTA PANGRATTATO

A spring-green soup with a lemony freshness and sweetness of asparagus, made more luxurious with chicken bone broth and a crisp pancetta crumb to finish. This is like spring in a bowl, the perfect starter before a lamb roast dinner!

SERVES 4
PREP TIME: 10 MINUTES
COOK TIME: 25 MINUTES

500g (1lb 2oz) asparagus, woody ends trimmed
2 tablespoons olive oil
1 small leek or onion, finely sliced
1 garlic clove, crushed
500ml (17fl oz) chicken bone broth
100ml (3½fl oz) double cream
Zest of ½ lemon, juice to taste
Sea salt and freshly ground black pepper

FOR THE PANGRATTATO
60g (2¼oz) pancetta, diced
1 small garlic clove, finely grated
40g (1½oz) stale breadcrumbs or panko
1 teaspoon lemon zest

PREP THE ASPARAGUS
Cut the tips off a handful of asparagus and set aside. Chop the remaining stalks into chunks.

COOK THE VEG
Heat the olive oil in a large saucepan. Add the leek with a pinch of salt and cook for 6–8 minutes until soft. Add the garlic and chopped asparagus stalks and cook for 2–3 minutes more.

SIMMER
Pour in the bone broth and 250ml (9fl oz) water, bring to a simmer and cook for 10–12 minutes until the asparagus is tender.

PREP THE ASPARAGUS TIPS
Meanwhile, bring a small pan of salted water to a boil and blanch the reserved asparagus tips for 1–2 minutes until bright and tender. Drain and set aside in a bowl of cold water to stop the cooking.

BLITZ THE SOUP
Blitz using a hand blender until smooth. Stir in the cream, lemon zest and a little lemon juice. Season to taste and warm through without boiling.

MAKE THE PANGRATTATO
For the pangrattato, heat a frying pan over medium heat. Add the pancetta and cook for 4–5 minutes until crisp. Stir in the garlic and breadcrumbs. Cook, stirring, for 3–4 minutes until golden and crunchy. Remove from the heat and mix in the lemon zest.

TO SERVE
Ladle the soup into bowls and top with asparagus tips and a generous spoonful of pangrattato.

GAZPACHO

One of our all-time family favourites, perfect for the height of summer. This version adds chilled bone broth, which gives the soup a subtle savoury depth without overwhelming its clean, fresh flavour. Before serving, let it sit in the fridge for a few hours to allow the flavour to mellow and develop.

SERVES 4
PREP TIME: 15 MINUTES
CHILL TIME: 2–3 HOURS

500g (1lb 2oz) ripe tomatoes, roughly chopped
1 red pepper, deseeded and chopped
½ cucumber (around 150g/5½oz), peeled and chopped
1 small red onion, chopped
1 garlic clove, crushed
250ml (9fl oz) chilled chicken bone broth
1–2 tablespoons red wine vinegar
50ml (1¾fl oz) extra virgin olive oil
Sea salt and freshly ground black pepper

TO SERVE
Drizzle of extra virgin olive oil
Extra chopped cucumber and tomato
Torn basil or flat-leaf parsley
Croutons (optional)

BLEND THE VEG
Put the tomatoes, red pepper, cucumber, onion and garlic into a blender with a good pinch of salt and a grind of pepper. Blend until mostly smooth.

ADD THE BONE BROTH AND BLEND AGAIN
Add the chilled bone broth, vinegar and olive oil. Blend again until completely smooth.

SEASON
Taste and adjust the seasoning. If it's too thick, add a little cold water.

CHILL
Chill for at least 2–3 hours, ideally longer, until properly cold and the flavours have had time to come together.

TO SERVE
Serve in bowls or mugs with your choice of garnish – a small drizzle of olive oil, some chopped veg for crunch, fresh herbs or a few croutons.

CLASSIC CREAM OF MUSHROOM SOUP

An old-school earthy soup, made from chestnut mushrooms, butter and slow-cooked onion, with chicken bone broth adding a glossy texture and more depth of flavour. Finish with a splash of cream and plenty of black pepper for a silky, steaming soup you'll be slurping every last drop of.

SERVES 4
PREP TIME: 10 MINUTES
COOK TIME: 25–30 MINUTES

40g (1½oz) unsalted butter
1 tablespoon olive oil
1 onion, finely diced
2 garlic cloves, crushed
500g (1lb 2oz) chestnut mushrooms, sliced
2 teaspoons fresh thyme leaves or 1 teaspoon dried
750ml (26fl oz) chicken bone broth
100ml (3½fl oz) double cream
Squeeze of lemon juice
Sea salt and freshly ground black pepper

TO SERVE (OPTIONAL)
Extra double cream
Chopped chives

SOFTEN THE ONION
Melt the butter with the olive oil in a heavy-based pan over medium heat. Add the onion and a pinch of salt and cook for 5–6 minutes until soft but not coloured.

COOK THE MUSHROOMS
Add the garlic, cook for 1–2 minutes, then tip in the mushrooms and thyme. Turn up the heat slightly and cook for 8–10 minutes until the mushrooms have released their moisture and started to brown.

ADD THE BONE BROTH
Pour in the bone broth, scraping up any bits at the bottom of the pan. Simmer gently for 10–12 minutes until everything is soft and well combined.

BLITZ THE SOUP
Use a hand blender to blitz until smooth, or leave a bit of texture if preferred.

ENRICH WITH CREAM
Stir in the cream, season with salt, plenty of black pepper and a few drops of lemon juice to lift it. Warm through but don't let it boil.

TO SERVE
Ladle into warm bowls. Swirl with a little extra cream, if you like, and scatter with chopped chives.

FENNEL & CRAB BISQUE

A fancier, silkier soupy bisque where sweet crab meat and aromatic fennel combine in a rich, brandy-kissed broth. Simple to make but with a real showstopper flavour, finish with a swirl of cream and a side of warm, crusty bread. Delicious!

SERVES 4
PREP TIME: 15 MINUTES
COOK TIME: 45 MINUTES

2 tablespoons olive oil
1 small fennel bulb (about 200g/7oz), finely sliced
1 banana shallot, finely chopped
1 carrot, finely chopped
2 garlic cloves, crushed
1 tablespoon tomato purée
50ml (1¾fl oz) brandy (or dry sherry)
500ml (17fl oz) fish bone broth
150ml (5fl oz) double cream
200g (7oz) white crab meat
Zest and juice of ½ lemon
Pinch of cayenne or paprika for warmth (optional)
Sea salt and white pepper

TO SERVE
Chopped fennel fronds
Extra double cream

SOFTEN THE VEG
In a heavy-based saucepan, heat the olive oil over medium heat. Add the fennel, shallot and carrot with a pinch of salt. Cook for 10–12 minutes, stirring often, until soft and fragrant but not coloured.

COOK OFF THE BRANDY
Stir in the garlic and tomato purée. Cook for 1–2 minutes, then pour in the brandy. Let it bubble for 1–2 minutes to burn off the alcohol.

SIMMER THE SOUP
Add the fish broth and 200ml (7fl oz) water. Simmer uncovered for 20 minutes until the vegetables are very soft and the broth is slightly reduced.

BLITZ THE SOUP
Use a hand blender to blend the soup until smooth. Stir in the cream and simmer for 2–3 minutes more.

ADD THE CRAB
Fold in half the crab meat and warm through gently for 1–2 minutes. Add the lemon zest and juice, and season with salt, white pepper and cayenne or paprika, if using.

TO SERVE
Ladle into warm bowls and top with fennel fronds, a drizzle of cream and the remaining crab meat.

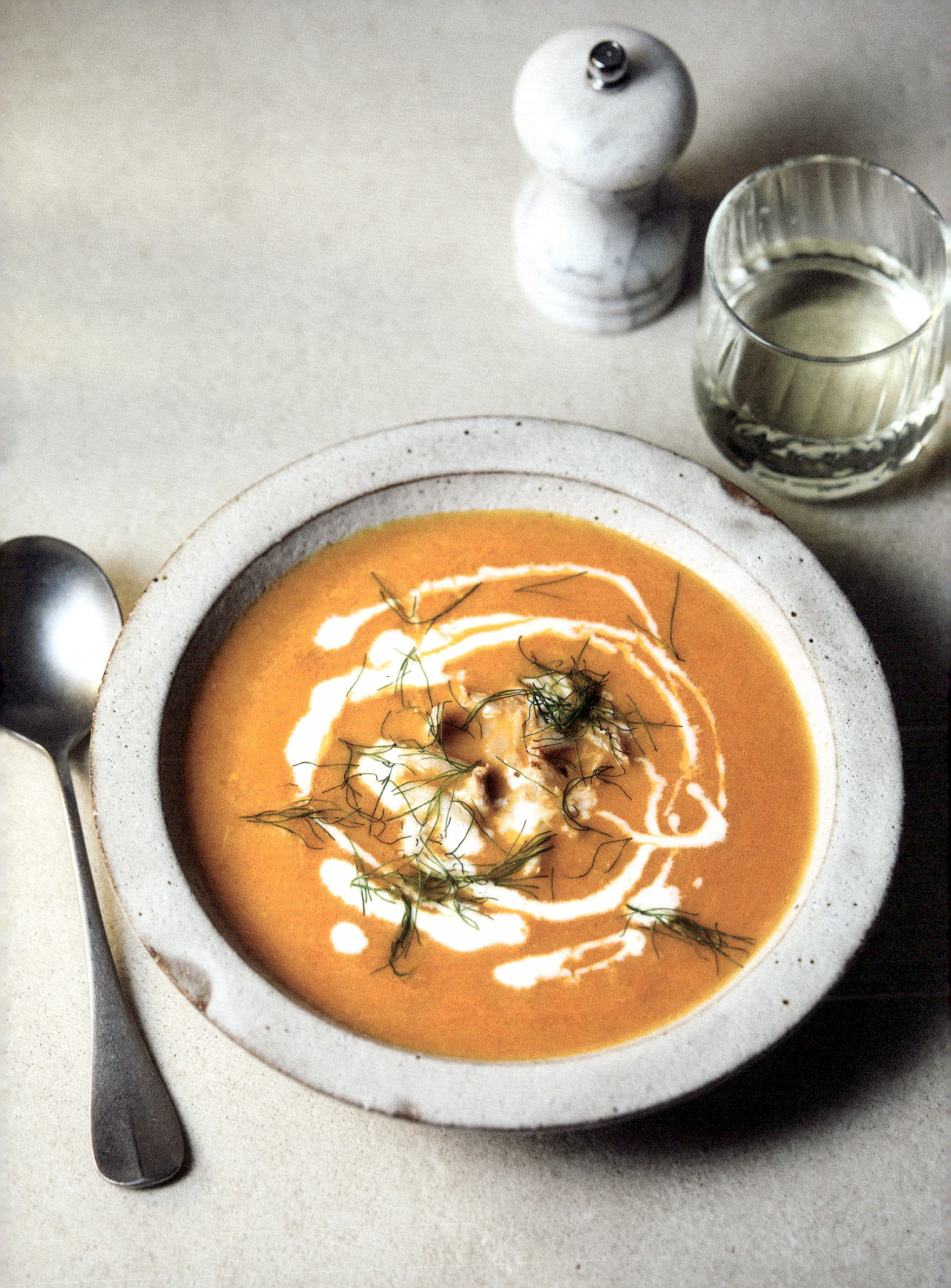

HARISSA BUTTERNUT SQUASH SOUP

This rich, autumnal soup layers the natural sweetness of roasted squash with smoky harissa and bone broth for warmth and richness. The tamari seeds on top finish it all off with a lovely savoury crunch.

SERVES 4
PREP TIME: 10 MINUTES
COOK TIME: 45 MINUTES

1 medium butternut squash (about 1kg/2lb 4oz), halved and deseeded
2 tablespoons olive oil, plus extra for roasting
1 onion, chopped
2 garlic cloves, crushed
1 tablespoon rose harissa paste
600ml (21fl oz) chicken bone broth
1 tablespoon lemon juice, or to taste
Sea salt and freshly ground black pepper

TO SERVE
40g (1½oz) pumpkin seeds
1 teaspoon olive oil
1 tablespoon tamari or soy sauce
Drizzle of extra virgin olive oil
Extra rose harissa paste

ROAST THE BUTTERNUT SQUASH
Preheat the oven to 200°C (180°C fan)/400°F/gas 6. Rub the cut sides of the squash with olive oil and season with salt and pepper. Place cut-side down on a baking tray and roast for 35–40 minutes until very tender.

ROAST THE PUMPKIN SEEDS
For the pumpkin seeds, mix them with the olive oil and tamari and pop them in the oven for 3–4 minutes until golden and sticky. Set aside until serving.

SOFTEN THE ONION
While the squash and seeds roast, heat 2 tablespoons of olive oil in a pan. Add the onion and cook for 6–8 minutes until soft. Stir in the garlic and harissa and cook for a further 1–2 minutes.

ADD THE ROASTED BUTTERNUT SQUASH
Scoop the flesh from the roasted squash and add to the pan. Pour in the bone broth, stir well and bring to a simmer. Cook for 5–6 minutes.

BLITZ THE SOUP
Blend with a hand blender until smooth. Stir in the lemon juice, season well and warm gently. Add some water if needed to loosen.

TO SERVE
Serve the soup hot, topped with the tamari seeds, a swirl of olive oil and some extra harissa if you like it spicy!

SRI LANKAN VEGETABLE & COCONUT SOUP

A warming, spice-infused coconut broth packed with seasonal vegetables, fresh curry leaves and soft onions. This soup only needs a short simmer to bring out its rich, comforting flavour. Serve with hot roti or flatbread to soak it all up.

SERVES 4
PREP TIME: 15 MINUTES
COOK TIME: 35 MINUTES

2 tablespoons coconut oil
1 teaspoon black mustard seeds
½ teaspoon fenugreek seeds
1 small cinnamon stick
10–12 fresh curry leaves
1 small onion, finely sliced
2 garlic cloves, finely chopped
1 teaspoon grated fresh ginger
1 green chilli, finely sliced
½ teaspoon ground turmeric
1 teaspoon ground coriander
½ teaspoon ground cumin
300ml (10½fl oz) chicken bone broth
1 x 400ml tin coconut milk
1 small sweet potato, peeled and cut into 1cm (½ inch) cubes
1 large carrot, diced
100g (3½oz) green beans, trimmed and halved
Juice of ½ lime
Sea salt

FOR THE COCONUT TOPPER (OPTIONAL)
½ teaspoon coconut oil
2 tablespoons coconut flakes
Pinch of salt
Small pinch of chilli flakes (optional)

TO SERVE
Warm roti or flatbread

FRY THE SPICES AND CURRY LEAVES
Heat the coconut oil in a large saucepan over medium heat. Add the mustard seeds, fenugreek, cinnamon stick and curry leaves. Let them crackle and pop for 1–2 minutes.

ADD THE BASE FLAVOURS
Add the sliced onion and cook for 5–6 minutes until soft and starting to brown. Stir in the garlic, ginger and chilli. Cook for 1–2 minutes.

ADD THE SPICES, BONE BROTH AND COCONUT MILK
Add the turmeric, coriander and cumin. Stir for 30 seconds, then pour in the bone broth and coconut milk.

COOK THE VEG
Bring to a gentle simmer, then add the sweet potato and carrot. Cook for 12–15 minutes until just tender. Blitz roughly with a hand blender so the soup is thick and creamy.

COOK THE GREEN BEANS
Add the green beans and cook for a final 4–5 minutes. Squeeze in the lime juice and season with salt.

MAKE THE COCONUT TOPPER
Heat a frying pan with the coconut oil. Add the coconut flakes with a pinch of salt and the chilli flakes. Cook for 2–3 minutes, stirring often, until golden.

TO SERVE
Spoon into bowls and scatter with the coconut topper, if using. Serve with warm roti for dipping, scooping and slurping.

HEARTY SOUPS & CHOWDERS

Bone broth is the ideal deep, savoury base for any wholesome, hearty soup. These are the recipes we reach for as soon as the weather starts to cool or we start to feel run down.

The hearty soups and chowders in this chapter are some of our favourites from around the world, showcasing the best of regional ingredients, methods and flavours.

Whether you prefer the thought of the deep, purple earthiness of a Beetroot Borscht or the creamy, smoky richness of a Cullen Skink, serve each with a generous helping of crusty bread to soak up every last spoonful.

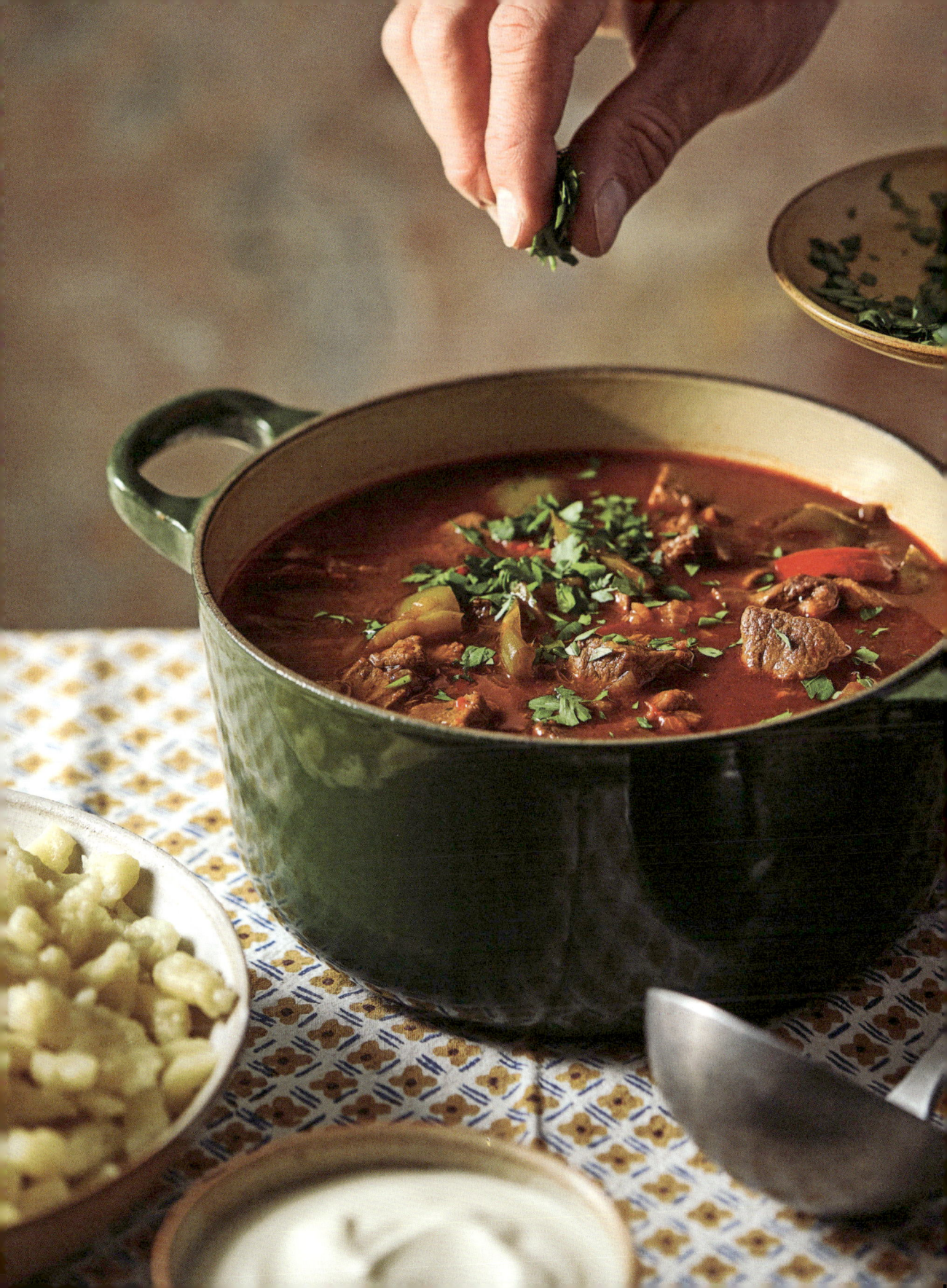

TUSCAN RIBOLLITA-STYLE MINESTRONE

A rustic, broth-based take on the Tuscan classic. Cannellini beans, greens and chunky veg simmered in bone broth, finished with chunks of fresh sourdough for extra thickness and depth – simple to make, yet deeply satisfying to eat.

SERVES 4
PREP TIME: 15 MINUTES
COOK TIME: 45 MINUTES

2 tablespoons olive oil
1 large onion, chopped
2 carrots, peeled and chopped into chunks
2 celery sticks, chopped
3 garlic cloves, finely chopped
1 tablespoon tomato purée
1 x 400g tin cannellini beans, drained
Small bunch of cavolo nero or curly kale, stalks removed, leaves roughly chopped
1 rosemary sprig
2 bay leaves
1 litre (35fl oz) beef bone broth
3 slices of stale sourdough or crusty bread, torn into rough chunks
Sea salt and freshly ground black pepper

TO SERVE
Extra virgin olive oil
Grated Parmesan or pecorino cheese

SOFTEN THE VEG
Heat the olive oil in a large saucepan over medium heat. Add the onion, carrot and celery and cook for 8–10 minutes until softened.

COOK THE GARLIC AND TOMATO PURÉE
Stir in the garlic and tomato purée and cook for 1–2 minutes until fragrant.

ADD THE BEANS, VEG AND LIQUID
Add the beans, cavolo nero, rosemary, bay leaves, bone broth and 500ml (17fl oz) water. Bring to a simmer.

SIMMER
Cook gently for 25–30 minutes until the greens are tender and the broth has deepened.

REMOVE THE HERBS AND SEASON
Remove the rosemary and bay leaves. Season generously with salt and pepper.

THICKEN WITH BREAD
Stir in the torn bread and let it sit in the broth for 1–2 minutes to soak slightly but not break down fully.

TO SERVE
Ladle into bowls and top with a drizzle of extra virgin olive oil and a grating of cheese.

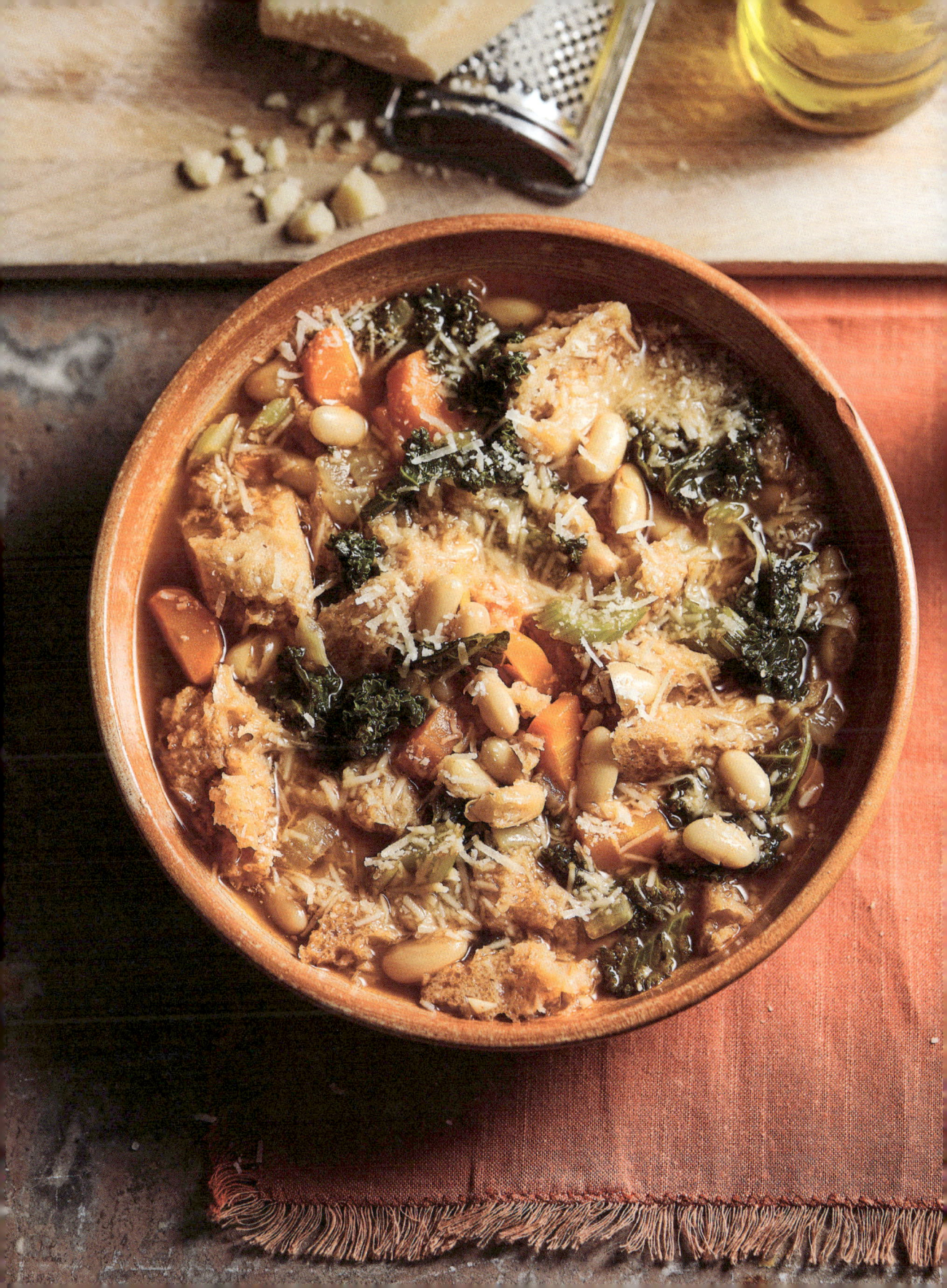

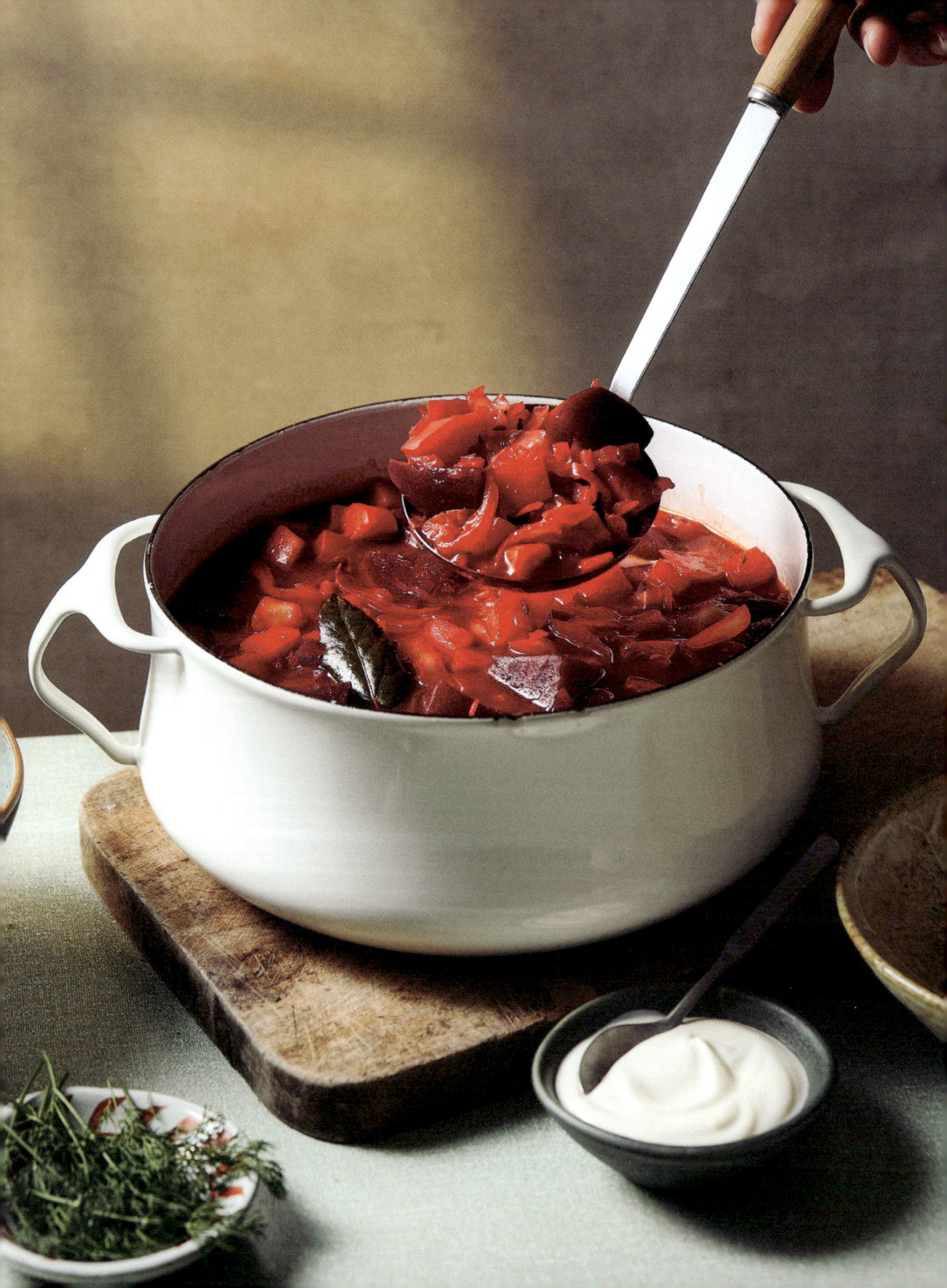

CHUNKY BEETROOT BORSCHT

This vibrant Eastern European classic is full of deep, earthy flavour with a nourishing, brothy twist. Traditionally slow-cooked and finely shredded, this version keeps the beetroot chunky and the broth silky and clear, while staying true to its roots with sweet vegetables, a touch of vinegar, fresh dill and a swirl of sour cream to finish.

SERVES 4
PREP TIME: 20 MINUTES
COOK TIME: 1 HOUR

1 tablespoon olive oil
1 onion, chopped
2 garlic cloves, crushed
1 tablespoon tomato purée
1 teaspoon caraway seeds
3 beetroot (about 400g/14oz), peeled and cut into chunks
2 carrots, peeled and cut into chunks
2 potatoes, peeled and cut into chunks
½ small white cabbage, sliced
1 litre (35fl oz) beef bone broth
1 bay leaf
1 tablespoon red wine vinegar, plus more to taste
Sea salt and freshly ground black pepper

TO SERVE
Sour cream
Chopped dill

SOFTEN THE ONION
Heat the oil in a large pot over medium heat. Add the onion and cook for 5–6 minutes until softened.

BUILD THE FLAVOUR
Stir in the garlic, tomato purée and caraway seeds and cook for 1–2 minutes.

ADD THE VEG
Add the beetroot, carrots, potatoes and cabbage to the pot. Stir well to coat in the flavour base.

ADD THE LIQUID
Pour in the bone broth and 500ml (17fl oz) water. Add the bay leaf and bring to a simmer.

COOK THE VEG UNTIL SOFT
Cover loosely and cook for 40–45 minutes until the vegetables are tender but still hold their shape.

ADD SOME ZING
Stir in the vinegar, then season generously with salt and pepper to taste.

TO SERVE
Ladle into bowls and serve hot, topped with a dollop of sour cream and a sprinkle of dill.

NORDIC SALMON & DILL CHOWDER

Inspired by Lohikeitto, Finland's beloved salmon soup, this is a lighter, brothier take on chowder that lets the flavour of the fish shine. Rich salmon, sweet root vegetables and delicate dill come together in a light bone broth enriched with just enough cream to feel luxurious, not heavy. Simple, soothing and best served with rye bread on the side, this dish is also delicious with trout instead of salmon.

SERVES 4
PREP TIME: 15 MINUTES
COOK TIME: 35 MINUTES, PLUS RESTING TIME

1 tablespoon butter
1 leek, halved and sliced
2 garlic cloves, crushed
2 potatoes (about 300g/10½oz), peeled and diced
1 carrot, diced
1 bay leaf
500ml (17fl oz) fish bone broth
300g (10½oz) skinless salmon fillet, cut into large chunks
150ml (5fl oz) double cream
Handful of dill, roughly chopped
Sea salt and ground white pepper

TO SERVE
Lemon wedges
Rye bread

SOFTEN THE LEEK
Melt the butter in a large saucepan over medium heat. Add the leek and garlic and cook for 5 minutes until softened but not coloured.

ADD THE REMAINING VEG AND SIMMER
Add the potatoes, carrot, bay leaf, bone broth and 500ml (17fl oz) water. Bring to a simmer.

COOK UNTIL TENDER
Cover loosely and cook for 20 minutes, or until the vegetables are just tender.

SIMMER THE SALMON
Add the salmon chunks and simmer gently for 5–6 minutes until just cooked through.

ENRICH WITH CREAM
Stir in the cream and most of the dill, then season well with salt and white pepper. Cook for 2–3 minutes further or until thickened slightly.

PREPARE TO SERVE
Remove from the heat and rest for 5 minutes before serving. Discard the bay leaf.

TO SERVE
Ladle into bowls and top with the remaining dill. Serve with lemon wedges and rye bread on the side.

SCOTCH BEEF & BARLEY BROTH

A hearty, slow-simmered Scottish classic made with tender chunks of beef, nutty pearl barley and root vegetables in a rich beef bone broth. Nourishing, simple and perfect for cold days.

SERVES 4
PREP TIME: 15 MINUTES
COOK TIME: 1 HOUR 30 MINUTES

1 tablespoon sunflower oil
400g (14oz) stewing beef, cut into bite-size pieces
1 onion, chopped
2 carrots, chopped
2 celery sticks, chopped
1 small swede, peeled and diced
2 garlic cloves, finely chopped
100g (3½oz) pearl barley, rinsed
1 bay leaf
1 teaspoon dried thyme
1 litre (35fl oz) beef bone broth
Sea salt and freshly ground black pepper

TO SERVE
Fresh parsley
Oatcakes or crusty bread

BROWN THE BEEF
Heat the oil in a large pot over medium heat. Add the beef and brown on all sides for 6–8 minutes. Remove and set aside.

ADD THE VEG
In the same pot, add the onion, carrots, celery, swede and garlic. Cook for 5–7 minutes until softened slightly.

COAT THE BEEF AND BARLEY
Return the beef to the pot along with the barley, bay leaf and thyme. Stir to coat.

ADD THE BONE BROTH
Pour in the beef bone broth and 500ml (17fl oz) water. Bring to a gentle simmer.

SIMMER, LOW AND SLOW
Skim off any foam that rises to the surface, then cover partially and simmer for 1 hour 15 minutes, stirring occasionally.

TEST IF READY
Check that the barley is tender and the beef is soft. If needed, cook for an extra 10–15 minutes. Season with salt and black pepper to taste.

TO SERVE
Remove the bay leaf, ladle into warm bowls and scatter with fresh parsley. Serve with oatcakes or crusty bread.

THE ULTIMATE FRENCH ONION SOUP

French Onion Soup is all about patience – slow-cooked onions that melt into a jammy, caramelised base, simmered with deeply savoury broth. Topped with golden, bubbling cheese toast, it's a timeless comfort food that rewards the time and love you put into it. Our kids love it as much as we do!

SERVES 4
PREP TIME: 15 MINUTES
COOK TIME: 1 HOUR 15 MINUTES

50g (1¾oz) unsalted butter
1 tablespoon olive oil
1kg (2lb 4oz) brown onions, thinly sliced
2 garlic cloves, finely chopped
1 teaspoon sugar
1 tablespoon plain flour
150ml (5fl oz) dry white wine
1 litre (35fl oz) beef bone broth
2 teaspoons Worcestershire sauce
1 bay leaf
1 teaspoon fresh thyme leaves or ½ teaspoon dried
Sea salt and freshly ground black pepper

TO SERVE
Good quality sourdough, sliced
150g (5½oz) Gruyère or Emmental cheese, grated
Extra thyme leaves (optional)

MELT THE BUTTER AND ADD THE ONIONS
Melt the butter with the olive oil in a large heavy-based pot over low heat. Add the onions, garlic and sugar.

CARAMELISE THE ONIONS
Cook slowly over a low heat for 35–40 minutes, stirring often, until the onions are deeply golden and caramelised. Don't rush this step, it builds the flavour.

ADD FLOUR
Stir in the flour and cook for 1 minute to thicken slightly.

COOK OFF THE WINE
Add the white wine and scrape up any brown bits from the bottom of the pan. Let it reduce for 2–3 minutes.

ADD THE BONE BROTH
Pour in the beef bone broth and 500ml (17fl oz) water, then add the Worcestershire sauce, bay leaf, thyme and a good pinch of salt and pepper.

SIMMER AWAY
Simmer gently for 25 minutes, partially covered. Remove the bay leaf and taste for seasoning.

MAKE YOUR GRILLED CHEESE
While the soup simmers, preheat the grill. Toast the sourdough on one side, flip, then top with cheese and grill again until bubbling and golden.

TO SERVE
Ladle the soup into bowls and float the cheesy toasts on top. Sprinkle with a few thyme leaves and get cosy.

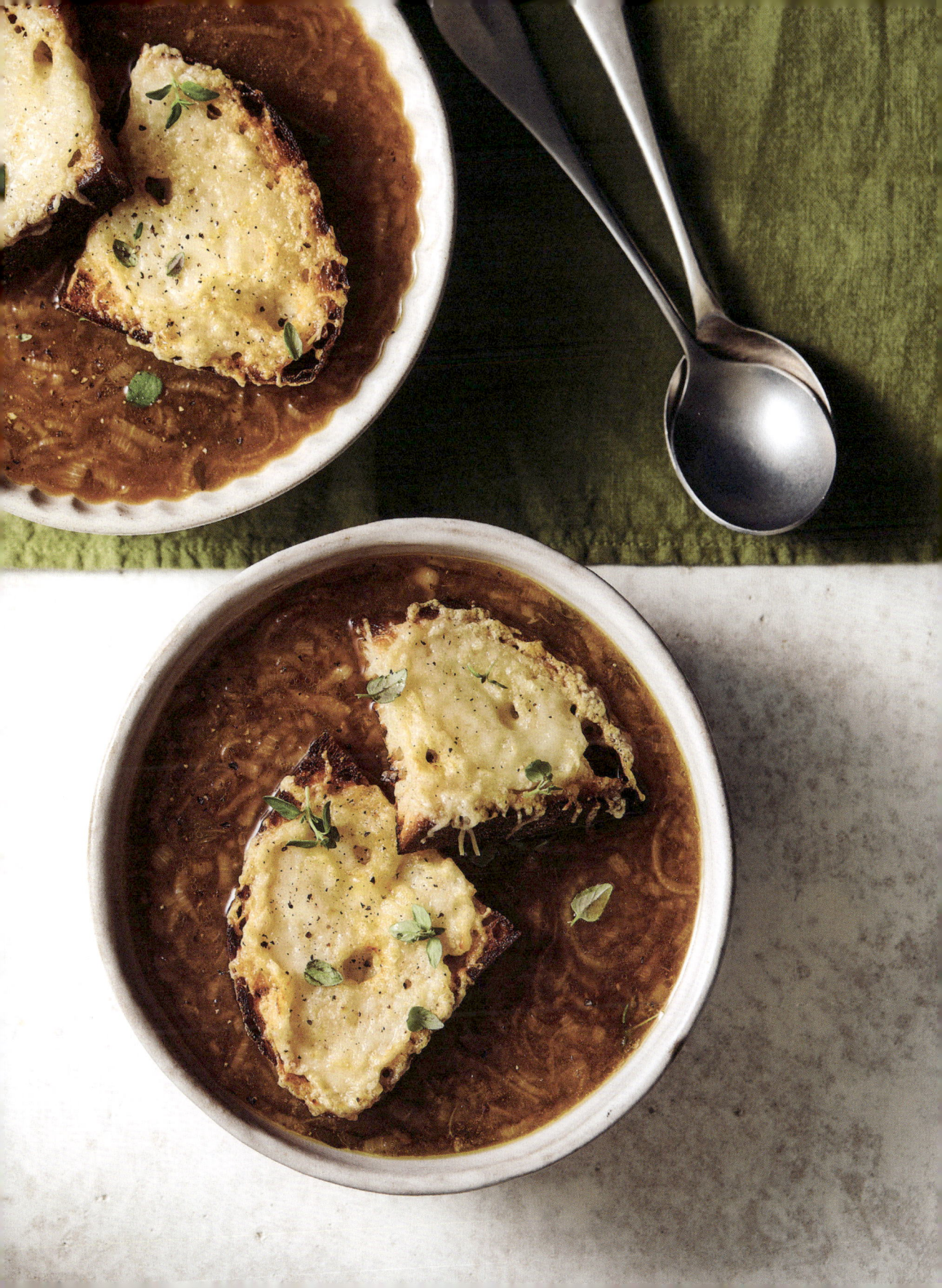

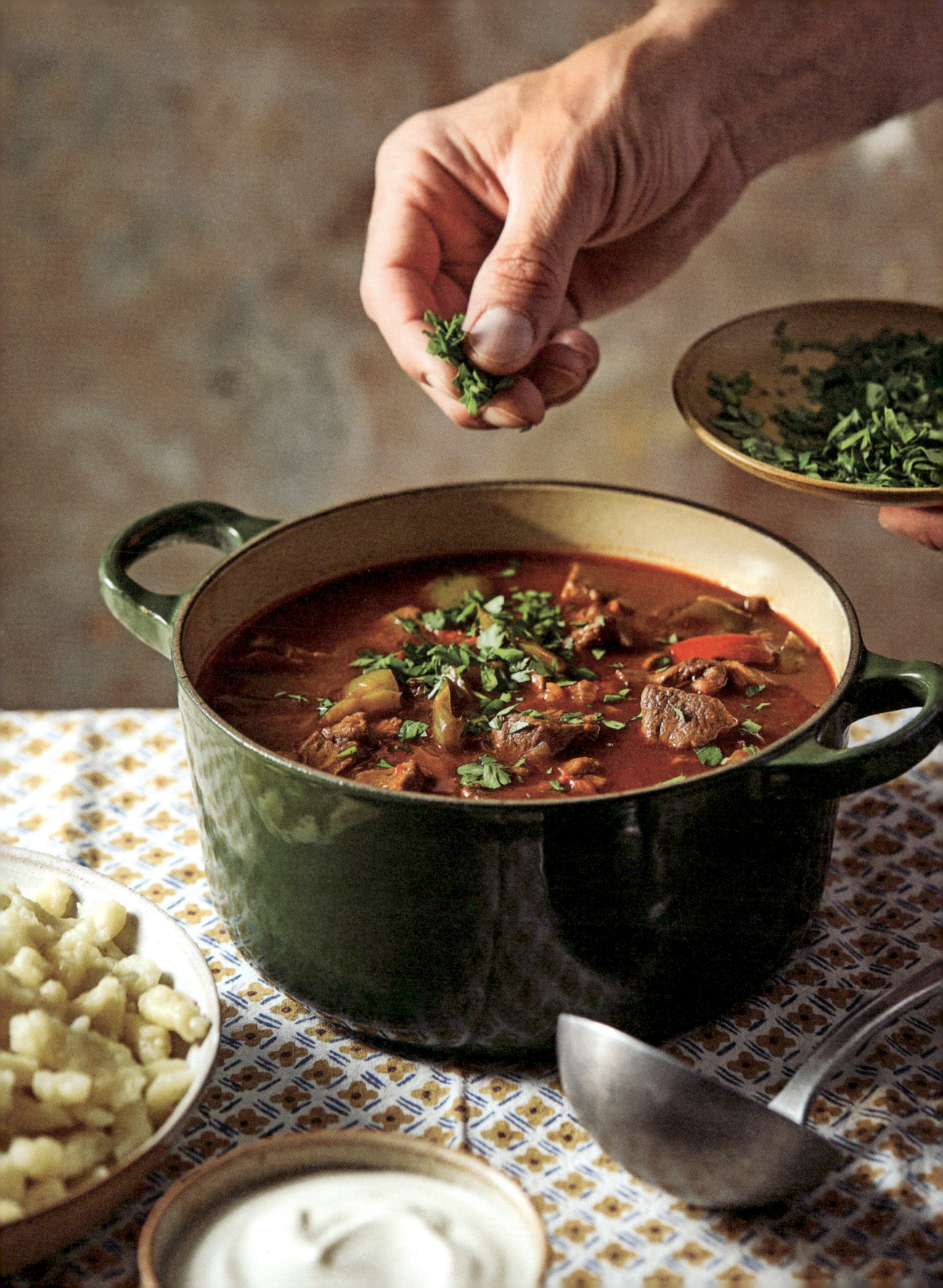

HUNGARIAN SMOKY BEEF GOULASH

A rich, paprika-heavy beef stew made brothy rather than thick, with tender chunks of meat, sweet peppers and a deep smoky warmth. This lighter, rustic take on the Hungarian classic is perfect when ladled over buttery noodles or served with crusty bread.

SERVES 4
PREP TIME: 20 MINUTES
COOK TIME: 2 HOURS

1 tablespoon sunflower oil
500g (1lb 2oz) stewing beef, cut into chunks
2 onions, thinly sliced
3 garlic cloves, finely chopped
2 teaspoons sweet Hungarian paprika
1 teaspoon smoked paprika
1 teaspoon caraway seeds (optional)
1 tablespoon tomato purée
1 green pepper, chopped
1 red pepper, chopped
1 bay leaf
1 litre (35fl oz) beef bone broth
Sea salt and freshly ground black pepper

TO SERVE
Chopped parsley or dill
Sour cream, to dollop (optional)
Buttered egg noodles
Mashed potato or crusty rye bread

BROWN THE BEEF
Heat the oil in a large, heavy-based pot over medium heat. Brown the beef in batches, 6–8 minutes total, then set aside.

SOFTEN THE ONIONS
To the same pot, add the onions and cook gently for about 10–12 minutes until deeply golden and soft.

ADD THE AROMATICS
Stir in the garlic, paprika (both sweet and smoked) and caraway seeds. Cook for 1 minute until fragrant.

COOK THE TOMATO PURÉE
Add the tomato purée and cook for another minute. Return the beef to the pot.

ADD THE VEG
Stir in the chopped peppers, bay leaf, bone broth and 250ml (9fl oz) water. Season lightly with salt and pepper.

SIMMER THE GOULASH
Bring to a simmer, partially cover and cook gently for 1 hour 30 minutes–2 hours until the beef is tender and the broth rich.

SEASON
Adjust the seasoning to taste. Remove the bay leaf.

TO SERVE
Spoon into bowls, garnish with parsley or dill and top with a spoon of sour cream. Serve with buttered egg noodles, mashed potato or crusty rye bread.

LEEK & MUSSEL CHOWDER IN A SOURDOUGH BOWL

This leek and mussel chowder blends creamy richness with briny freshness, packed with sweet leeks and tender mussels. Served in a hollowed-out sourdough loaf, it's hearty, nourishing and quite sophisticated too! Ideal for cooler days when you want something comforting with a touch of indulgence.

SERVES 4
PREP TIME: 20 MINUTES
COOK TIME: 25 MINUTES

1kg (2lb 4oz) fresh mussels, cleaned and beards removed
250ml (9fl oz) dry white wine
1 tablespoon olive oil
Knob of butter
2 leeks, halved lengthways and finely sliced
2 garlic cloves, finely chopped
500ml (17fl oz) fish bone broth
1 bay leaf
150ml (5fl oz) double cream
2 teaspoons Dijon mustard
Sea salt and freshly ground black pepper

TO SERVE
4 small round sourdough loaves
Chopped chives or parsley

STEAM THE MUSSELS
In a large lidded pot, combine the mussels and white wine. Cover, bring to a high heat and steam for 3–4 minutes until the mussels have opened. Discard any that stay shut.

TAKE THE MUSSELS OUT OF THEIR SHELLS
Strain the mussels through a fine-mesh sieve over a bowl to reserve the cooking liquor. Set the mussels aside to cool slightly, then remove most from their shells, keeping a few whole for garnish.

SOFTEN THE VEG
In another large pan, heat the olive oil and butter over medium heat. Add the sliced leeks and garlic and sauté gently for 8–10 minutes until soft and sweet but not coloured.

SIMMER AWAY
Pour in the reserved mussel liquor (leaving behind any gritty sediment) and the bone broth. Add the bay leaf and a pinch of salt. Simmer for 10 minutes.

ENRICH WITH CREAM
Stir in the cream and mustard, then return the shelled mussels to the pot. Warm through gently for 2–3 minutes. Adjust the seasoning with salt and pepper.

MAKE YOUR SOURDOUGH BOWL
Hollow out the sourdough loaves to form bowls (reserving the torn-out bread).

TO SERVE
Ladle the hot chowder into each 'bowl', top with a few mussels in their shells and a scattering of chives or parsley. Serve immediately, with the torn-out bread on the side for dunking.

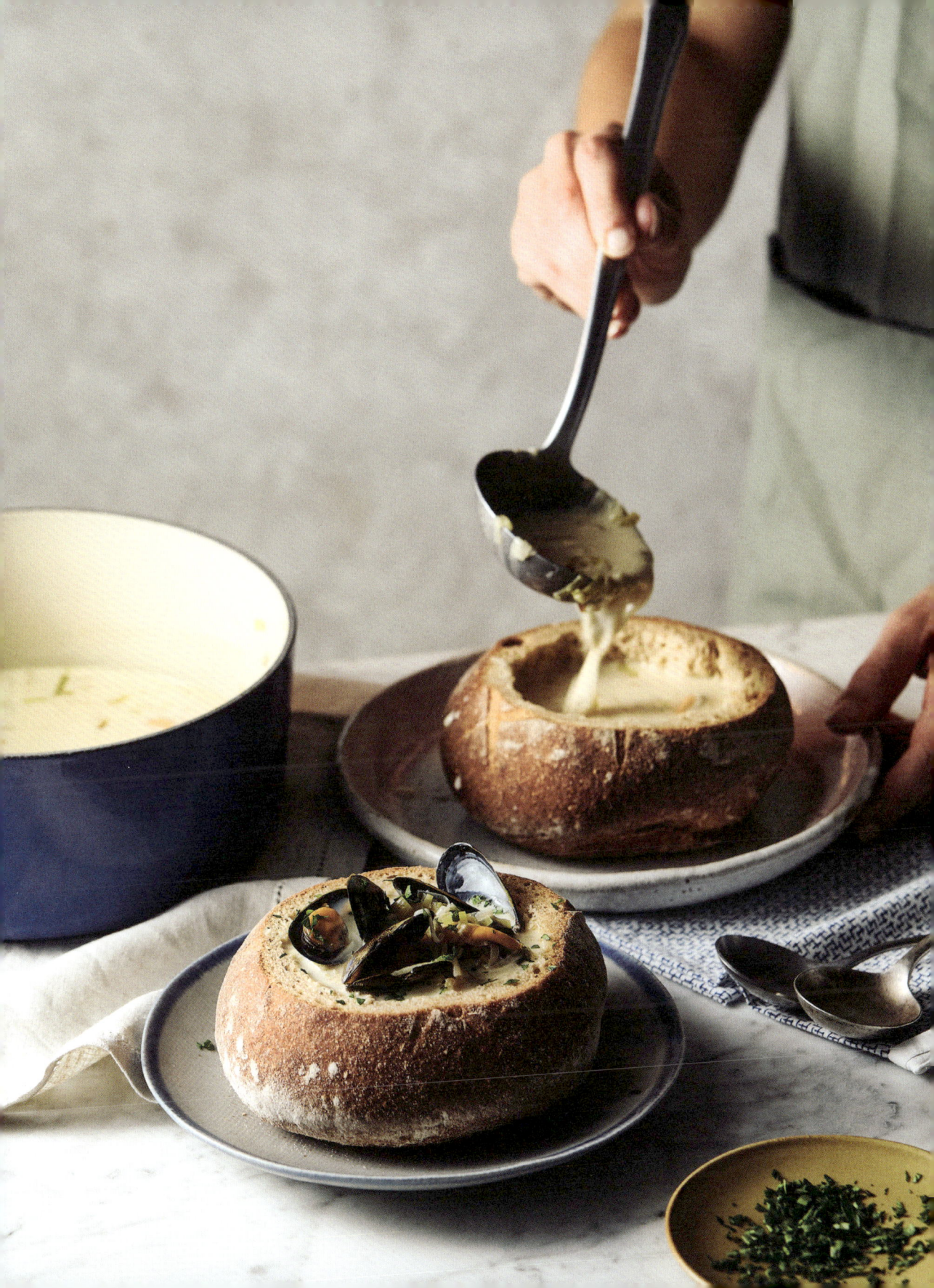

ITALIAN PESTO & GNOCCHI SOUP

Pillowy gnocchi floating in a fragrant, pesto-infused bone broth? We're sold. Every mouthful of this crowd pleaser is packed with fresh and comforting flavour. Quick to make but full of soul, this soup is perfect for any day you need a little lift. Serve with a drizzle of extra virgin olive oil and a generous scattering of Parmesan.

SERVES 4
PREP TIME: 10 MINUTES
COOK TIME: 20 MINUTES

1 tablespoon olive oil
1 small onion, finely chopped
2 garlic cloves, minced
1 litre (35fl oz) chicken bone broth
100g (3½oz) green beans, trimmed and halved
100g (3½oz) peas (fresh or frozen)
300g (10½oz) potato gnocchi (fresh or store-bought)
4 tablespoons prepared basil pesto (or check out our homemade pesto recipe in Cheat's Ratatouille on page 122)
80ml (2½fl oz) double cream
Sea salt and freshly ground black pepper

TO SERVE
Basil leaves
Drizzle of extra virgin olive oil
Grated Parmesan cheese (optional)

SOFTEN THE ONION
Heat the olive oil in a large pot over medium heat. Add the onion and garlic and cook for 5 minutes until softened.

ADD THE BONE BROTH
Pour in the bone broth and bring to a gentle simmer.

COOK THE GREENS
Stir in the green beans and peas and cook for 3–4 minutes until just tender.

COOK THE GNOCCHI
Add the gnocchi and cook according to the packet instructions until they float and are tender, usually 2–3 minutes.

ADD THE PESTO AND CREAM
Stir through the pesto and cream and cook for 1–2 minutes further. Season with salt and black pepper to taste.

TO SERVE
Ladle into bowls and garnish with fresh basil, a drizzle of good-quality olive oil and a generous grating of Parmesan.

CULLEN SKINK
(SCOTTISH SMOKED HADDOCK CHOWDER)

A Scottish classic that's as comforting as it gets. Smoky haddock, tender potatoes and leeks come together in a silky broth that's gently enriched with milk. Lightly mashing some of the potatoes gives the soup its signature thickness without losing the chunks that make it feel rustic and nourishing.

SERVES 4
PREP TIME: 10 MINUTES
COOK TIME: 30 MINUTES

1 tablespoon olive oil
1 small onion, finely chopped
1 leek, halved lengthways and thinly sliced
1 garlic clove, minced
300g (10½oz) floury potatoes, peeled and diced small
500ml (17fl oz) fish bone broth
300ml (10½fl oz) whole milk
300g (10½oz) smoked haddock fillets (skin on or off)
80ml (2½fl oz) double cream
1 tablespoon butter
Sea salt and ground white pepper

TO SERVE
Chopped chives or parsley (optional)
Crusty bread or sourdough

SOFTEN THE VEG
Heat the olive oil in a large pot over medium heat. Add the onion, leek and garlic with a pinch of salt and cook for 5–6 minutes until softened but not coloured.

ADD THE POTATOES AND BONE BROTH
Stir in the diced potatoes, pour in the bone broth and 250ml (9fl oz) water and bring to a gentle simmer. Cover loosely and cook for 10–12 minutes or until the potatoes are soft.

MASH SLIGHTLY
Use a potato masher to gently crush some of the potatoes in the pot – just enough to thicken the soup while keeping some chunks intact.

POACH THE HADDOCK
Pour in the milk and lay the haddock into the pan. Simmer gently for 6–8 minutes until the fish is just cooked through. Lift the fish out with a slotted spoon and set aside.

FINISH THE SOUP
Stir in the cream and butter. Flake the haddock into large chunks and gently fold it back into the soup. Season with salt and white pepper to taste.

TO SERVE
Ladle into bowls and top with a little chopped parsley or chives if using. Best served with warm crusty bread or sourdough.

BROTHY VEGETABLES

Vegetables love broth. Whether it's a splash in the roasting tray or a slow braise on the hob, bone broth adds richness and a savoury depth to even the simplest veg. It brings out their natural sweetness, softens edges and helps level-up humble side dishes and mains alike.

Whether you're looking for a delicious new Sunday roast side dish (we'd recommend the Oven-Braised Red Cabbage with Horseradish Cream) or an indulgent weekend breakfast (check out the Boozy Beef Mushrooms on Toast), these recipes are a celebration of how much you can do with a few simple vegetables and a splash of bone broth.

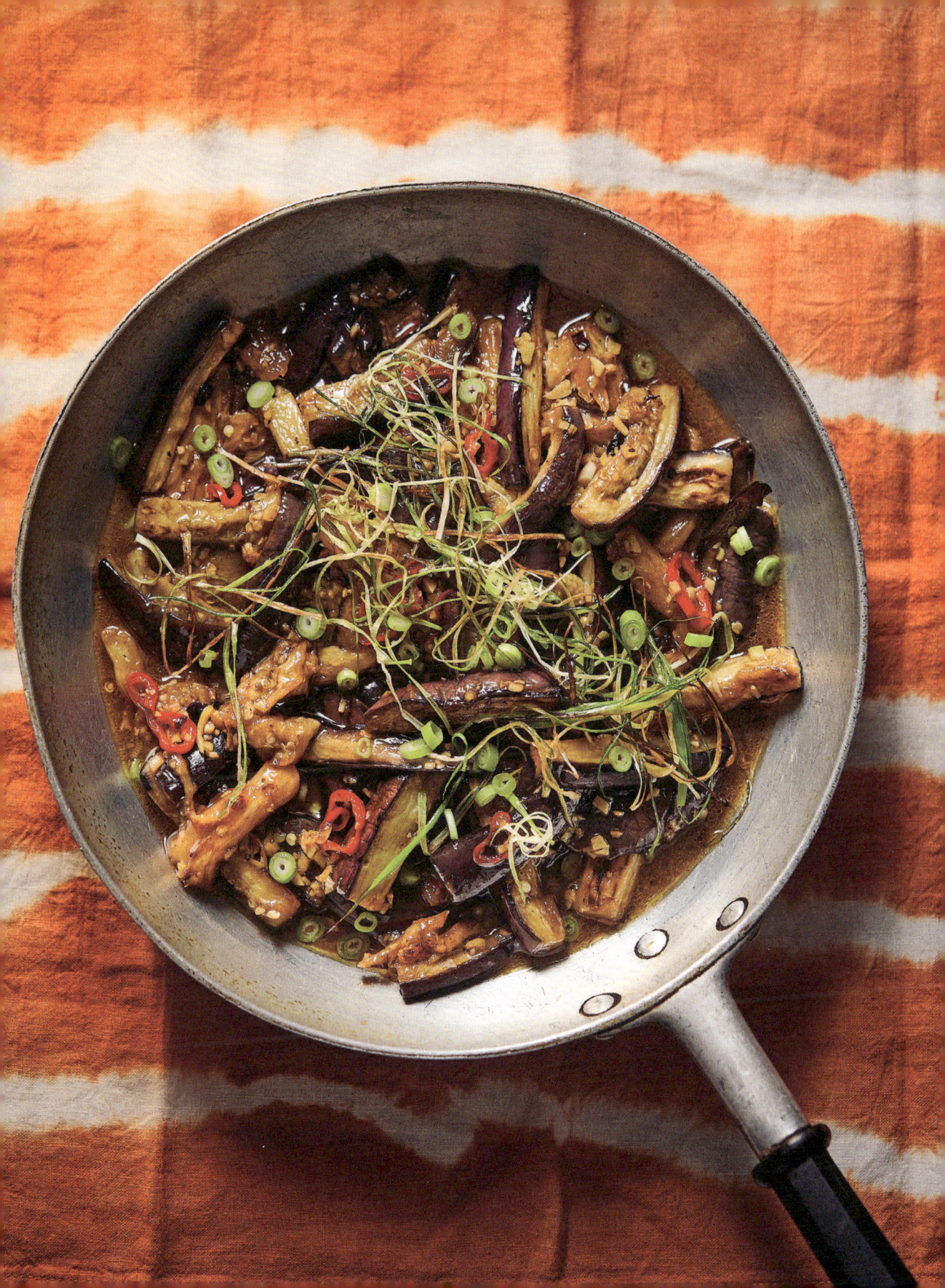

SUMAC-SPICED TOMATOES & GREEN BEANS

This dish brings together tart, spiced tomatoes and crisp green beans in a light, savoury broth. The splash of bone broth adds depth and rounds out the flavours, without weighing it down. Sumac gives it a tangy finish that makes this dish the perfect side dish – it's especially good with lamb or roast chicken or even flaky white fish. Serve warm or at room temperature.

SERVES 4
PREP TIME: 10 MINUTES
COOK TIME: 25 MINUTES

1 tablespoon olive oil
2 garlic cloves, finely sliced
1 teaspoon ground cumin
1 teaspoon ground coriander
½ teaspoon chilli flakes (optional)
300g (10½oz) cherry tomatoes, halved
1 teaspoon sugar
250ml (9fl oz) chicken bone broth
250g (9oz) green beans, trimmed
Small bunch of parsley, roughly chopped
1 tablespoon sumac
Sea salt and freshly ground black pepper

TO SERVE
Drizzle of extra virgin olive oil

COOK THE GARLIC
In a wide frying pan, heat the olive oil over medium heat. Add the garlic and cook for 1–2 minutes until just golden.

ADD THE SPICES
Stir in the cumin, coriander and chilli flakes, if using. Toast for 30 seconds until fragrant.

SOFTEN THE TOMATOES
Add the cherry tomatoes, sugar and a pinch of salt. Cook for 5–6 minutes, stirring occasionally, until the tomatoes start to soften and release their juices.

ADD THE BONE BROTH
Pour in the bone broth and green beans and bring to a gentle simmer. Let it bubble for 10–12 minutes until the tomatoes have collapsed further and the broth has reduced slightly.

SEASON
Season with black pepper and more salt to taste. Scatter with the chopped herbs and sprinkle generously with sumac.

TO SERVE
Drizzle over some good-quality olive oil, and tuck in.

CREAMED SHALLOTS & GARLIC WITH PANGRATTATO

This dish brings a heady richness and delicious sweetness from slow-cooked shallots and garlic in a glossy bone broth and cream sauce. If you're planning to make this as a side for your Sunday roast, be warned that it may just steal the show.

SERVES 4
PREP TIME: 10 MINUTES
COOK TIME: 35 MINUTES

- 1 tablespoon olive oil
- 30g (1oz) unsalted butter
- 600g (1lb 5oz) banana shallots, peeled and halved lengthways
- Small bulb of garlic, cloves separated and peeled
- 75ml (2½fl oz) dry white wine (or extra broth if you prefer)
- 250ml (9fl oz) chicken bone broth (or beef if you prefer deeper flavour)
- 1 bay leaf
- 4 thyme sprigs
- 150ml (5fl oz) double cream
- 1 teaspoon sherry vinegar or white balsamic
- Small knob of cold butter (optional)
- Sea salt and freshly ground black pepper

FOR THE PANGRATTATO
- 1 tablespoon olive oil
- 1 small garlic clove, crushed
- 1 thick slice of sourdough or rustic bread, torn into crumbs
- Zest of ½ lemon (optional)

START THE BRAISE
Heat 1 tablespoon of olive oil and the butter in a wide-based frying pan. Tip in the shallots and garlic, reserving one clove, season with salt and pepper and let them gently colour for 5 minutes.

ADD LIQUIDS AND AROMATICS
Pour in the white wine and simmer for 2–3 minutes to reduce slightly. Add the bone broth, bay leaf and 3 thyme sprigs. Cover loosely and cook over low heat for 15–20 minutes, turning occasionally, until the shallots are very soft and the broth has mostly reduced.

INFUSE THE CREAM
While the shallots are braising, gently warm the double cream in a small saucepan with a smashed garlic clove and a sprig of thyme. Let it infuse for 10 minutes on the lowest heat, then strain and set aside.

REDUCE AND FINISH THE SAUCE
Remove the bay leaf and thyme from the shallots. Turn the heat to medium-high and let the broth reduce until almost sticky. Pour in the infused cream and simmer gently for 5–7 minutes until thickened. Stir in the sherry vinegar. Take off the heat and swirl in a final knob of cold butter if you want an extra silky finish.

MAKE THE PANGRATTATO
While the cream sauce is reducing, heat 1 tablespoon of olive oil in a small frying pan. Add the crushed garlic and breadcrumbs, seasoning with salt. Cook, stirring often, until golden and crisp. Stir through the lemon zest, if using.

TO SERVE
Add a crack of black pepper and sprinkle on the pangrattato at the end for extra crunch.

CHEAT'S RATATOUILLE

Think of this as the unfussy cousin of traditional ratatouille. No careful layering, no standing over the hob, just a pick-and-mix of summer veg baked slowly in a rich tomato and bone broth base. It's a one-dish, throw-it-all-in kind of recipe that still creates deep flavour. Add a spoonful of fresh basil pesto at the end for an extra dollop of 'je ne sais quoi'.

SERVES 4
PREP TIME: 15 MINUTES, PLUS 15–30 MINUTES RESTING
COOK TIME: 1 HOUR 30 MINUTES

- 3 tablespoons olive oil
- 3 garlic cloves, thinly sliced
- 1 teaspoon fennel seeds
- 1 teaspoon dried thyme
- 1 x 400g tin chopped tomatoes
- 250ml (9fl oz) chicken bone broth
- 1 aubergine, chopped into bite-sized chunks
- 2 courgettes, chopped
- 2 red peppers, chopped
- 1 large red onion, chopped
- Sea salt and freshly ground black pepper

FOR THE BASIL PESTO
- Small bunch of basil
- 1 garlic clove
- Zest of 1 lemon
- 3 tablespoons olive oil
- 1 tablespoon toasted pine nuts
- Pinch of salt

PREHEAT THE OVEN
Set your oven to 200°C (180°C fan)/400°F/gas 6. Use a wide, shallow baking dish (about 30 x 22cm/12 x 8½ inches) so the broth reduces well and the vegetables can roast, not stew.

MAKE THE BASE
Heat 2 tablespoons of the olive oil in a pan over medium heat. Add the sliced garlic, fennel seeds and thyme. Let them sizzle gently for a minute or two, then pour in the chopped tomatoes and bone broth. Season with salt and pepper and simmer for 5–10 minutes until slightly thickened.

TOSS THE VEG
Tip the aubergine, courgettes, red peppers and red onion into the baking dish. Drizzle with 1 tablespoon olive oil and season lightly. Pour the hot tomato and broth mixture over the top and toss everything to coat.

BAKE COVERED AND UNCOVERED
Cover the dish tightly with foil and bake for 45 minutes. Remove the foil and return to the oven for another 30 minutes until the top is golden and the sauce is rich and reduced.

REST THE DISH
Take the ratatouille out of the oven and let it sit for 15–30 minutes. This helps the sauce thicken and makes it easier to serve.

MAKE THE PESTO
While it rests, blitz the basil, garlic, lemon zest, olive oil, pine nuts and a pinch of salt in a small blender or food processor until roughly combined. Add a splash more oil if you like it looser.

TO SERVE
Spoon the ratatouille onto plates, then drizzle with the fresh pesto. Leftovers are great cold or reheated the next day.

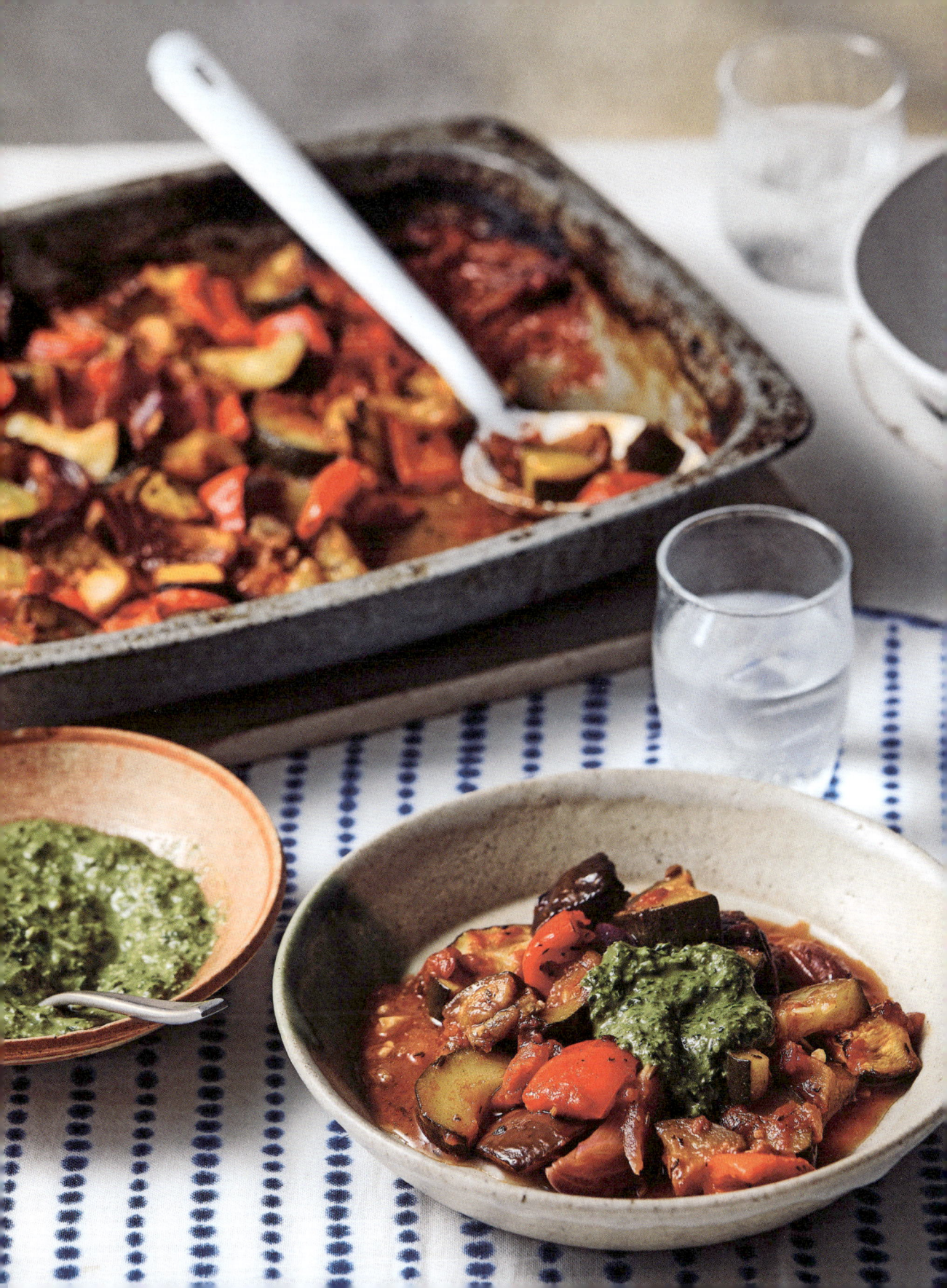

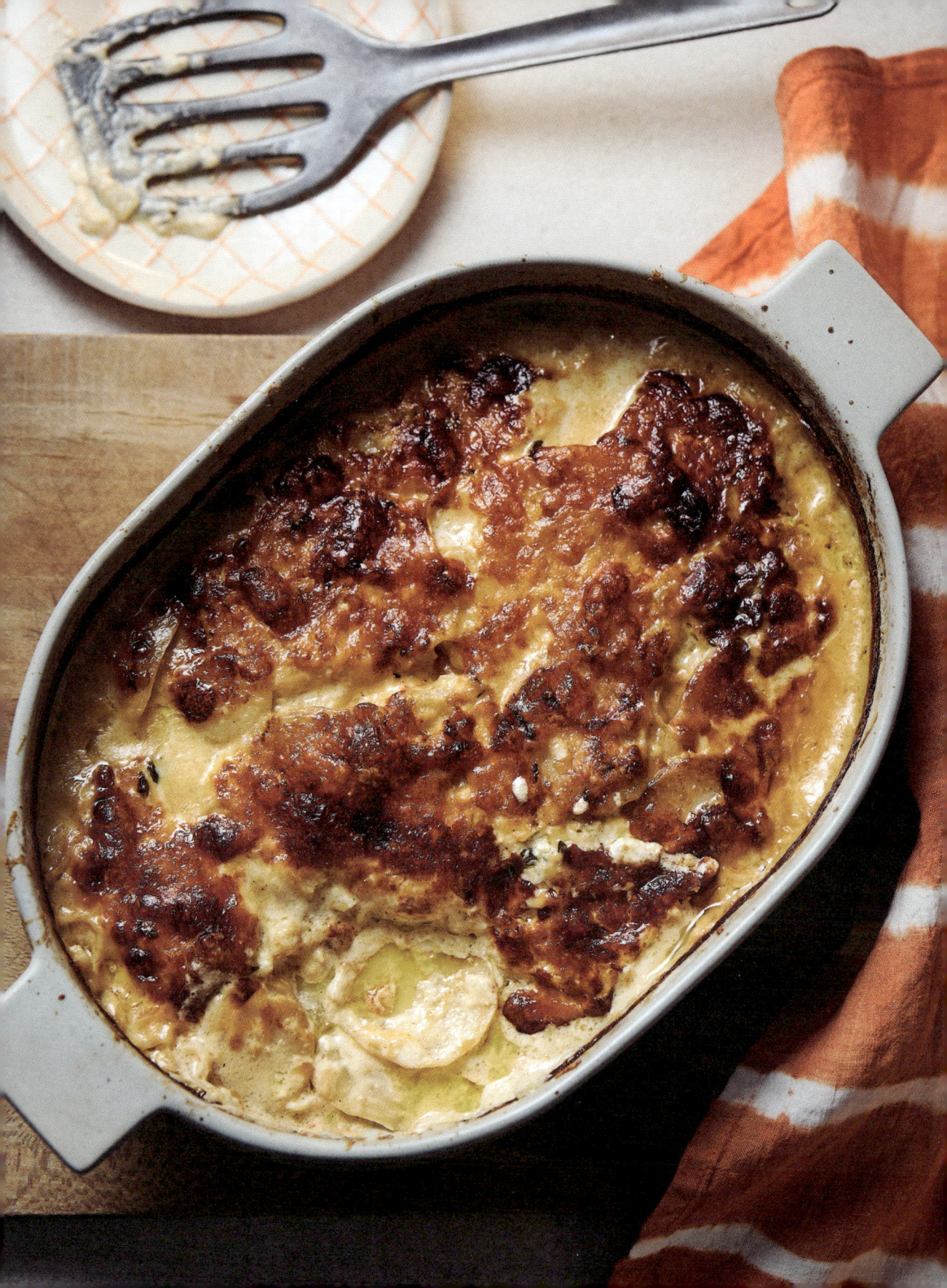

'BOULANGOISE'
(BOULANGÈRE MEETS DAUPHINOISE)

If you've ever been torn between the earthy flavours of Pommes Boulangère and the decadent creaminess of Gratin Dauphinoise, you will never have to compromise again! Our Sunday family favourite takes the guilt out of a guilty pleasure by grounding all that delicious, cheesy richness with sweet onions and savoury broth. There will be no leftovers.

SERVES 4
PREP TIME: 25 MINUTES, PLUS 10 MINUTES RESTING
COOK TIME: 1 HOUR 20 MINUTES

1 tablespoon unsalted butter, for greasing
300ml (10½fl oz) beef bone broth
2 garlic cloves, finely chopped
2 teaspoons fresh thyme leaves or 1 teaspoon dried
150ml (5fl oz) double cream
800g (1lb 12oz) floury potatoes (such as Maris Piper), peeled and thinly sliced (2mm/$\frac{1}{16}$ inch, ideally with a mandoline)
1 large onion, finely sliced
60g (2¼oz) Gruyère or Comté cheese, grated
30g (1oz) mature Cheddar cheese, grated
25g (1oz) Parmesan cheese, finely grated
Sea salt and freshly ground black pepper

PREHEAT THE OVEN
Set your oven to 200°C (180°C fan)/400°F/gas 6. Lightly butter a medium baking dish (about 20 × 30cm/8 x 12 inches).

REDUCE THE BONE BROTH
In a small saucepan, bring the bone broth to the boil and reduce it by roughly one-third (down to around 200ml/7fl oz). Add the garlic and thyme, then take off the heat and stir in the cream. Season with salt and plenty of black pepper.

BUILD THE DISH
Arrange half the potato slices in overlapping layers in the base of the dish. Scatter over half the onion and a mix of the Gruyère and Cheddar. Repeat with the remaining potatoes, onion and most of the remaining cheese (reserving some Parmesan for the top).

POUR IN THE LIQUID
Slowly pour the hot broth and cream mixture over the layers. It should come about three-quarters of the way up the potatoes.

BAKE COVERED
Cover loosely with foil and bake for 45 minutes.

FINISH UNCOVERED
Remove the foil, sprinkle over the remaining Parmesan, then bake for a further 20–30 minutes until golden, bubbling and tender.

REST BEFORE SERVING
Let the dish sit for at least 10 minutes before slicing. This allows the layers to set a little and intensifies the flavour.

TO SERVE
Serve alongside any rich meat, such as roasted rib of beef, with plenty of greens and lashings of red wine gravy.

SPRING GREENS WITH GARLIC & LEMON

Fast, simple and full of flavour, these humble greens punch well above their weight. The lemon and garlic brighten the dish, while the broth gives it backbone. You can serve this as a side to any roast dinner, but particularly roast pork or gammon, or turn it into a light lunch with added grains or a soft-boiled egg.

SERVES 4
PREP TIME: 10 MINUTES
COOK TIME: 20 MINUTES

1 large bag (about 300–350g/10½–12oz) of pre-chopped spring greens or Swiss chard
500ml (17fl oz) beef bone broth
3 garlic cloves, thinly sliced
Zest of 1 lemon
Pinch of chilli flakes (optional)
2 tablespoons olive oil, plus more to finish
Juice of ½ lemon, to taste
Fine sea salt and freshly ground black pepper

TO SERVE (OPTIONAL)
Toasted pine nuts, crushed hazelnuts or a spoonful of crème fraîche

BLANCH THE GREENS
Bring a large pot of salted water to the boil. Drop in the greens and blanch for 30 seconds, then transfer straight into a bowl of iced water. This locks in their colour and helps them cook evenly later.

INFUSE THE BONE BROTH
Pour the bone broth into a medium saucepan and add the sliced garlic, lemon zest and chilli flakes, if using. Warm gently over low heat for 5–10 minutes so the flavours infuse without boiling. Set aside.

SAUTÉ AND BRAISE
In a large frying pan, heat the olive oil over medium heat. Add the blanched greens and a small pinch of salt. Stir for 2–3 minutes until they start to soften.

ADD THE INFUSED BONE BROTH
Pour in the warm broth mixture. Simmer uncovered for 5–7 minutes, or until the greens are tender and the broth has reduced slightly.

FINISH AND SEASON
Turn off the heat. Stir in the lemon juice and a final drizzle of olive oil (or a knob of butter if preferred). Taste and adjust with more salt, pepper or lemon juice, if needed.

TO SERVE
To dress it up even further, top with toasted pine nuts, hazelnuts or a spoonful of crème fraîche just before serving.

OVEN-BRAISED RED CABBAGE WITH HORSERADISH CREAM

Transform a humble red cabbage into a show-stopping centrepiece thanks to rich beef bone broth, fragrant star anise and some fun, fancy finishing touches of toasted hazelnuts and horseradish cream.

SERVES 4
PREP TIME: 20 MINUTES
COOK TIME: 1 HOUR 45 MINUTES–2 HOURS 15 MINUTES

1 tablespoon butter or olive oil
1 red onion, thinly sliced
1 small red cabbage (about 800g/1lb 12oz), core removed, finely sliced
1 apple (e.g. Braeburn or Gala), peeled and sliced
250ml (9fl oz) beef bone broth
3 tablespoons apple cider vinegar
1 tablespoon brown sugar or maple syrup
2 whole star anise
Sea salt and freshly ground black pepper

FOR THE HORSERADISH CREAM
100g (3½oz) crème fraîche
1 tablespoon prepared horseradish
Pinch of salt

TO SERVE
25g (1oz) toasted hazelnuts, roughly chopped
½ apple, thinly sliced or julienned
Small handful of parsley or chervil (optional)

PREHEAT THE OVEN
Set your oven to 160°C (140°C fan)/325°F/gas 2–3.

COOK THE ONION
In a large ovenproof casserole dish, melt the butter or oil over medium heat. Add the red onion and cook for 3–4 minutes until softened.

ADD THE CABBAGE AND AROMATICS
Stir in the red cabbage and cook for a further 3–4 minutes. Add the sliced apple, beef bone broth, 2 tablespoons of the apple cider vinegar, the brown sugar, star anise and a pinch of salt and pepper.

START THE BRAISE
Cover tightly with a lid or foil and braise in the oven for 1 hour 30 minutes–2 hours, stirring once halfway through. The cabbage should be silky and the broth mostly reduced.

SET THE BRAISED RED CABBAGE ASIDE
When ready, remove from the oven. Discard the star anise. Transfer the cabbage to a serving dish using a slotted spoon.

THICKEN THE BRAISING LIQUID
Place the braising liquid back on the hob over medium heat. Add an extra tablespoon of vinegar and simmer for 5–7 minutes to reduce to a light glaze. Spoon over the cabbage.

PREPARE THE HORSERADISH CREAM
In a small bowl, mix the crème fraîche with the horseradish and a pinch of salt.

TO SERVE
Finish the dish with toasted hazelnuts, raw apple slices and small spoonfuls of the horseradish cream. Sprinkle with parsley or chervil, if using, to finish.

BOOZY BEEF MUSHROOMS ON TOAST

This is breakfast dialled up to the max. Glistening layers of mushrooms cooked in boozy, beefy broth, piled onto golden, pan-fried sourdough. Luxurious, umami and utterly delicious. What more could you want?

SERVES 4
PREP TIME: 10 MINUTES
COOK TIME: 25 MINUTES

400g (14oz) mixed mushrooms (e.g. chestnut, oyster, shiitake, portobello), torn or thickly sliced
1 tablespoon olive oil, plus extra for the toast
30g (1oz) unsalted butter, plus extra for the toast
2 shallots, finely sliced
2 garlic cloves, finely chopped
100ml (3½fl oz) good-quality fortified wine (Madeira, Marsala or dry sherry)
250ml (9fl oz) beef bone broth
1 teaspoon Worcestershire sauce
1 tablespoon wholegrain mustard (optional)
2 teaspoons fresh thyme leaves or 1 teaspoon dried
1 teaspoon lemon juice
Knob of cold butter
4 thick slices of day-old sourdough
Sea salt and freshly ground black pepper

TO SERVE
Handful of chopped herbs (parsley, chives or tarragon)

DRY-FRY THE MUSHROOMS
Heat a large, dry frying pan over medium-high heat. Add the mushrooms and cook without oil, stirring occasionally, for about 6–8 minutes until they release their liquid and begin to brown. Transfer to a bowl.

BUILD THE BASE
Add the olive oil and butter to the same pan. Sauté the shallots for 3–4 minutes until soft, then add the garlic and cook for 1 more minute. Return the mushrooms to the pan.

DEGLAZE WITH FORTIFIED WINE
Pour in the wine and let it bubble and reduce for 2–3 minutes. Scrape up any browned bits from the bottom of the pan to deepen the flavour.

ADD BONE BROTH AND SIMMER
Add the beef bone broth, Worcestershire sauce, mustard (if using) and thyme. Simmer for 5–7 minutes until the liquid has reduced and thickened slightly.

FINISH THE SAUCE
Stir in a squeeze of lemon juice and a final knob of butter off the heat to give the sauce a silky texture. Taste and adjust the seasoning with salt and pepper.

FRY THE TOAST
In a separate pan, fry the sourdough slices in a little olive oil or butter over medium heat until golden and crisp on both sides.

TO SERVE
Spoon the mushrooms and sauce generously over the fried toast. Scatter with chopped fresh herbs and gobble it up immediately.

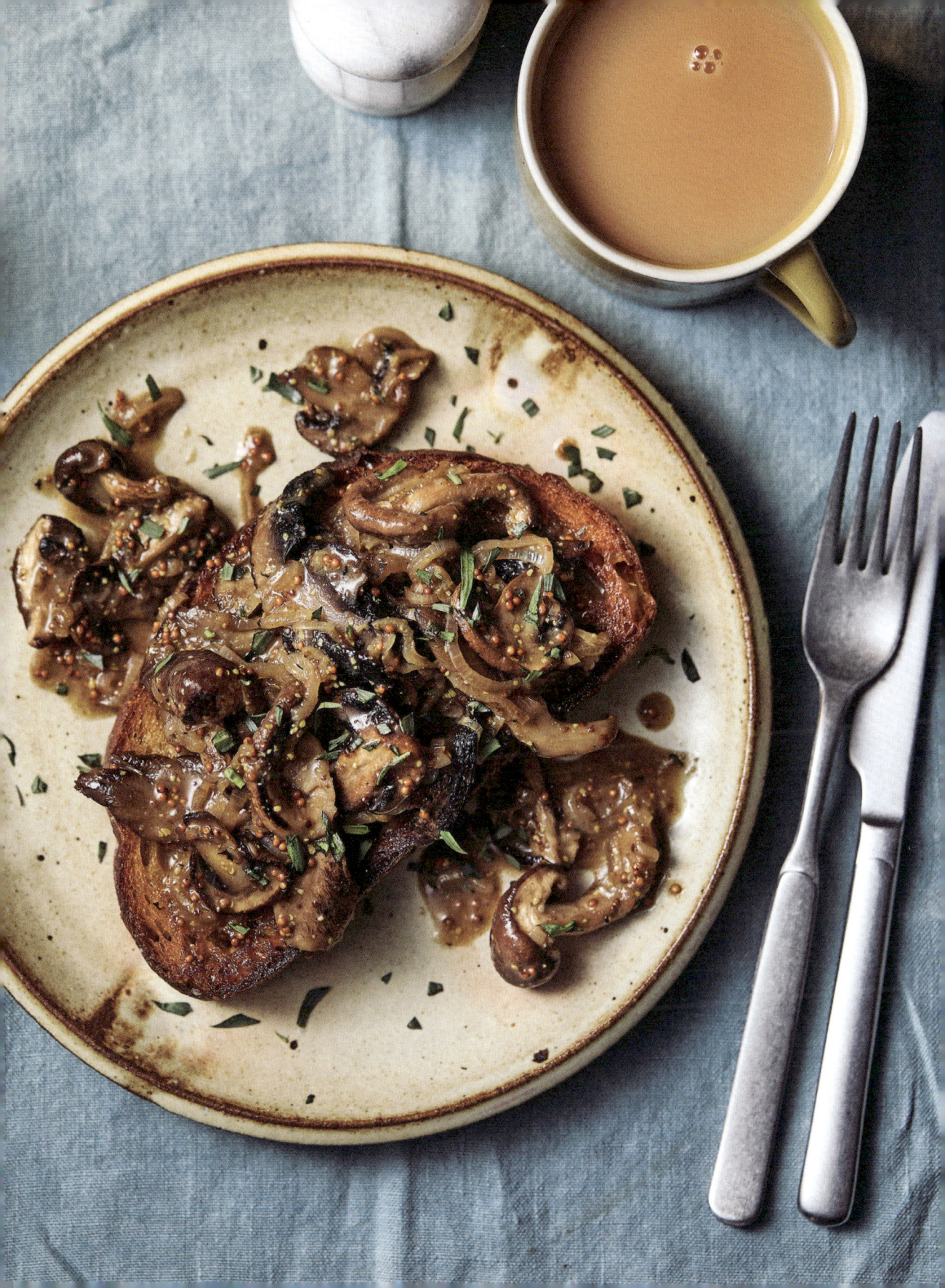

FONDANT POTATOES

These potatoes have it all – golden and crisp on top, soft and buttery inside. Cooking them slowly in bone broth adds savoury depth and gives you a glossy, spoonable sauce at the end. They're a bit of a show-off side dish but still use just a handful of ingredients. Make sure your potatoes are roughly the same size so they cook evenly.

SERVES 4
PREP TIME: 10 MINUTES
COOK TIME: 45–50 MINUTES

- 4 large floury potatoes (Maris Piper or King Edward)
- 2 tablespoons neutral oil (vegetable or sunflower)
- 50g (1¾oz) unsalted butter
- 2 garlic cloves, crushed
- 2 thyme sprigs
- 500ml (17fl oz) chicken or beef bone broth (depending on what you're serving them with)
- Sea salt and freshly ground black pepper

PREPARE THE POTATOES
Peel the potatoes and trim the ends to make barrel shapes. Cut each one in half across the middle so you have eight thick cylinders. Rinse briefly under cold water and pat very dry.

SEAR THE POTATOES
Heat the oil in a wide, heavy-based frying pan over medium heat. Add the potatoes, flat-side down, and cook for about 5–6 minutes until deep golden brown. Flip and brown the other flat side for another 5–6 minutes. Don't rush this, the crust is key.

ADD THE BUTTER AND AROMATICS
Add the butter, garlic and thyme to the pan. Let the butter foam and baste the potatoes for 1–2 minutes.

POUR OVER THE BONE BROTH
Carefully pour in the warm bone broth. It should come about halfway up the sides of the potatoes. Season well with salt and pepper.

COVER AND SIMMER
Cover loosely with a lid or foil, reduce the heat to low and simmer gently for 25–30 minutes until the potatoes are tender all the way through. Baste once or twice as they cook.

REDUCE THE LIQUID TO A SAUCE
Remove the lid and increase the heat slightly to reduce the remaining liquid to a glossy sauce, basting again to coat. Discard the thyme and garlic.

TO SERVE
Serve hot, with the buttery broth spooned over the top. Ideal with any roast meats, or as the star of the plate next to some fresh seasonal greens.

CREAMY MUSTARD-GLAZED FENNEL

This dish transforms humble fennel bulbs into a delectable, aromatic side dish, coated in a silky mustard cream. Enriched by bone broth, the result is a perfectly balanced dish of aniseed sweetness, tangy sharpness and savoury depth that feels equally at home beside roast chicken or a pan-seared fish fillet.

SERVES 4
PREP TIME: 10 MINUTES
COOK TIME: 40 MINUTES

3 fennel bulbs, trimmed, outer layer removed, cut into wedges (roots intact to hold shape)
1 tablespoon olive oil
25g (1oz) unsalted butter
100ml (3½fl oz) dry white wine (or use more broth)
250ml (9fl oz) chicken bone broth
1 bay leaf
2–3 sprigs of fresh thyme
Sea salt and freshly ground black pepper

FOR THE CREAMY MUSTARD GLAZE
150ml (5fl oz) double cream
1½ tablespoons Dijon mustard
1 teaspoon wholegrain mustard
1 teaspoon honey
1 teaspoon sherry vinegar or lemon juice, to finish

TO SERVE (OPTIONAL)
Fennel fronds, finely chopped
Cracked black pepper
Lemon zest

START THE FENNEL BRAISE
In a wide frying pan, heat the olive oil and butter over medium heat. Add the fennel wedges, cut-side down, and cook for about 5–7 minutes, turning occasionally, until lightly golden. Season with salt and pepper.

ADD LIQUIDS AND AROMATICS
Pour in the white wine and let it bubble for 2–3 minutes to reduce slightly. Add the chicken bone broth, bay leaf and thyme. Cover loosely with a lid or foil and simmer gently for about 20–25 minutes, turning the fennel once or twice, until tender and most of the liquid has reduced to a glossy coating.

MAKE THE MUSTARD CREAM
Meanwhile, in a small saucepan, gently warm the double cream with both mustards and honey. Stir to combine and cook over very low heat for 5–10 minutes until smooth and slightly thickened. Season to taste.

GLAZE AND FINISH
Remove the bay leaf and thyme from the fennel pan. Pour in the mustard cream and swirl gently to coat the fennel. Simmer together for 3–5 minutes until the sauce is thick and silky. Add a splash of sherry vinegar or lemon juice to brighten.

TO SERVE
Transfer the fennel to a warm serving dish, spoon over the creamy mustard glaze and finish with a sprinkle of fennel fronds, cracked black pepper and a little lemon zest.

BRAISED AUBERGINE WITH SPRING ONION

This silky aubergine dish is braised in a rich glaze made with soy sauce and bone broth, then finished with a crispy onion topping. Fragrant, deep and delicious, even the fussy eaters in our household who 'don't like aubergines' end up licking their plates.

SERVES 4
PREP TIME: 20 MINUTES, PLUS AUBERGINE SALTING
COOK TIME: 25 MINUTES

FOR THE BRAISED AUBERGINE
3 aubergines (about 750g/1lb 10oz), cut into thick batons (about 2 x 6cm/¾ x 2½ inches)
3 tablespoons neutral oil (vegetable or sunflower), plus extra if needed
4 garlic cloves, finely chopped
1 thumb-sized piece of fresh ginger, finely chopped
2 spring onions, white and green parts separated and finely sliced
1 red chilli, finely sliced (optional)
½ teaspoon doubanjiang or fermented black beans (optional, for added depth)

FOR THE BRAISING SAUCE
150ml (5fl oz) beef bone broth
1½ tablespoons soy sauce
1 tablespoon oyster sauce (or hoisin for a vegetarian version)
1 teaspoon Chinese black vinegar (or rice vinegar)
½ teaspoon sugar
1 teaspoon cornflour mixed with 1 tablespoon cold water

FOR THE CRISPY SPRING ONION TOPPING
2 spring onions, cut into fine matchsticks
3 tablespoons neutral oil (vegetable or sunflower)
Pinch of salt

TO SERVE (OPTIONAL)
Drizzle of sesame oil or crispy chilli oil

REDUCE THE BONE BROTH
Pour the broth for the braising sauce into a small pan. Simmer gently until reduced to about 100ml (3½fl oz), then set aside.

PREP AND STEAM THE AUBERGINES
Sprinkle the aubergine batons lightly with salt and set aside for 10–15 minutes. Pat dry with kitchen paper. Steam the aubergines for 8–10 minutes until just tender but still holding their shape.

CRISP THE SPRING ONIONS
Soak the matchstick spring onions for the crispy topping in iced water for 5 minutes to curl. Drain and pat dry. Heat the neutral oil in a small pan. Fry the spring onion matchsticks for 1–2 minutes until golden and crisp. Remove to kitchen paper and sprinkle with salt.

SEAR THE AUBERGINES
In a large non-stick frying pan or wok, heat 2 tablespoons of the oil. Add the aubergines in a single layer and sear over medium-high heat until golden on each side. Remove and set aside.

BUILD THE FLAVOUR BASE
In the same pan, and adding a little more oil if needed, gently fry the garlic, ginger, spring onion whites and chilli (if using) for 1–2 minutes. If using doubanjiang or fermented black beans, stir in and fry briefly.

BRAISE THE AUBERGINES
Return the aubergines to the pan. Add the reduced bone broth, soy sauce, oyster sauce, vinegar and sugar. Simmer uncovered for 6–8 minutes until slightly reduced. Stir in the cornflour slurry and cook for 1–2 more minutes until the sauce thickens and coats the aubergine.

TO SERVE
Transfer the aubergine to a serving dish. Scatter over the crispy spring onions and the sliced spring onion greens. Optionally, finish with a drizzle of sesame oil or crispy chilli oil.

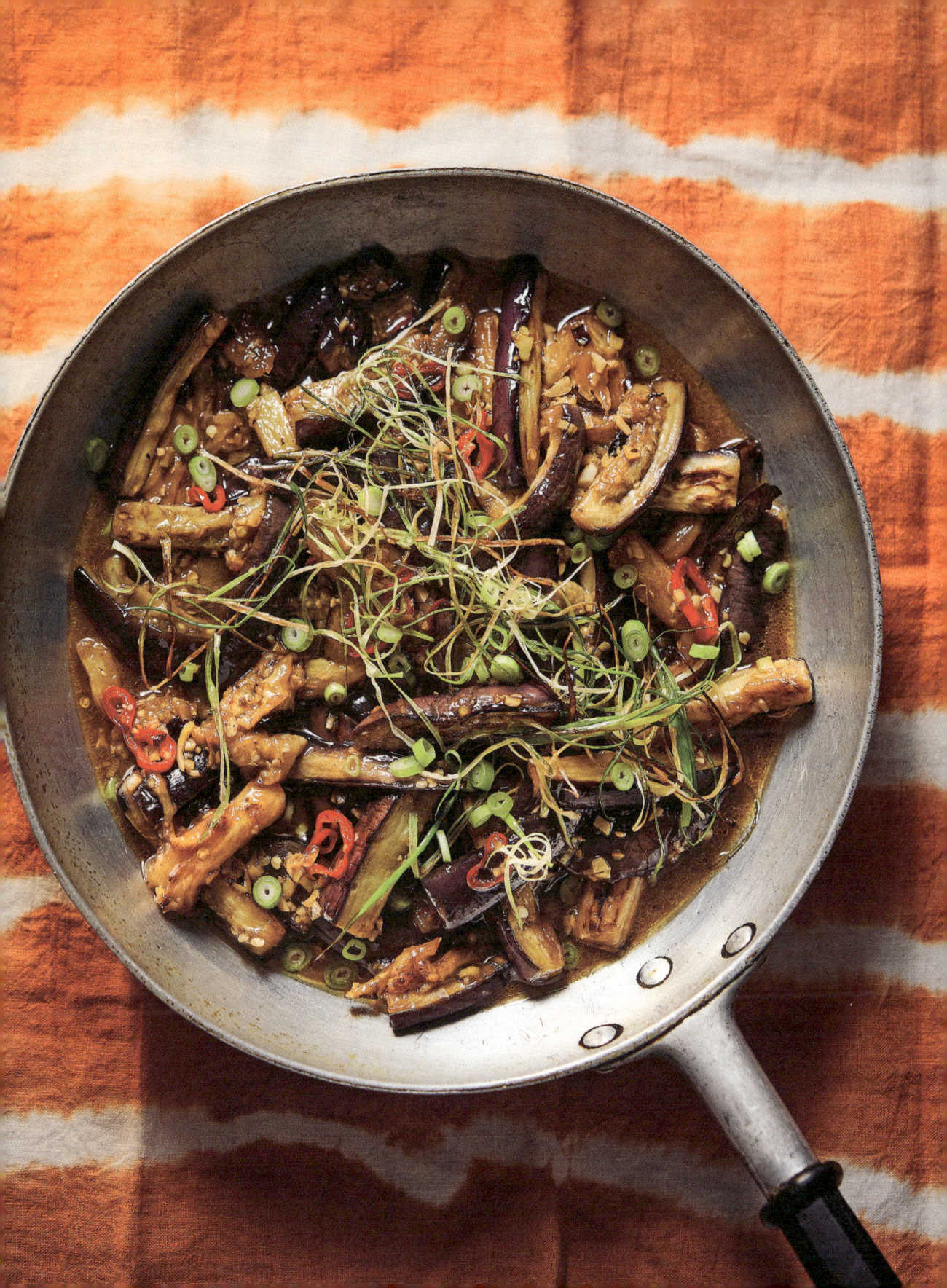

RICE, GRAINS & PULSES

Rice, grains and pulses can sometimes feel tricky to get right – undercooked, overcooked, too much water, not enough flavour. This chapter is designed to help you cut the guesswork and get perfectly cooked grains, deliciously melty beans and flavour-packed rice every time, with the help of broth.

From simple sides like Perfect Puy Lentils, to mains like One-Pan Prawn Jambalaya where rice is the hero ingredient, or our must-try Bristol Baked Beans with Pork Belly, get ready to transform the way you think about – and cook – these humble staples.

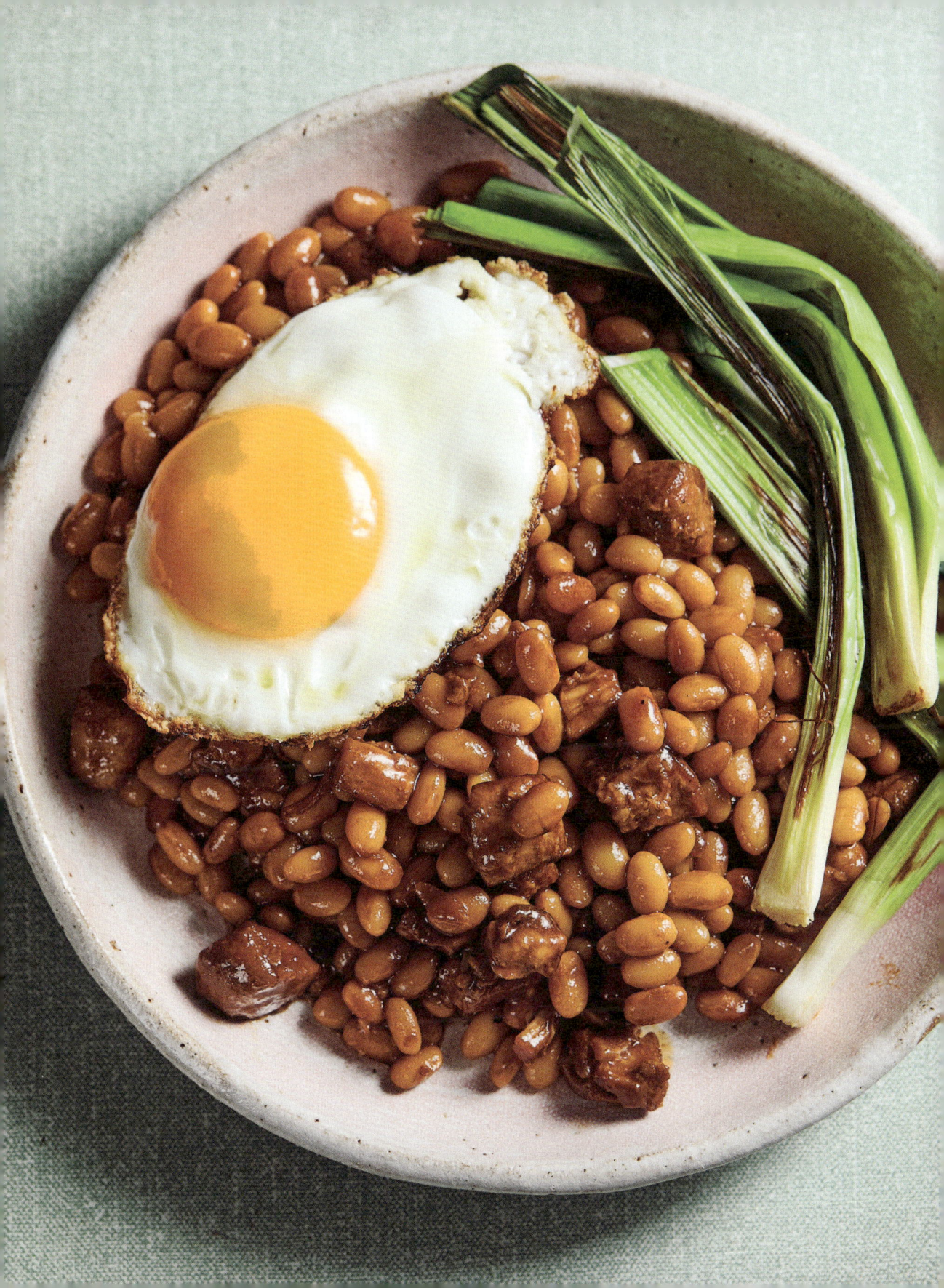

ULTIMATE FLUFFY RICE

Light, fluffy grains with just the right bite. This is your go-to method for perfect rice every time – no draining, no burnt pans. Just a lid, low heat and a timer. We've swapped water for bone broth to add depth, extra nutrition and savoury flavour.

SERVES 4
PREP TIME: 2 MINUTES
COOK TIME: 12 MINUTES, PLUS 10 MINUTES RESTING

200g (7oz) basmati rice
Small knob of butter or a drizzle of vegetable oil
½ teaspoon fine sea salt
500ml (17fl oz) chicken bone broth

RINSE THE RICE
Rinse the rice in a fine-mesh sieve under cold running water for about 1–2 minutes until the water runs clear. This removes excess starch and helps prevent it from clumping. Drain very well.

COAT THE RICE
Melt a knob of butter in a medium saucepan. Add the drained rice and salt and cook for 1–2 minutes until coated in the butter and slightly toasted.

COOK THE RICE
Add the bone broth. Set over medium heat and bring to a gentle boil. As soon as it starts boiling, put a tight-fitting lid on the pan, turn the heat down to very low and cook undisturbed for 12 minutes.

LET THE RICE STEAM
Turn off the heat and leave the lid on. Let it sit for 10 minutes to steam – don't lift the lid early or the rice will end up undercooked.

TO SERVE
Fluff gently with a fork and serve with your favourite main.

FOOLPROOF COUSCOUS

This is our go-to couscous recipe when plain won't do. Golden sultanas and sun-dried tomatoes bring a subtle sweet-savoury balance to the umami broth. It's great alongside grilled meats, spiced veg or as part of a mezze spread.

SERVES 4
PREP TIME: 10 MINUTES
COOK TIME: 5 MINUTES

200g (7oz) couscous
1 tablespoon olive oil
30g (1oz) raisins or sultanas
40g (1½oz) sun-dried tomatoes, finely chopped
Large pinch of salt
250ml (9fl oz) chicken bone broth
Small handful of flat-leaf parsley, finely chopped
Small handful of mint leaves, finely chopped
Squeeze of lemon juice

PREPARE THE COUSCOUS
Place the couscous in a heatproof bowl with the olive oil, raisins, sun-dried tomatoes and a pinch of salt. Stir to coat the grains and distribute the ingredients evenly.

HEAT THE BONE BROTH
Put the bone broth in a saucepan over high heat and bring to the boil.

COVER THE COUSCOUS
Add the hot bone broth to the couscous, stir quickly and cover with a lid. Leave to steam for 5 minutes.

FLUFF THE COUSCOUS
Uncover and fluff gently with a fork, breaking up any clumps and dispersing the fruit and tomatoes evenly. Fold in the chopped parsley and mint and a squeeze of lemon juice.

TO SERVE
Spoon warm onto plates or add chopped salad veg and pop it in the fridge to enjoy as a speedy lunch.

PERFECT PUY LENTILS

These little dark green lentils truly punch above their weight! They hold their shape beautifully and absorb all the flavour as they cook. Simmered in bone broth with some additional flavour boosters like garlic and thyme, they make a sumptuous side or base for roast veg, fish or slow-cooked meats.

SERVES 4
PREP TIME: 5 MINUTES
COOK TIME: 35–40 MINUTES, PLUS RESTING

3 tablespoons olive oil
1 small onion, diced
1 carrot, diced
1 celery stick, diced
1 garlic clove, diced
200g (7oz) Puy lentils, rinsed
1 bay leaf
1 thyme sprig or a pinch of dried thyme
600ml (21fl oz) chicken or vegetable bone broth
1 teaspoon red wine vinegar or lemon juice (optional)
Sea salt and freshly ground black pepper

TO SERVE
Drizzle of extra virgin olive oil

SOFTEN THE BASE VEG
Heat a large saucepan with the olive oil over medium heat. Once hot, add the diced onion, carrot, celery and garlic with a pinch of salt and cook for 4–5 minutes or until starting to soften.

ADD THE LENTILS AND BROTH
Add the lentils, bay leaf and thyme. Pour over the bone broth and bring to the boil.

SIMMER THE LENTILS
Reduce the heat to a gentle simmer and cook, covered, for 25–30 minutes, or until the lentils are tender but still hold their shape.

REST THE LENTILS
Once cooked, let the lentils rest for 10 minutes before serving. Discard the bay and thyme. Stir through the red wine vinegar and taste for seasoning.

TO SERVE
Drizzle with olive oil just before serving.

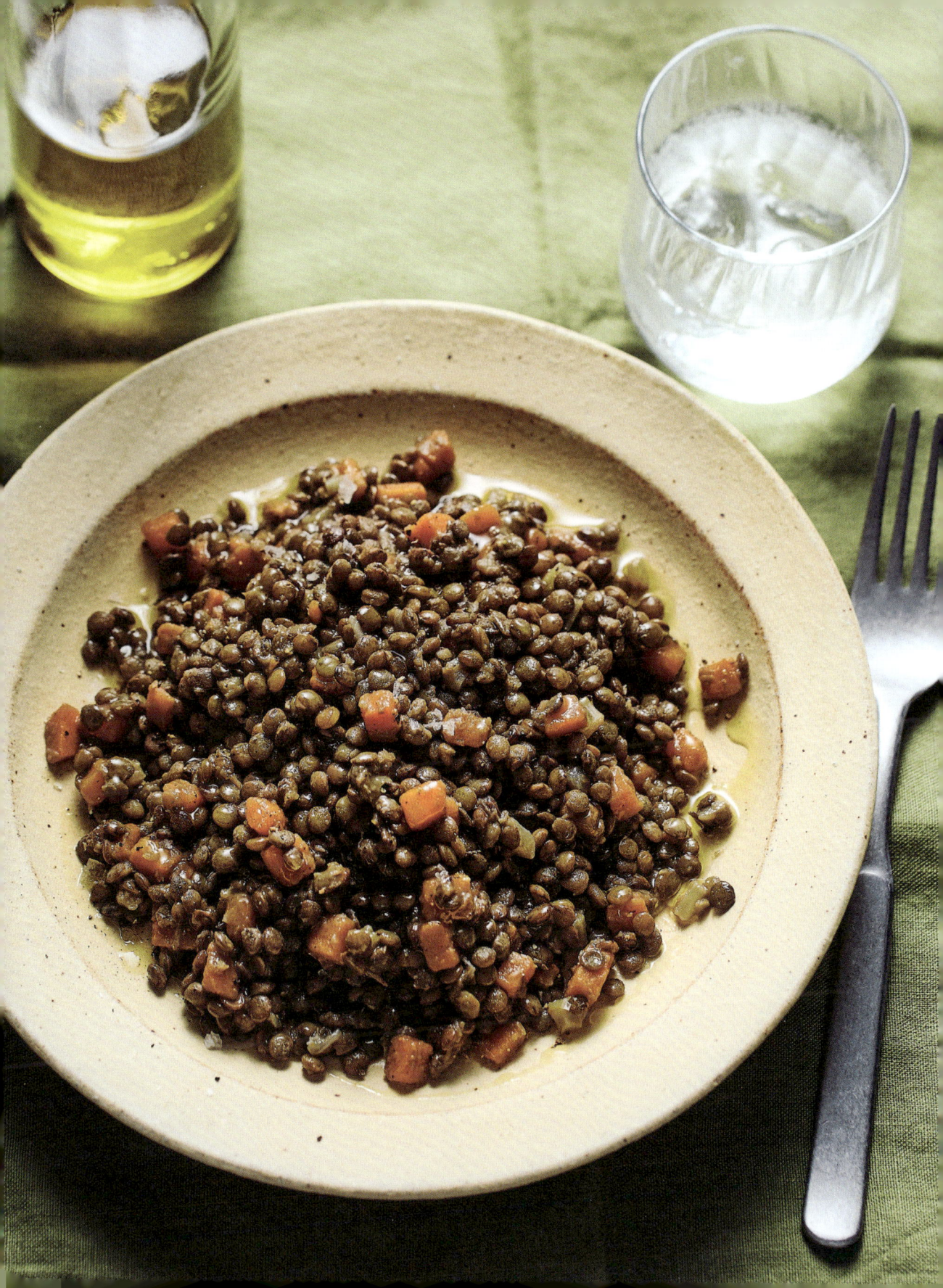

CARAMELISED ONION FREEKEH PILAF

Sweet, slow-cooked onions stirred through nutty freekeh – this is a side dish that doesn't hold back. Bone broth lifts the grains, giving savoury depth to every bite, and a scattering of herbs and toasted pine nuts brings freshness and texture.

SERVES 4
PREP TIME: 10 MINUTES
COOK TIME: 45 MINUTES

2 tablespoons olive oil
Knob of butter
2 large onions, thinly sliced
1 teaspoon sugar
1 garlic clove, finely chopped
1 teaspoon ground cumin
200g (7oz) cracked freekeh, rinsed
500ml (17fl oz) chicken bone broth
Sea salt and freshly ground black pepper

TO SERVE
Small handful of flat-leaf parsley, roughly chopped
1 tablespoon toasted pine nuts
Squeeze of lemon juice

SOFTEN THE ONIONS
Heat the olive oil and butter in a large frying pan over medium-low heat. Add the onions with a pinch of salt and cook slowly for 20–25 minutes, stirring occasionally, until soft, golden and starting to caramelise.

COOK UNTIL JAMMY
Sprinkle over the sugar and continue to cook for another 5 minutes, until dark (but not burnt) and jammy.

ADD YOUR GARLIC AND SPICE
Stir in the garlic and cumin and cook for 1–2 minutes until fragrant.

MIX THE FREEKEH THROUGH THE ONIONS
Add the rinsed freekeh and stir to coat in the onion mixture.

ADD THE BONE BROTH
Pour in the bone broth and bring to the boil. Reduce the heat to very low, cover and simmer for 15–18 minutes, or until the liquid is absorbed and the freekeh is tender with a little bite.

LEAVE IT TO STEAM
Remove from the heat and let it sit, covered, for 5 minutes to steam.

TO SERVE
Fluff with a fork, season well with salt and pepper and stir through the parsley and pine nuts. Add a squeeze of lemon juice to add extra zing before serving.

FASOLIA
(LAMB & WHITE BEAN STEW)

A hearty Lebanese-style stew made with white beans, tender lamb and a rich tomato and bone broth base. It's a simple, filling dish you can leave gently bubbling away while you get on with other things – or pour yourself a glass of wine and take a moment for yourself. Your call.

SERVES 4
PREP TIME: 20 MINUTES
COOK TIME: 2 HOUR 30 MINUTES

2 tablespoons olive oil
500g (1lb 2oz) diced lamb shoulder (boneless)
1 large onion, finely chopped
3 garlic cloves, minced or finely chopped
1 tablespoon tomato purée
1 teaspoon ground allspice
½ teaspoon ground cinnamon
¼ teaspoon freshly ground black pepper
1 bay leaf
500ml (17fl oz) chicken bone broth
2 x 400g tins white beans, drained and rinsed
Juice of ½ lemon
Sea salt

TO SERVE
Small handful of parsley or coriander, chopped

SEAR THE LAMB
Put the olive oil in a large pot over medium heat and brown the lamb in batches until nicely coloured. Set aside.

BUILD THE BASE
To the same pot, add the chopped onion and a pinch of salt. Cook gently for 10–12 minutes until soft and golden. Stir in the chopped garlic and tomato purée. Cook for a further 2–3 minutes until it darkens slightly.

ADD SPICES AND DEGLAZE
Stir in the allspice, cinnamon, black pepper and bay leaf. Return the lamb to the pot and stir everything together. Pour in the bone broth and 500ml (17fl oz) water, scraping up any sticky bits from the bottom of the pan.

SIMMER GENTLY
Bring to a gentle simmer and cook for about 1 hour 30 minutes, partially covered, until the lamb is tender. Add the beans and cook for a further 20–30 minutes to allow them to absorb flavour and soften into the broth.

FINISH THE STEW
Season to taste with salt, then stir in the lemon juice to brighten everything.

TO SERVE
Scatter over the fresh herbs just before serving and grab a spoon to dig in.

POLENTA QUATTRO FORMAGGI
(FOUR CHEESE POLENTA)

A staple of northern Italy, polenta is traditionally a simple, hearty classic, but this four-cheese version dials up the indulgence. Simmered with bone broth and melted cheese, it turns into a velvety, spoonable dish that's equal parts comfort and luxury. Serve it as a standout side or give it the spotlight as a main.

SERVES 4
PREP TIME: 5 MINUTES
COOK TIME: 35–40 MINUTES

1 litre (35fl oz) chicken bone broth
200g (7oz) polenta (coarse, stone-ground)
1 tablespoon butter
50g (1¾oz) Gorgonzola cheese, crumbled
50g (1¾oz) Taleggio cheese, chopped
50g (1¾oz) Parmesan cheese, grated
50g (1¾oz) mozzarella, grated
Sea salt and freshly ground black pepper

BOIL THE BONE BROTH
Bring the bone broth to the boil in a heavy-based saucepan.

WHISK IN THE POLENTA
Reduce the heat to low and slowly pour in the polenta in a steady stream, whisking continuously to prevent lumps.

COOK THE POLENTA
Cook the polenta over low heat for 30–35 minutes, stirring regularly with a wooden spoon, until thick, soft and pulling away from the sides of the pan.

STIR IN THE BUTTER AND CHEESE
Remove from the heat and stir in the butter and all four cheeses until completely melted and creamy.

SEASON TO PERFECT
Season with salt and a generous amount of black pepper, to taste.

TO SERVE
Serve immediately while soft or pour into a tray to cool and set for grilling or baking later.

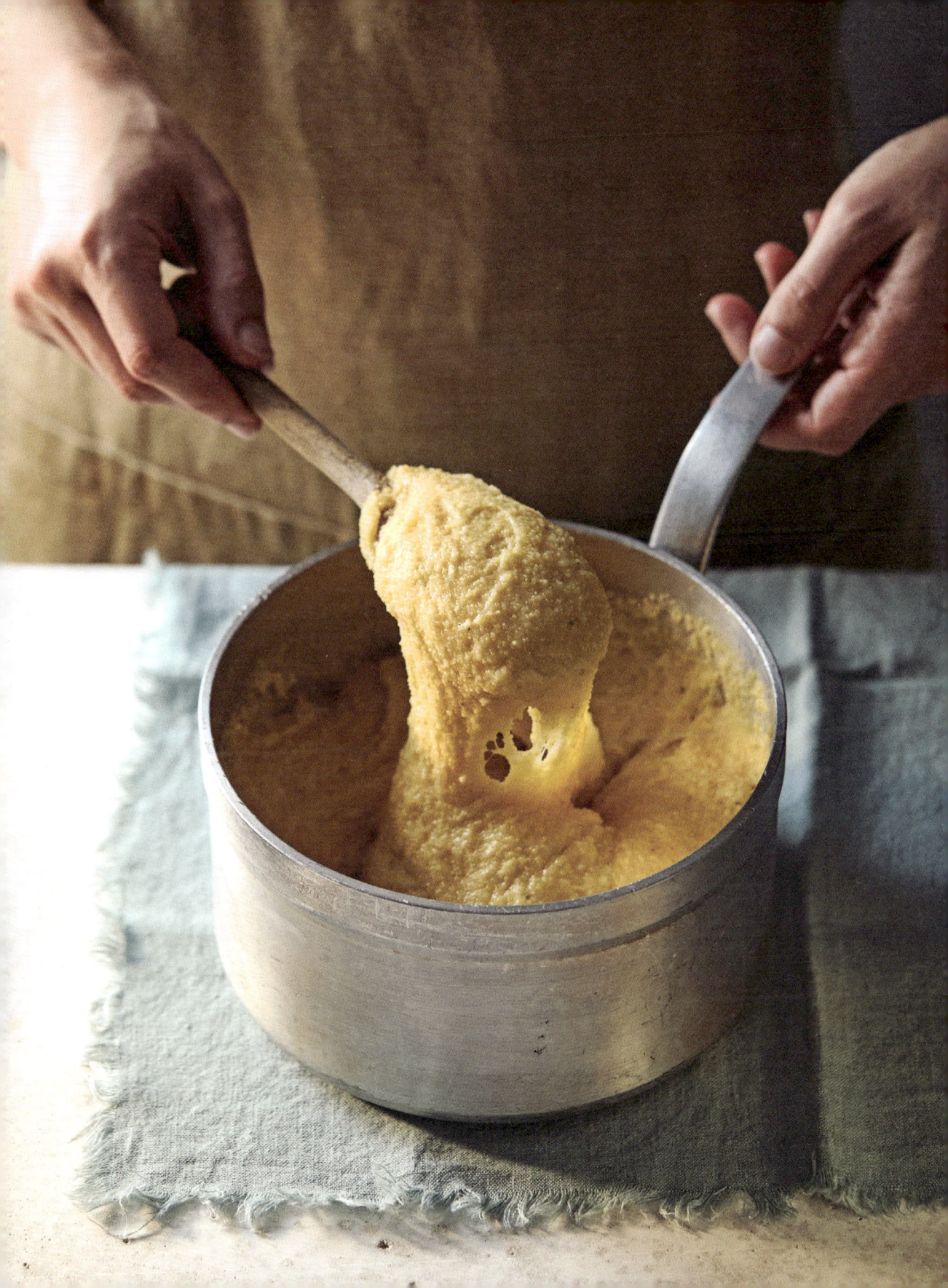

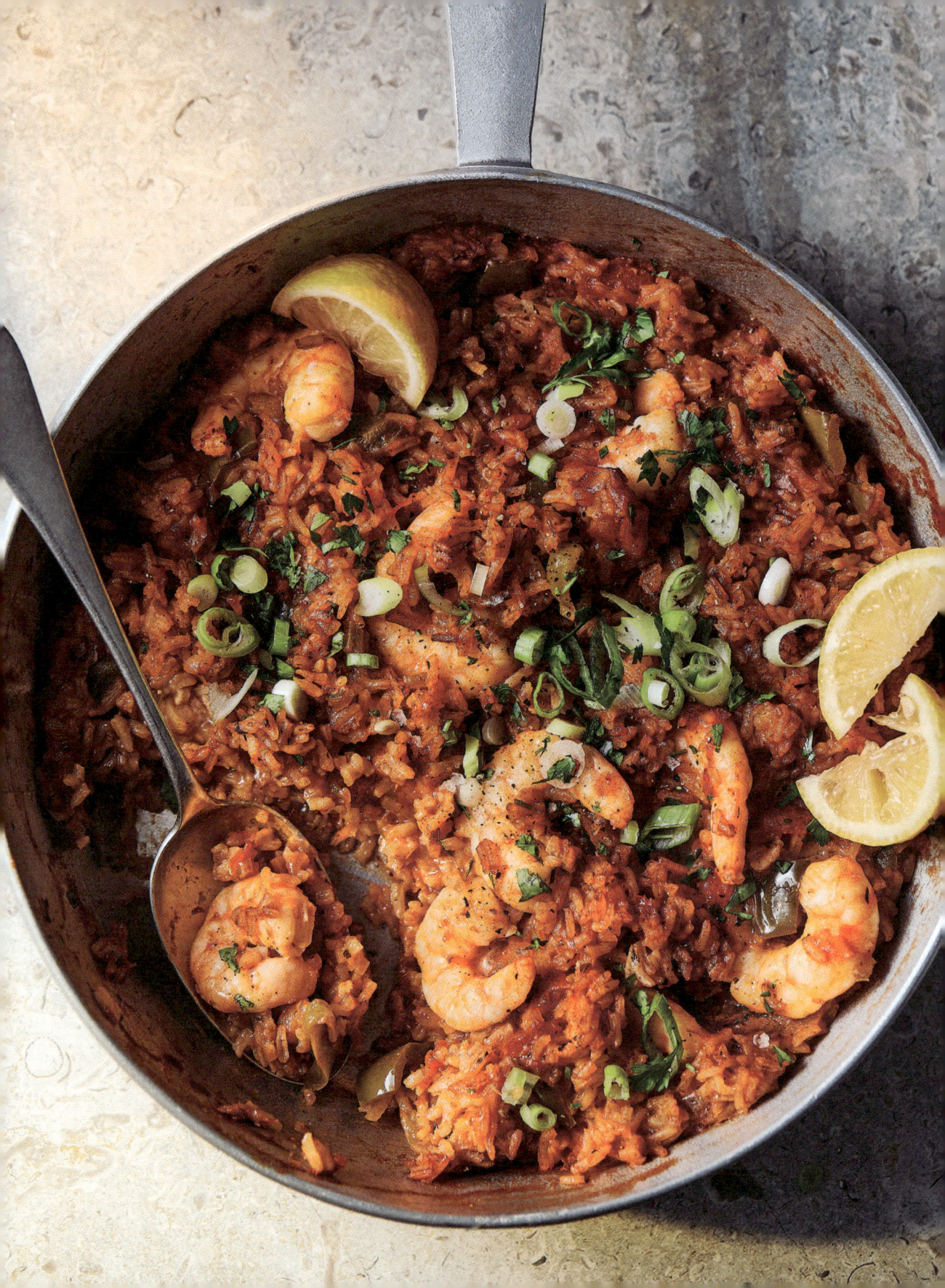

ONE-PAN PRAWN JAMBALAYA

All the punchy flavour of a classic jambalaya, none of the constant stirring. This oven-baked version gives you fluffy, spicy rice with rich bone broth depth and sweet, tender prawns. It's a one-pan wonder that brings big flavour with minimal effort.

SERVES 4
PREP TIME: 15 MINUTES
COOK TIME: 40 MINUTES

1 tablespoon olive oil
1 small onion, finely chopped
1 celery stick, finely chopped
1 green pepper, chopped
2 garlic cloves, finely chopped
1 teaspoon smoked paprika
1 teaspoon dried oregano
½ teaspoon dried thyme
½ teaspoon cayenne pepper, or to taste
1 tablespoon tomato purée
200g (7oz) long-grain rice
1 × 400g tin chopped tomatoes
400ml (14fl oz) fish bone broth
250g (9oz) raw prawns, peeled and deveined
Sea salt and freshly ground black pepper

TO SERVE
1 spring onion, sliced
Small handful of parsley, chopped
Lemon wedges
Hot sauce

SOFTEN THE VEG
Preheat the oven to 200°C (180°C fan)/400°F/gas 6. Heat the olive oil in a large casserole dish over medium heat. Add the onion, celery and green pepper and cook for 6–8 minutes until softened.

ADD THE CREOLE SPICES
Stir in the garlic, smoked paprika, oregano, thyme and cayenne and cook for 1–2 minutes until fragrant. Stir in the tomato purée and cook for 1 minute more.

ADD THE RICE, TOMATOES AND BONE BROTH
Tip in the rice and stir to coat it in the spicy oil and vegetables. Add the chopped tomatoes and bone broth, season generously with salt and pepper and bring to a simmer.

BAKE UNTIL TENDER
Cover the pan tightly with a lid or foil and bake for about 25–30 minutes until the rice is just tender and the liquid mostly absorbed.

COOK THE PRAWNS
Remove from the oven, stir in the raw prawns, re-cover and let sit for 5–7 minutes. The residual heat will gently cook the prawns until pink and tender.

TO SERVE
Scatter over the spring onion and parsley, then serve with lemon wedges and a generous splash of hot sauce on the side.

ARROZ CALDOSO
(BROTHY RICE WITH WILD MUSHROOMS)

Somewhere between a risotto and a stew, this is comfort food the Spanish way – brothy, savoury and best eaten slowly, with a spoon. Made with wild mushrooms and bone broth, it's earthy, rich and full of depth. It's softer than paella, with a richness that lingers long after the last bite.

SERVES 4
PREP TIME: 10 MINUTES
COOK TIME: 40 MINUTES

1 litre (35fl oz) beef bone broth
2 tablespoons olive oil
1 small onion, finely chopped
2 garlic cloves, finely chopped
1 teaspoon sweet smoked paprika
1 teaspoon chopped fresh thyme
1 teaspoon chopped fresh rosemary
500g (1lb 2oz) mixed wild mushrooms, torn or chopped
100ml (3½fl oz) dry white wine
250g (9oz) short-grain rice (such as Calasparra or Arborio)
Sea salt and freshly ground black pepper

TO SERVE
Chopped parsley
Drizzle of extra virgin olive oil

WARM THE BONE BROTH
Heat the beef bone broth in a medium saucepan until hot and gently bubbling.

SOFTEN THE ONIONS
Heat the olive oil in a wide, heavy-based pan over medium heat. Add the onion and cook gently for 5–6 minutes until soft and translucent.

COOK THE MUSHROOMS
Stir in the garlic, paprika and fresh herbs, followed by the mushrooms. Cook for 5–8 minutes until the mushrooms are golden and their moisture has mostly evaporated.

COOK OFF THE WINE
Pour in the white wine and let it bubble for 1–2 minutes, scraping up any bits from the bottom of the pan.

COAT THE RICE
Stir in the rice and cook for 1–2 minutes to coat it in the oil and flavours.

ADD THE BONE BROTH
Begin adding the hot bone broth, two ladles at a time, stirring regularly. Keep the mixture at a simmer and continue adding broth as it's absorbed, much like making risotto.

FINISH COOKING THE RICE
After about 25 minutes, the rice should be tender but loose and brothy. If it's a bit thick, add some boiled water to thin it out. Season generously with salt and pepper.

TO SERVE
Serve in shallow bowls, scattered with parsley and finished with a drizzle of olive oil, if desired.

RUSTIC FRENCH CASSOULET

A slow-cooked, peasant-style dish from the south of France, cassoulet is all about comfort. Layers of white beans, sausage and pork, simmered together in a deeply savoury bone broth until bubbling and golden – this dish truly showcases the best of both beans and broth.

SERVES 4
PREP TIME: 30 MINUTES
COOK TIME: 2 HOURS 45 MINUTES–3 HOURS 15 MINUTES, PLUS RESTING

2 tablespoons olive oil
1 onion, finely chopped
2 carrots, diced
2 celery sticks, diced
4 garlic cloves, crushed
2 bay leaves
1 tablespoon tomato purée
1 teaspoon fresh thyme leaves or ½ teaspoon dried
400g (14oz) pork shoulder, cut into chunks
300g (10½oz) Toulouse sausage, thickly sliced
1 × 400g tin white beans (haricots), drained
500ml (17fl oz) chicken bone broth
Sea salt and freshly ground black pepper

FOR THE CRISPY BREADCRUMBS
75g (2½oz) fresh white breadcrumbs
1 tablespoon olive oil

TO SERVE
Green salad
Crusty baguette

SOFTEN THE VEG
Preheat the oven to 180°C (160°C fan)/350°F/gas 4. Heat the olive oil in a large Dutch oven or deep ovenproof pot. Add the onion, carrot and celery and cook for 8–10 minutes until soft and golden.

ADD THE GARLIC AND HERBS
Stir in the garlic, bay leaves, tomato purée and thyme and cook for 1–2 minutes until fragrant.

BROWN THE PORK
Add the pork shoulder and cook for about 5–6 minutes until browned on all sides. Remove and set aside.

BROWN THE SAUSAGES
Add the sausage to the pot, searing for 2–3 minutes or until brown.

ADD THE PORK AND BEANS
Return the pork to the pan along with the beans. Pour in the bone broth and 500ml (17fl oz) water until just covered. Season with salt and pepper and bring to a gentle simmer.

PUT IN THE OVEN
Cover with a lid and transfer to the oven. Cook for 2 hours–2 hours 30 minutes, stirring once or twice, until the beans are tender and the pork is falling apart.

CRISP THE BREADCRUMBS
In a small bowl, mix the breadcrumbs with the olive oil. Remove the pot from the oven, uncover and scatter the breadcrumbs over the top. Return to the oven uncovered for 20–30 minutes until golden and crusty. Leave to rest for 10 minutes before serving.

TO SERVE
Serve simply, with a green salad on the side and plenty of buttered baguette for mopping and scooping.

FEIJOADA
(BRAZILIAN BLACK BEAN STEW)

A soulful, smoky Brazilian stew made with black beans, savoury pork cuts and spiced sausage, simmered slowly in bone broth until thick and rich? Yes please. Traditionally served with rice, orange slices and garlicky greens, we think this bean dish is absolutely irresistible.

SERVES 4
PREP TIME: 20 MINUTES
COOK TIME: 1 HOUR 45 MINUTES–2 HOURS 15 MINUTES

2 tablespoons olive oil
1 onion, finely chopped
3 garlic cloves, finely chopped
1 bay leaf
1 teaspoon smoked paprika
½ teaspoon ground cumin
½ teaspoon dried oregano
150g (5½oz) streaky bacon, chopped
200g (7oz) pork shoulder, cut into 2–3cm (¾–1¼ inch) chunks
200g (7oz) smoked sausage (like kielbasa or chorizo), sliced
1 x 400g (14oz) tin of black beans
750ml (26fl oz) beef bone broth
Sea salt and freshly ground black pepper

TO SERVE
Steamed rice
Sautéed greens
Orange wedges
Coriander

SOFTEN THE ONIONS
Heat the olive oil in a large heavy-based pot over medium heat. Add the onion and cook for 5–7 minutes until softened and lightly golden.

ADD THE AROMATICS
Add the garlic, bay leaf, smoked paprika, cumin and oregano. Cook for 1–2 minutes until fragrant.

BROWN THE MEAT
Stir in the bacon and cook for 3–4 minutes until starting to crisp, then add the pork shoulder and sausage. Cook until browned on all sides, about 6–8 minutes.

SIMMER
Add the black beans, bone broth and enough water to cover everything by a few centimetres (about 500ml/17fl oz). Bring to the boil, then reduce the heat to low and simmer gently, partially covered, for 1 hour 30 minutes–2 hours, or until the meat is tender and the stew is thick. Stir occasionally and top up with more water if needed.

SEASON
Season generously with salt and pepper and remove the bay leaf. The broth should be rich and slightly glossy, with tender chunks of meat throughout.

TO SERVE
Serve hot with rice, sautéed greens and orange wedges, with a sprinkle of coriander to finish.

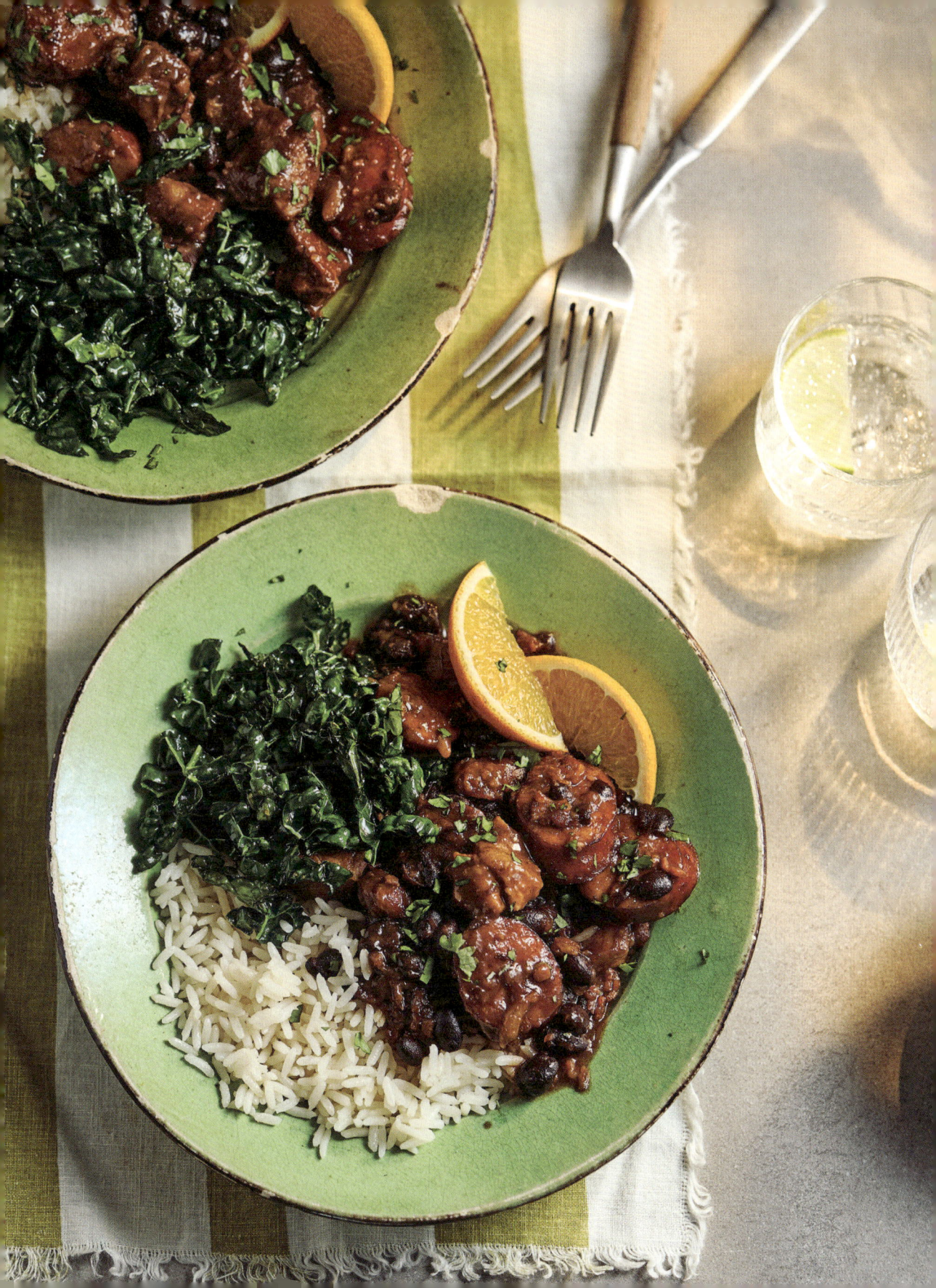

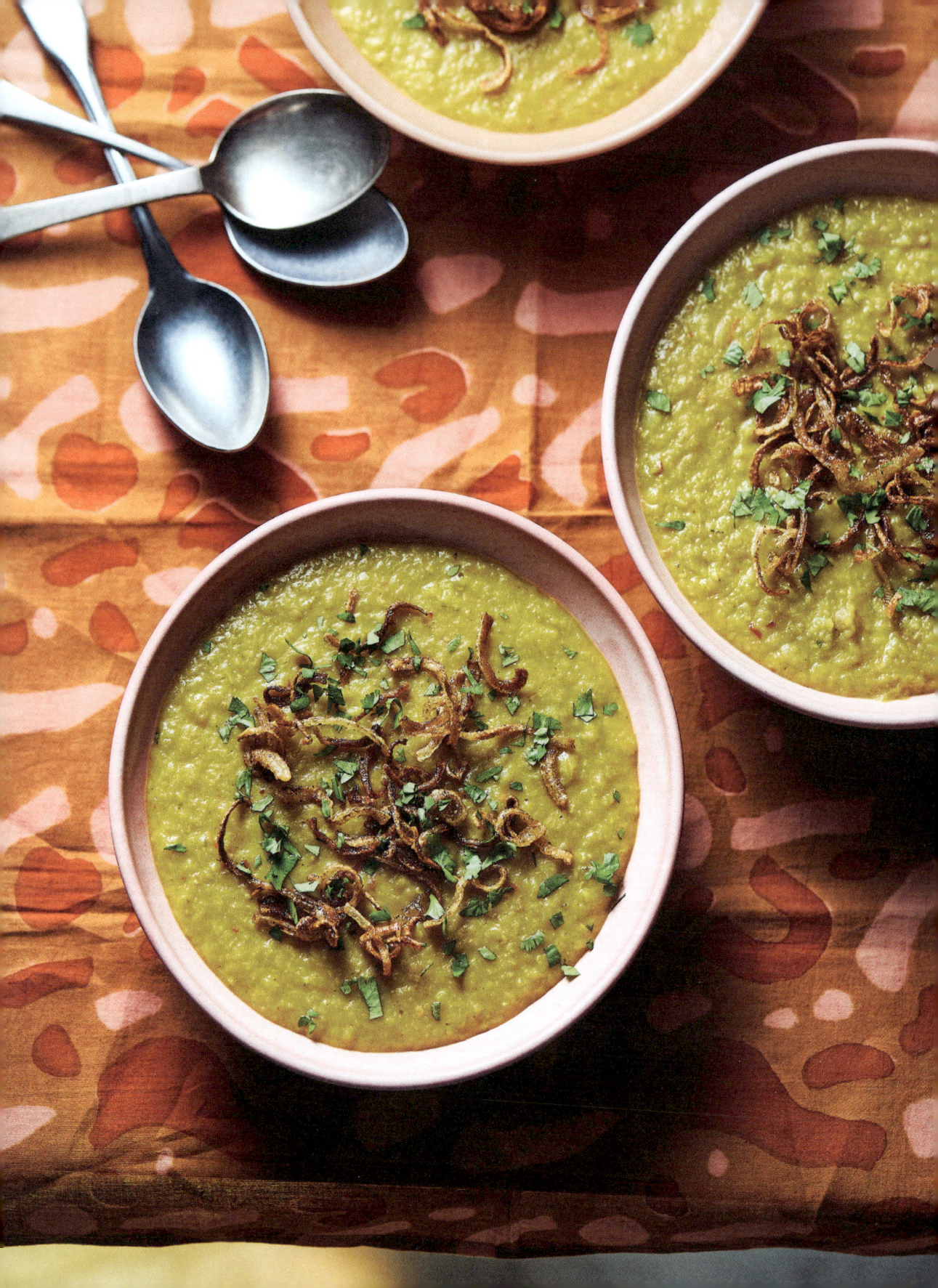

RED DAAL WITH CRISPY ONIONS

This is one of those dishes everyone asks for again. Built on store cupboard ingredients, lifted with warm spices and given depth with savoury chicken bone broth, it's an all-round winner. Forget hours of simmering, this one-pot is wonderfully quick and easy, works well for weeknights and even better as leftovers.

SERVES 4
PREP TIME: 10 MINUTES
COOK TIME: 35 MINUTES

1 tablespoon coconut oil or ghee
1 onion, finely chopped
3 garlic cloves, minced
1 thumb-sized piece of fresh ginger, grated
1 teaspoon ground turmeric
1 teaspoon ground cumin
1 teaspoon ground coriander
½ teaspoon chilli flakes (optional)
200g (7oz) red lentils, rinsed
750ml (26fl oz) chicken bone broth
200ml (7fl oz) full-fat coconut milk
Juice of ½ lemon
Sea salt

FOR THE GARAM MASALA CRISPY ONIONS

1 tablespoon neutral oil (sunflower or avocado work well)
1 large onion, thinly sliced
Pinch of salt
½ teaspoon garam masala

TO SERVE (OPTIONAL)
Chopped coriander

START WITH THE CRISPY ONIONS
Heat the oil in a frying pan over medium heat. Add the onion and a pinch of salt and cook slowly, stirring often, for about 10–15 minutes until golden and crisp. Stir in the garam masala in the final minute, then transfer to kitchen paper.

BUILD THE BASE
In a large saucepan, heat the coconut oil or ghee over medium heat. Add the chopped onion and cook for 5–7 minutes until soft. Stir in the garlic, ginger, turmeric, cumin, coriander and chilli flakes. Let the spices sizzle for 30–60 seconds to bring out their flavour.

COOK THE DAAL
Add the rinsed lentils, bone broth and coconut milk. Bring to a gentle simmer and cook uncovered for 20–25 minutes, stirring occasionally. The lentils should break down and the mixture should thicken into a creamy texture.

SEASON
Add a splash more water or broth if it gets too thick. Season with salt and finish with lemon juice to brighten the flavour.

TO SERVE
Spoon the daal into bowls and top generously with the garam masala onions. Scatter over fresh coriander, if using. This also works beautifully as a side or sharer alongside other Indian dishes (check out our Comfort Cooking chapter on pages 178–209 for more inspiration).

RISOTTO BIANCO

A timeless Italian favourite that's all about technique and quality ingredients. This creamy, smooth and rich risotto can be rustled up in less than half an hour. Bone broth replaces water to give subtle, savoury depth, making it perfectly satisfying on its own or as a base for seasonal vegetables, seafood or poultry.

SERVES 4
PREP TIME: 5 MINUTES
COOK TIME: 25 MINUTES

1 litre (35fl oz) chicken bone broth
2 tablespoons olive oil
50g (1¾oz) unsalted butter
1 small onion, finely chopped
1 garlic clove, finely chopped
300g (10½oz) Arborio rice
100ml (3½fl oz) dry white wine
50g (1¾oz) Parmesan cheese, finely grated
Sea salt and freshly ground black pepper

WARM THE BONE BROTH
Put the chicken bone broth in a medium saucepan over low heat just to keep warm.

SWEAT THE VEG
Heat the olive oil and half the butter in a large pan over medium heat. Add the onion and garlic and cook gently for 5 minutes until soft and translucent but not coloured.

COAT THE RICE
Stir in the rice and cook for 2 minutes, coating each grain with the fat.

ADD THE WHITE WINE
Pour in the white wine and stir until mostly absorbed.

ADD THE BONE BROTH
Add a ladle of warm bone broth to the rice and stir until absorbed. Continue adding the broth, one ladle at a time, stirring frequently and allowing it to absorb before adding more broth.

FINISH THE RISOTTO
After 18–20 minutes, the rice should be creamy but with a slight bite to the centre. Remove from the heat and stir in the remaining butter and the Parmesan. Season to taste with salt and pepper.

REST
Cover and rest for 2 minutes before serving.

TO SERVE
Delicious on its own, stir through fresh blanched asparagus or top with our rich Ossobuco alla Milanese (see page 222).

CONGEE WITH SLICED PORK BELLY

Congee, an age-old Asian rice porridge, is gaining popularity in the UK and rightly so. Our version is made with chicken bone broth, which gives the porridge a savoury backbone, extra nutrition and keeps it light yet sustaining.

SERVES 4
PREP TIME: 15 MINUTES
COOK TIME: 1 HOUR–1 HOUR 35 MINUTES

200g (7oz) jasmine rice or pudding rice
1.5 litres (52fl oz) chicken bone broth
1 thumb-sized piece of fresh ginger, sliced
2 spring onions (white part only)
Sea salt

FOR THE PORK BELLY
1 tablespoon neutral oil (vegetable or sunflower) or sesame oil
400g (14oz) sliced pork belly (5mm/¼ inch thick)
2 tablespoons light soy sauce
1 tablespoon Shaoxing wine or dry sherry
1 teaspoon soft brown sugar
1 teaspoon Chinese five-spice powder
1 garlic clove, crushed

TO SERVE
2–4 tablespoons crispy chilli oil
2 spring onions (green tops), finely sliced
Small handful of coriander, chopped (optional)
4 soft-boiled eggs (optional)

RINSE AND TOAST THE RICE
Rinse the rice thoroughly under cold water until the water runs mostly clear. For added depth of flavour, dry-toast the rinsed rice in a large saucepan over medium heat for 2–3 minutes, stirring regularly, until it smells slightly nutty but doesn't colour.

START THE CONGEE
Add the chicken bone broth, 250ml (9fl oz) water, the sliced ginger and the white parts of the spring onions to the pan with the toasted rice. Bring to the boil, then immediately reduce to a low simmer.

SIMMER UNTIL CREAMY
Cook the congee uncovered for 60–90 minutes, stirring occasionally to prevent sticking. Add a little more broth or water as needed to keep it loose and silky. The rice should break down completely, giving the congee a smooth, creamy texture. Season to taste with sea salt. Remove the ginger and spring onion before serving.

CRISP THE PORK BELLY
While the congee simmers, heat the oil in a large non-stick frying pan over medium-high heat. Add the sliced pork belly in a single layer and cook for 4–5 minutes until starting to brown and crisp at the edges.

GLAZE THE PORK
Turn the heat to medium and add the soy sauce, Shaoxing wine, sugar, five-spice and garlic. Let it bubble and reduce for 6–10 minutes, turning the pork as the glaze thickens and clings. Set aside and keep warm.

TO SERVE
Ladle the hot congee into warm bowls. Spoon over the sticky pork belly slices, drizzle with crispy chilli oil and garnish with spring onion greens, coriander and soft-boiled eggs, if using.

BRISTOL BAKED BEANS WITH CRISPY PORK BELLY

Bristol Baked Beans are our West Country take on the classic Boston Baked Beans, using cider instead of molasses. A generous helping of bone broth adds richness and body to the sauce, making these beans heaps heartier and more nourishing than the tinned kind.

SERVES 4
PREP TIME: 20 MINUTES (EXCLUDING BEAN SOAKING)
COOK TIME: 3 HOURS–3 HOURS 30 MINUTES

200g (7oz) pork belly, skin removed and cut into 2–3cm (¾–1¼ inch) cubes (optional, but recommended)
Small pinch of smoked paprika, plus extra for the base (optional)
1 tablespoon olive oil or beef dripping
1 onion, finely chopped
2 garlic cloves, minced
1 tablespoon tomato purée
1 tablespoon English mustard or Dijon
1 tablespoon brown sugar
500g (1lb 2oz) dried haricot beans, soaked overnight (or use flageolet or cannellini)
330ml (11¼fl oz) dry cider
400ml (14fl oz) beef bone broth
1 teaspoon apple cider vinegar
Sea salt and freshly ground black pepper

FOR THE ROAST LEEKS OR SHALLOTS (OPTIONAL)
Drizzle of olive oil
4 small leeks or 6 banana shallots, trimmed and halved lengthways
Fresh thyme (optional)

TO SERVE
Drizzle of extra virgin olive oil
Sourdough, jacket potatoes or a fried egg

PREPARE THE PORK BELLY (IF USING)
Pat the pork belly dry with kitchen paper. Season with salt, pepper and a small pinch of smoked paprika. Set aside while you prep the rest of the base.

COOK THE BASE
Preheat the oven to 170°C (150°C fan)/350°F/gas 4. In a large ovenproof pot or Dutch oven, heat the olive oil or beef dripping over medium heat. Add the onion and garlic, cooking until softened and starting to turn golden. Add the pork belly cubes and brown them on all sides. Stir in the tomato purée, mustard, brown sugar and paprika, if using. Cook for 1 minute. Pour in the cider and bring to a simmer. Let it reduce by about one-third.

ADD THE BEANS AND BONE BROTH
Add the soaked and drained beans. Pour in the bone broth and stir to combine. Add the apple cider vinegar and season with salt and pepper. Bring to a gentle simmer on the hob.

BAKE LOW AND SLOW
Cover the pot with a lid and transfer to the oven. Bake for 2 hours 30 minutes–3 hours, or until the beans are soft and the sauce is rich and thick. Remove the lid for the last 30 minutes if you want a stickier finish.

ROAST THE SHALLOTS OR LEEKS
While the beans bake, preheat a small roasting tray with a drizzle of olive oil. Toss the halved leeks or shallots with salt, pepper and the thyme, if using. Roast at 180°C (160°C fan)/350°F/gas 4 for 30–40 minutes until tender and lightly caramelised. Baste once or twice with the oil during cooking.

TO SERVE
Spoon the beans into shallow bowls and top with the roast leeks or shallots. Add a drizzle of olive oil or extra broth if needed. Serve with sourdough, jacket potatoes or a fried egg on top.

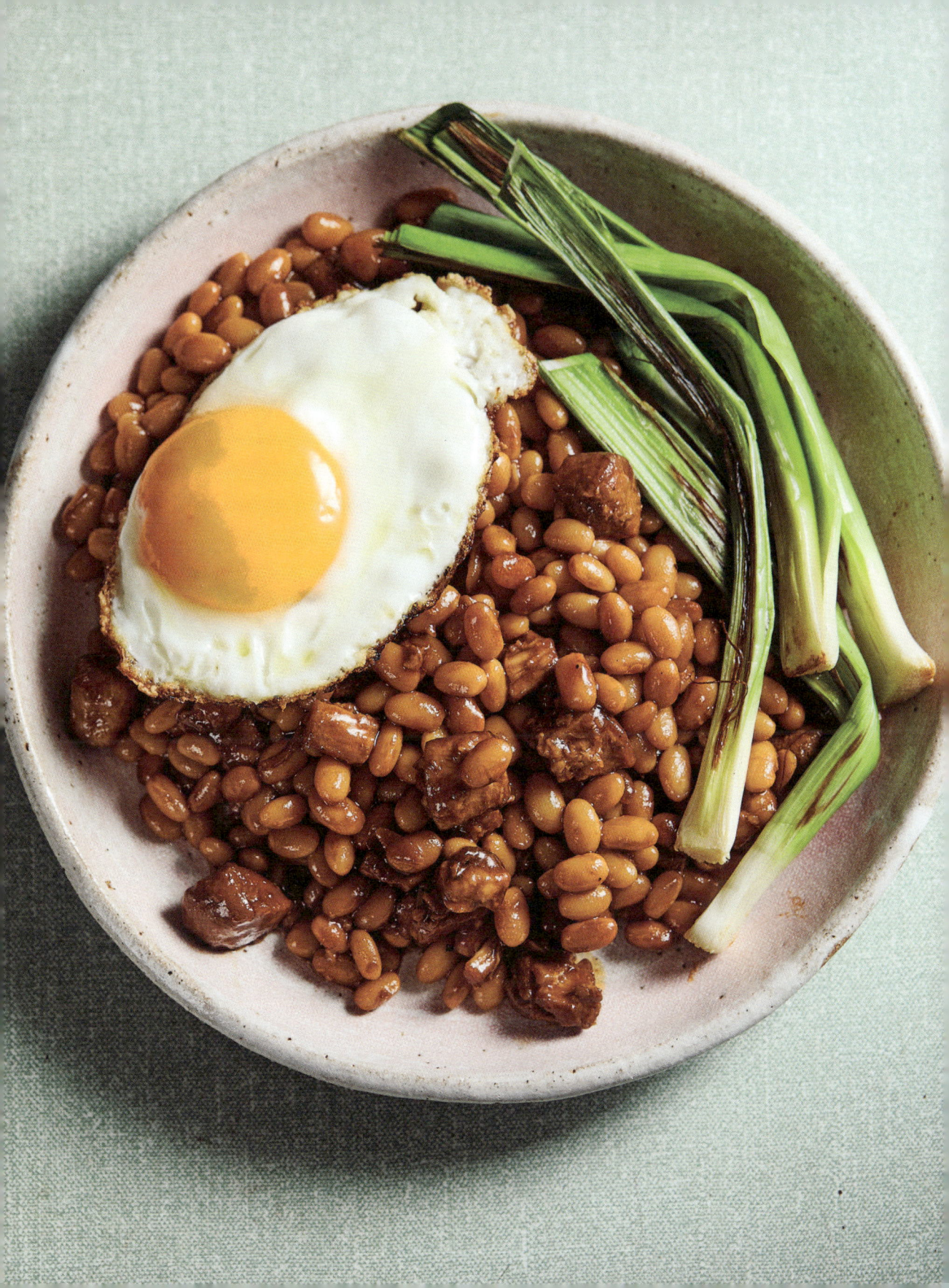

PASTA & NOODLES

Pasta and noodles are in a world of their own – comforting, hearty and endlessly varied. From a perfect-every-time One-Pot Puttanesca to an aromatic Malaysian Monkfish Laksa, the crowd-pleasing dishes in this chapter each have broth at their heart and are guaranteed to become family favourites in no time.

While we don't consider ourselves Ramen experts, we've added in an unmissable Instant Ramen Upgrade so that you can level up your noodle cup with extra flavour and nourishment, without compromising on convenience. Straightforward enough for a speedy lunch, but tasty enough to feel like a treat.

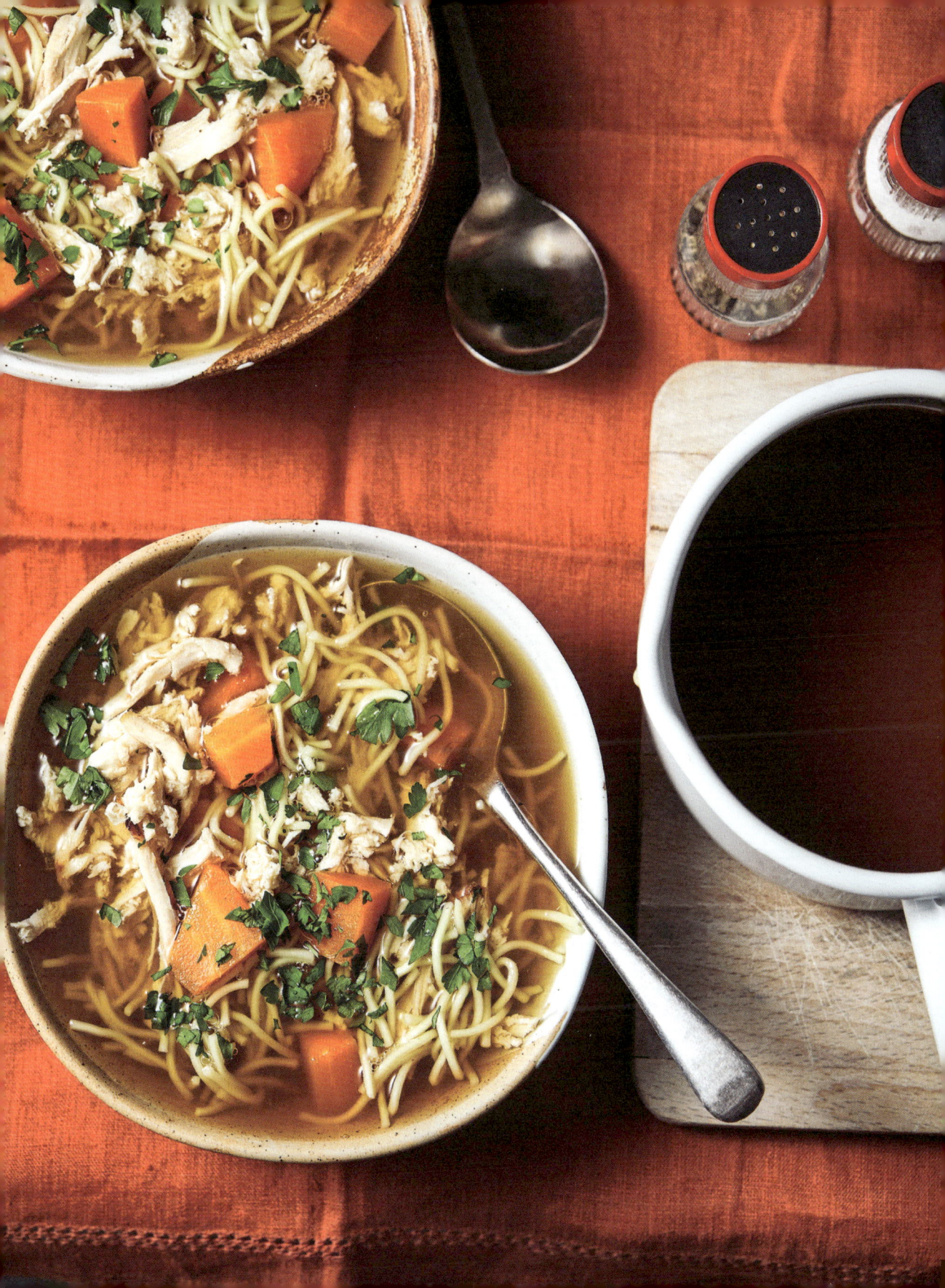

TORTELLINI IN BRODO

This is a simple, comforting Italian classic that relies on having a really good broth. We use ready-made tortellini for ease, but the quality of the broth is what takes it up a notch. Serve as a main with some crusty bread or a fresh tomato salad on the side.

SERVES 4
PREP TIME: 5 MINUTES
COOK TIME: 20 MINUTES

1.5 litres (52fl oz) beef bone broth
1 garlic clove, smashed
1 bay leaf
1 Parmesan rind (optional)
400–500g (14oz–1lb 2oz) fresh meat-filled tortellini (the best you can find!)
Sea salt and freshly ground black pepper

TO SERVE
Grated Parmesan
Drizzle of extra virgin olive oil

INFUSE THE BONE BROTH
Put the bone broth in a large saucepan with the garlic, bay leaf and Parmesan rind, if using. Bring to a gentle simmer and cook for 15 minutes to infuse.

REMOVE THE AROMATICS
Taste the broth and season with salt and pepper. Remove the garlic, bay leaf and Parmesan rind with a slotted spoon.

BOIL THE TORTELLINI
Add the tortellini to the hot broth and cook for 2–4 minutes, or according to the packet instructions, until just tender and floating. Be careful not to overcook the tortellini – they should be just soft with a bit of bite.

TO SERVE
Ladle into warm bowls and finish with grated Parmesan and a drizzle of good olive oil.

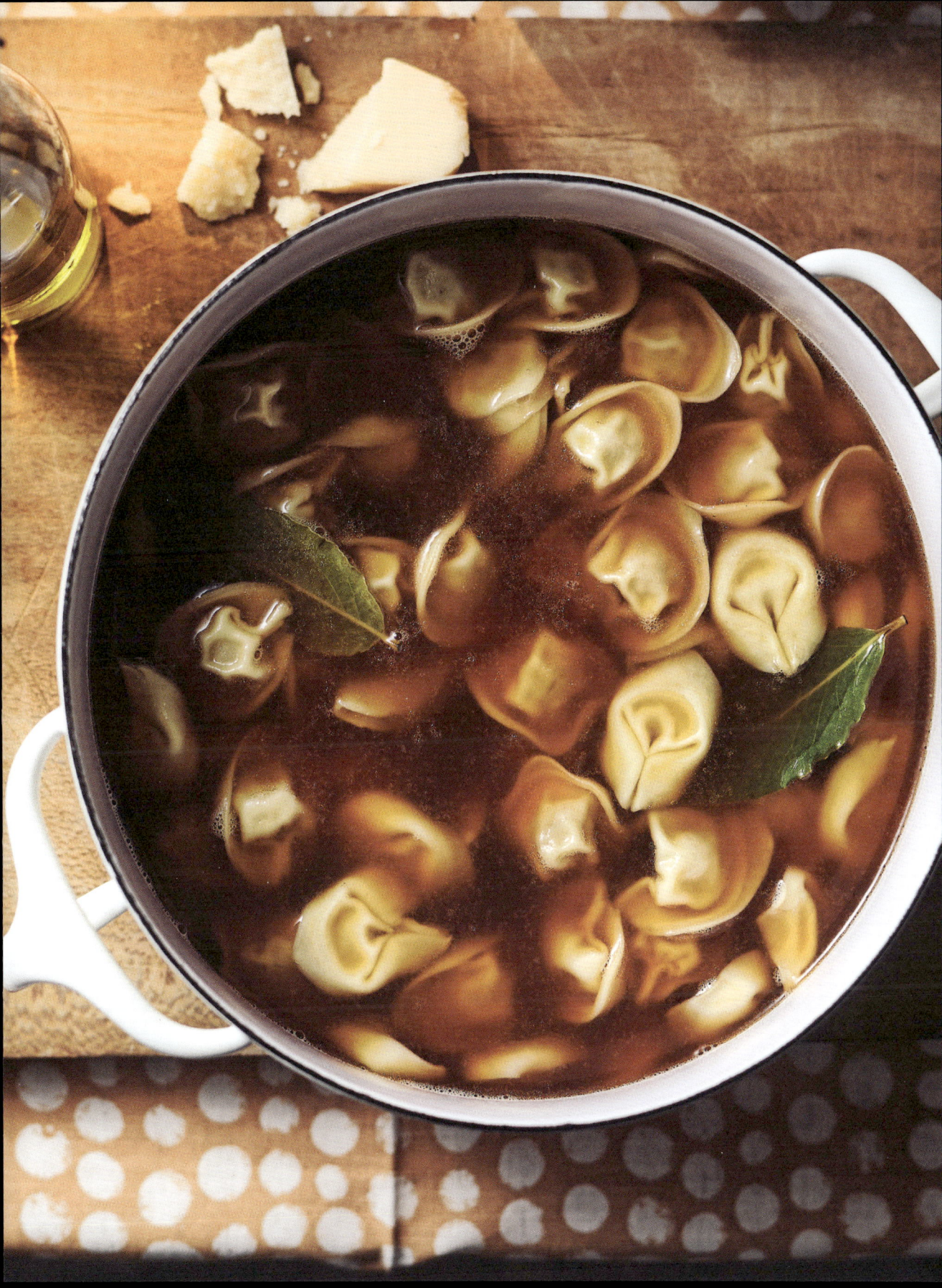

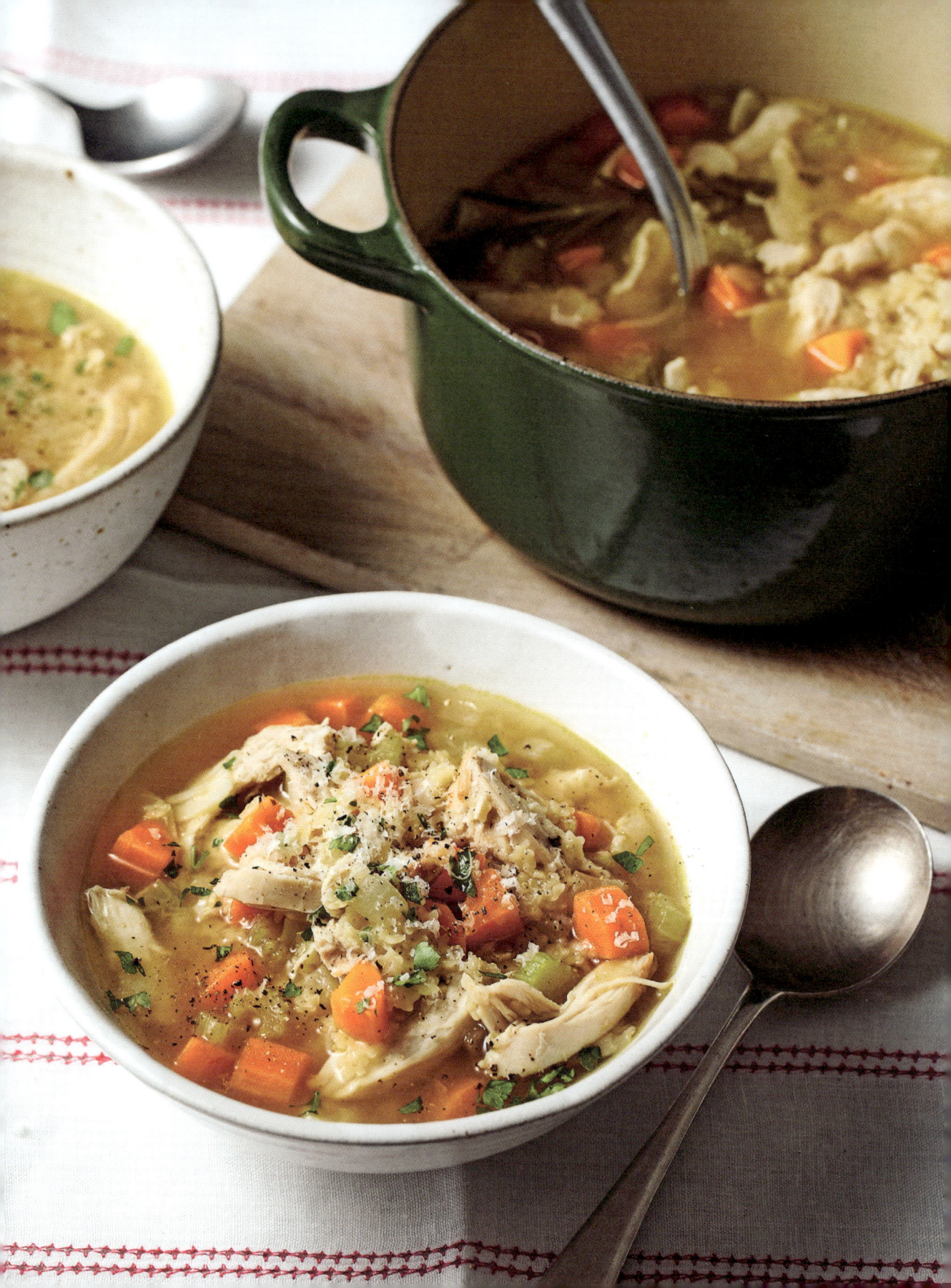

ITALIAN PENICILLIN SOUP

This is our go-to soup when someone's feeling under the weather. It's a simple chicken soup, but with boosted flavour thanks to rich bone broth. You can add orzo or rice, but this version is served with stelline pasta – shaped like tiny stars – which makes it a great choice for little ones.

SERVES 4
PREP TIME: 10 MINUTES
COOK TIME: 30 MINUTES

1 tablespoon olive oil
1 small onion, finely chopped
2 celery sticks, diced
2 carrots, diced
4 garlic cloves, thinly sliced
1 rosemary sprig
1.2 litres (40fl oz) chicken bone broth
100g (3½oz) stelline (little star pasta)
200g (7oz) cooked shredded chicken
Juice of ½ lemon
Sea salt and freshly ground black pepper

TO SERVE
Small bunch of flat-leaf parsley, finely chopped
Grated Parmesan cheese

COOK YOUR SOFFRITTO
Heat the olive oil in a large saucepan over medium-low heat. Add the onion, celery and carrot with a pinch of salt and cook for 15–20 minutes until soft but not coloured. The longer you cook the soffritto, the better the flavour of the soup.

ADD YOUR GARLIC AND HERBS
Add the garlic and rosemary and cook for another 1–2 minutes until fragrant.

ADD THE BONE BROTH
Pour in the chicken bone broth and bring to a gentle simmer.

COOK THE STELLINE
Add the stelline and cook for 6–8 minutes until tender.

FINISH THE SOUP
Stir in the shredded chicken and lemon juice, season well with salt and pepper and cook for a further 2–3 minutes to warm through. Remove the rosemary sprig.

TO SERVE
Stir through the parsley and ladle into bowls. Cover liberally with grated Parmesan.

BAKED RIGATONI WITH AUBERGINE

Combine the cosiness of a weeknight pasta bake with the indulgence of a classic Aubergine Parmigiana and you'll create this hearty winner. Using beef bone broth gives the finished dish a slow-cooked flavour, with creamy mozzarella, tomato and savoury aubergine in every bite.

SERVES 4
PREP TIME: 25 MINUTES (INCLUDING AUBERGINE DRAINING)
COOK TIME: 1 HOUR, PLUS RESTING TIME

2 aubergines (about 600–700g), cut into 1–2cm cubes
3 tablespoons olive oil
300g (10½oz) rigatoni or penne rigate
Fine sea salt

FOR THE TOMATO AND BROTH SAUCE
2 tablespoons olive oil
2 garlic cloves, finely sliced
½ teaspoon chilli flakes (optional)
1 tablespoon tomato purée
2 x 400g (14oz) tins chopped tomatoes
250ml (9fl oz) beef bone broth
1 teaspoon sugar
1 teaspoon dried oregano
Small bunch of basil, leaves torn
Sea salt and freshly ground black pepper

FOR THE CHEESE
2 x 125g (4½oz) mozzarella balls, torn into chunks
50g (1¾oz) Parmesan or pecorino, grated, plus extra for topping

TO SERVE
Olive oil or chilli oil
Fresh basil leaves

PREP THE AUBERGINES
Place the cubed aubergines in a colander, toss with a good pinch of salt and leave to drain for 30 minutes. This draws out excess moisture and helps them roast more evenly. Pat them dry with a clean tea towel.

ROAST THE AUBERGINES
Preheat the oven to 220°C (200°C fan)/425°F/gas 7. Spread the aubergines out on a baking tray, toss with olive oil and roast for 25–30 minutes, turning once, until golden and soft.

COOK THE PASTA
Bring a large pan of salted water to the boil. Cook the rigatoni for 2 minutes less than the packet says. Drain and set aside.

MAKE THE SAUCE
In a wide pan, heat 2 tablespoons of olive oil over low heat. Add the garlic and chilli flakes, letting them gently infuse the oil for 2–3 minutes without browning. Stir in the tomato purée and cook for 1–2 minutes. Add the chopped tomatoes, bone broth, sugar and oregano. Season with salt and pepper. Simmer uncovered for 15–20 minutes, stirring occasionally, until slightly thickened. Stir in the aubergines and torn basil.

ASSEMBLE THE BAKE
Preheat the oven to 200°C (180°C fan)/400°F/gas 6. In a large bowl, mix the drained pasta with the sauce, half the mozzarella and half the Parmesan. If it's looking a little dry, add a splash more bone broth. Spoon half the mixture into a baking dish, tuck in a few extra chunks of mozzarella, then add the rest of the pasta. Top with the remaining mozzarella and a layer of Parmesan.

BAKE AND REST
Bake for 25–30 minutes until bubbling and golden on top. Let sit for 5–10 minutes before serving to allow the cheese and sauce to settle.

TO SERVE
Drizzle with a little olive oil or chilli oil and scatter with a few basil leaves for an extra pop of colour.

ONE-POT PUTTANESCA

This take on Spaghetti Puttanesca is bold and savoury. Instead of boiling the pasta in water, we cook the pasta directly in a beef bone broth sauce, which reduces down and catches on the pan, creating golden, crisp edges. The result? A rich, umami and deeply satisfying all-in-one-pot dish – anchored by the depth of proper bone broth.

SERVES 4
PREP TIME: 10 MINUTES
COOK TIME: 25 MINUTES

- 3 tablespoons olive oil
- 6 anchovy fillets in oil, plus 1 teaspoon of the anchovy oil from the tin
- 3 garlic cloves, finely sliced
- ½ teaspoon chilli flakes (optional)
- 1 teaspoon tomato purée
- 100g (3½oz) pitted black olives, crushed or roughly chopped
- 2 tablespoons capers, drained
- 50ml (1¾fl oz) dry white wine or vermouth
- 1 x 400g (14oz) tin chopped tomatoes
- 500ml (17fl oz) beef bone broth
- 320g (11¼oz) dried spaghetti (ideally bronze-cut)
- Sea salt and freshly ground black pepper

TO SERVE
- Extra virgin olive oil
- Parsley
- Lemon zest

START THE BASE
Heat the olive oil and anchovy oil in a wide frying pan or shallow casserole dish over medium heat. Add the garlic, anchovy fillets and chilli flakes. Cook for 2 minutes until the anchovies dissolve and the garlic is soft but not browned.

BUILD FLAVOUR
Add the tomato purée and cook for about 30 seconds until darkened slightly. Add the olives and capers, cook for 1 minute more, then pour in the white wine. Let it bubble for 1–2 minutes until mostly evaporated.

ADD THE TOMATOES AND BONE BROTH
Stir in the chopped tomatoes and bring to a simmer. Pour in the beef bone broth and stir to combine.

COOK THE PASTA
Add the spaghetti, fanning it out evenly. Press it gently into the sauce as it softens, using tongs to bend and nest it into the pan. Keep the sauce at a lively simmer, uncovered.

SIMMER AND REDUCE
Cook for 12–15 minutes, stirring occasionally to prevent sticking. The pasta should be nearly cooked and most of the liquid reduced to a thick sauce. Taste and adjust the seasoning.

LET IT BROWN
Reduce the heat slightly and let the bottom of the pan begin to catch and brown in places. Don't stir too often – you want some crispness to develop on the base. Once you see slight browning and the pasta is tender, remove from the heat and let it rest for 2 minutes.

TO SERVE
Drizzle with high-quality olive oil and scatter over fresh parsley and a little lemon zest. Serve in shallow bowls, making sure to include the crisped bits from the bottom of the pan.

LINGUINE ALLE VONGOLE
(PASTA WITH CLAMS)

This dish is all about balance – the brininess of the clams, the heat of garlic and chilli and the richness of the sauce that clings to every strand of pasta. Using bone broth is a creative way to elevate an already delicious dish, adding extra depth and flavour. It comes together fast, so have everything prepped before you start.

SERVES 4
PREP TIME: 15 MINUTES
COOK TIME: 15 MINUTES

300g (10½oz) dried linguine
2 tablespoons olive oil
2 garlic cloves, finely sliced
1 small dried red chilli or a pinch of chilli flakes
150ml (5fl oz) dry white wine
100ml (3½fl oz) fish bone broth
1kg (2lb 4oz) fresh clams, scrubbed
Small bunch of parsley, finely chopped
Zest of 1 lemon
Sea salt and freshly ground black pepper

COOK THE PASTA
Bring a large pot of salted water to the boil and cook the linguine until just shy of al dente, around 1–2 minutes less than the packet says. Reserve a mug of pasta water before draining.

COOK THE GARLIC AND CHILLI
While the pasta cooks, heat the olive oil in a wide-based frying pan over medium heat. Add the garlic and chilli and cook gently for 1–2 minutes until fragrant but not browned.

REDUCE THE WINE AND BONE BROTH
Turn up the heat slightly and pour in the white wine and bone broth. Let it bubble for 2–3 minutes to cook off the alcohol and reduce slightly.

COOK THE CLAMS
Add the clams, cover with a lid and cook for 4–5 minutes, shaking the pan once or twice, until all the clams have opened. Discard any that stay shut.

MIX THE PASTA THROUGH
Add the drained pasta straight into the pan along with a splash of the reserved pasta water. Toss everything together for 1–2 minutes so the linguine finishes cooking and absorbs the sauce.

SEASON
Stir in most of the parsley and lemon zest. Season with black pepper and a little salt if needed (although the clams may be salty enough on their own).

TO SERVE
This dish waits for no one – get it from pan to plate fast while the clams are juicy and the pasta silky, then sprinkle over the remaining parsley and lemon zest.

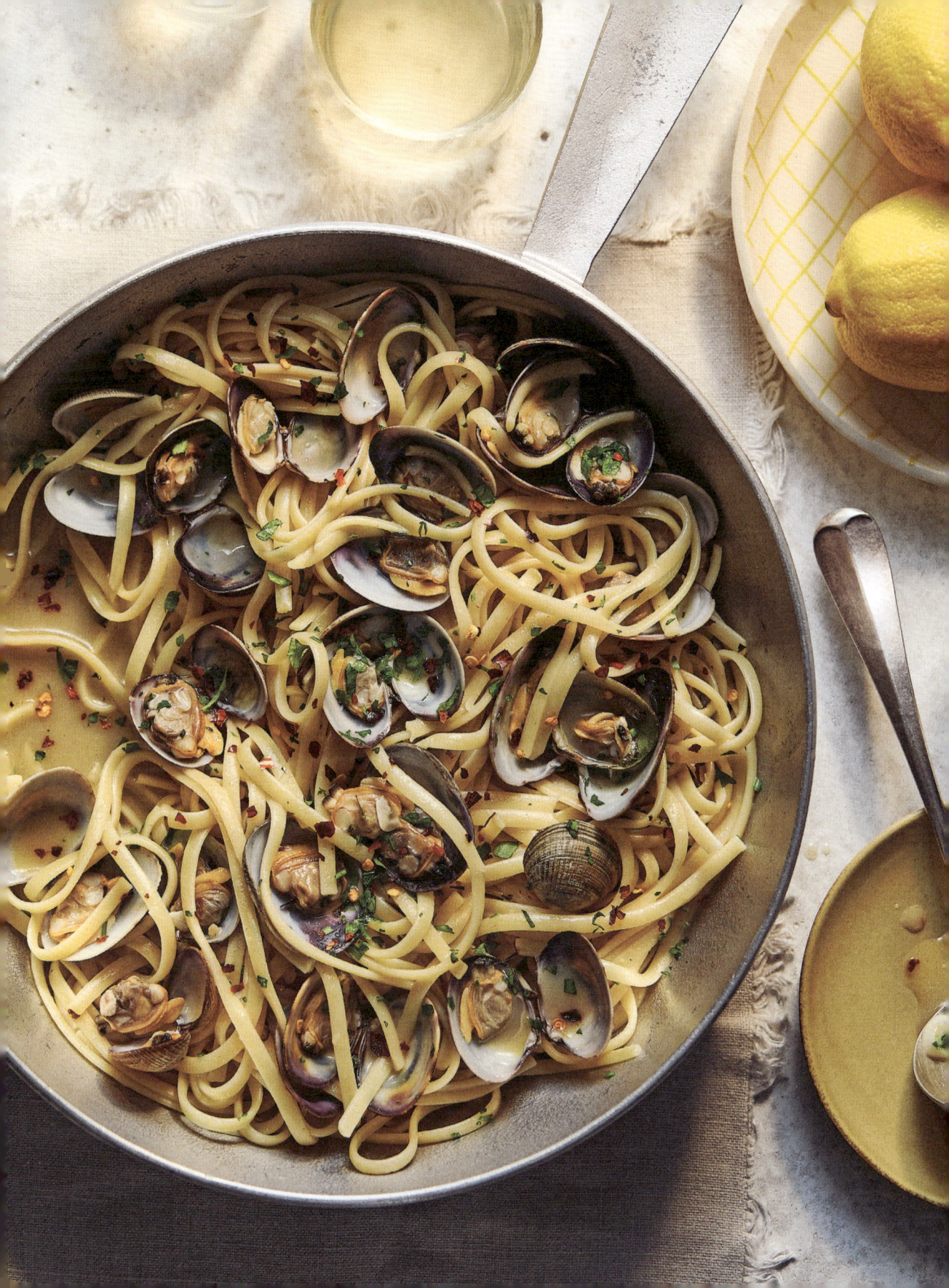

YOUVETSI
(GREEK ORZO WITH LAMB)

A traditional Greek dish where slow-cooked lamb melts into a tomato-rich broth, finished in the oven with orzo that soaks up all the flavour. We use lamb shoulder for its tenderness and bone broth to add richness. This is a one-pot meal that delivers huge amounts of flavour, despite very little hands-on cooking time.

SERVES 4
PREP TIME: 20 MINUTES
COOK TIME: 2 HOURS 30 MINUTES

2 tablespoons olive oil
700g (1lb 9oz) lamb shoulder, cut into large chunks
1 onion, finely chopped
3 garlic cloves, finely sliced
1 tablespoon tomato purée
1 x 400g (14oz) tin chopped tomatoes
500ml (17fl oz) beef bone broth
1 cinnamon stick
2 bay leaves
200g (7oz) orzo
Sea salt and freshly ground black pepper

TO SERVE
Grated kefalotyri (or Parmesan cheese)
Handful of chopped parsley

BROWN THE LAMB
Preheat the oven to 180°C (160°C fan)/350°F/gas 4. Heat the olive oil in a large casserole dish over a medium-high heat. Season the lamb with salt and pepper, then brown in batches until well coloured all over. Remove the lamb from the pan and set aside.

COOK THE ONIONS
Turn the heat down slightly and add the onion and garlic. Cook for 5–7 minutes until soft and fragrant. Stir in the tomato purée and cook for another 1–2 minutes.

BRAISE THE LAMB
Return the lamb to the pan along with the chopped tomatoes, bone broth, 250ml (9fl oz) water, cinnamon stick and bay leaves. Bring to a simmer, then cover with a lid (or tin foil) and put in the oven for 1 hour 30 minutes.

ADD THE ORZO
After 1½ hours, check the lamb – it should be tender. Stir in the orzo and a splash more water if it's looking dry. Cover and return to the oven.

BAKE THE ORZO
Bake for 30–35 minutes, uncovering for the last 10 minutes so the top can brown slightly. Stir once or twice to prevent the orzo sticking to the bottom. The orzo should be cooked through and the sauce thick and rich.

SEASON AND REST
Remove the bay leaves and cinnamon stick. Taste and adjust the seasoning. Let it sit for 5 minutes before serving.

TO SERVE
Spoon into bowls and sprinkle with the grated cheese and chopped parsley. Delicious with a bowl of olives and a glass of wine on the side.

TAGLIOLINI AL TARTUFO
(PASTA WITH WHITE TRUFFLE)

This classic Italian dish is all about simple ingredients brought together to make them sing. Traditionally, the sauce is loosened with a splash of rich broth rather than just pasta water, which adds a subtle savoury depth. Using bone broth here brings out the rich, earthy flavour of the truffle while keeping the sauce light and glossy.

SERVES 4
PREP TIME: 5 MINUTES
COOK TIME: 10 MINUTES

300g (10½oz) fresh tagliolini (or tagliatelle)
40g (1½oz) unsalted butter
2 teaspoons truffle paste
20g (¾oz) pecorino cheese, grated
75ml (2½fl oz) chicken bone broth
Sea salt

TO SERVE
Fresh truffle, to shave over (optional but excellent), or use a good-quality truffle oil
Extra grated pecorino cheese

BOIL THE PASTA
Bring a large pot of salted water to the boil and cook the pasta until just al dente, usually 2–3 minutes for fresh tagliolini.

MAKE THE TRUFFLE BUTTER
While the pasta cooks, melt the butter gently in a wide pan over low heat. Stir in the truffle paste and keep warm – you don't want it to bubble or fry, just melt.

ADD THE PASTA
Add the drained pasta to the truffle butter along with the grated cheese and the chicken bone broth. Toss or stir continuously over a low heat for 1–2 minutes until the sauce emulsifies and clings to the pasta.

ADJUST THE CONSISTENCY AND SEASONING
Add a splash more bone broth if you need to adjust the consistency. Taste and adjust the seasoning as necessary.

TO SERVE
Divide between warm bowls and either shave fresh truffle over the top or drizzle over a good-quality truffle oil. Grate over a little bit more pecorino to finish.

INSTANT RAMEN UPGRADE

Instant Ramen may usually be reserved as a guilty pleasure, but with a few simple tweaks it can be transformed into a much heartier, more wholesome meal. Using bone broth instead of plain water gives the soup real depth of flavour and added nutrition too, while fresh toppings add texture and flavour.

SERVES 1
PREP TIME: 5 MINUTES
COOK TIME: 10 MINUTES

1 egg
400ml (14fl oz) chicken bone broth
1 garlic clove, finely sliced
1 packet of instant ramen noodles
1 teaspoon dark soy sauce
1 teaspoon sesame oil
½ ramen seasoning sachet
60g (2¼oz) baby spinach leaves

TO SERVE
50g (1¾oz) shredded cooked chicken (optional)
1 spring onion, sliced
1 small carrot, julienned or thinly sliced
Sriracha, to taste

SOFT BOIL THE EGG
Bring a small saucepan of water to a gentle boil. Carefully lower in a room temperature egg and cook for 6½ minutes. Immediately transfer to a bowl of cold water to stop the cooking. Once cool, peel and set aside.

INFUSE THE BONE BROTH
Bring the bone broth to a gentle boil in a saucepan. Add the garlic and simmer for 2 minutes to infuse.

COOK THE NOODLES
Add the instant Ramen noodles and cook according to the packet instructions, usually 2–3 minutes, until just tender.

SEASON
Stir in the soy sauce, sesame oil and half of the seasoning sachet (don't add it all or it will be too salty). Add the baby spinach and cook for the last minute until wilted.

TO SERVE
Pour the soup and noodles into a bowl. Top with the soft-boiled egg, shredded chicken (if using), spring onion and the raw carrot. Drizzle with Sriracha for some extra heat.

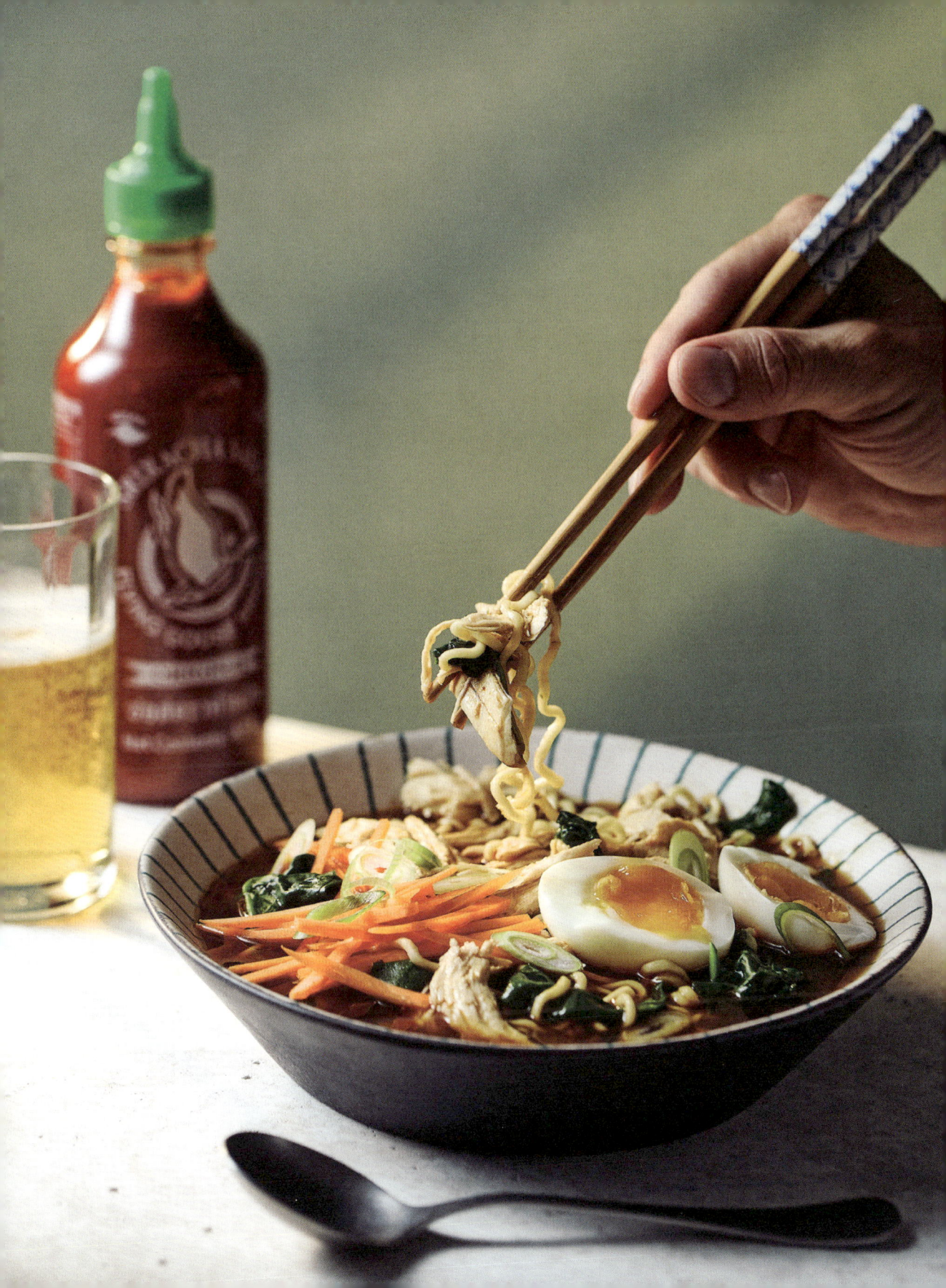

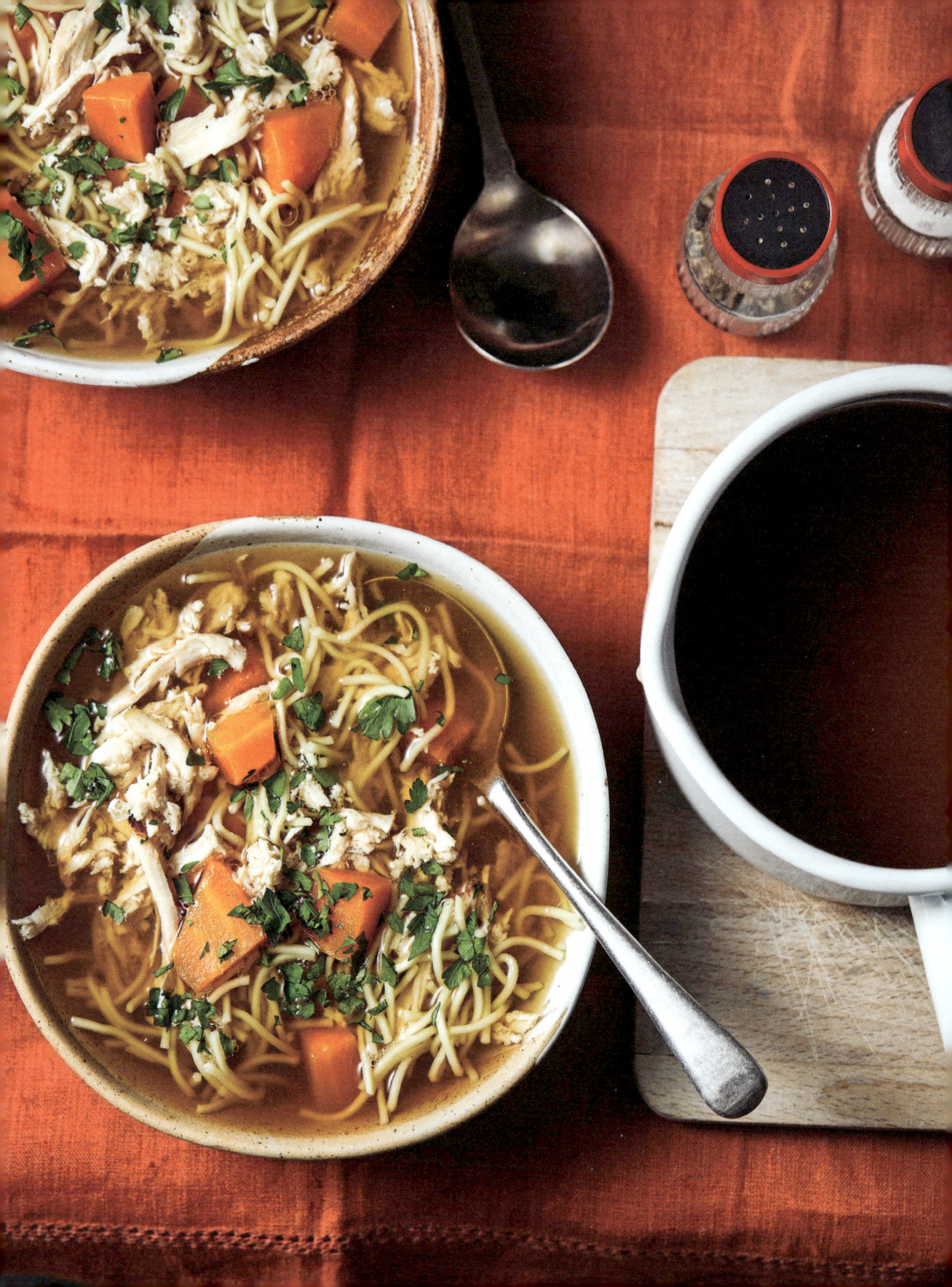

ROSÓŁ
(CLASSIC POLISH NOODLE SOUP)

Rosół is a traditional Polish chicken noodle soup cherished for its clear, fragrant broth and tender chicken. Using ready-made chicken bone broth as the base makes this recipe quicker, but just as comforting, and topping with shredded cooked chicken adds the heartiness you want, without the long simmer.

SERVES 4
PREP TIME: 15 MINUTES
COOK TIME: 45 MINUTES

1.5 litres (52fl oz) chicken bone broth
2 large carrots, peeled and roughly chopped
1 large parsnip, peeled and roughly chopped
1 onion, peeled and halved
2 celery sticks, halved
1 small leek, cleaned and halved
4 garlic cloves, peeled and crushed
Handful of whole black peppercorns
2 bay leaves
150g (5½oz) egg noodles or kluski noodles
250g (9oz) shredded cooked chicken
Sea salt

TO SERVE
Chopped parsley

SIMMER THE VEG
In a large pot, combine the chicken bone broth, carrots, parsnip, onion, celery, leek, garlic, peppercorns and bay leaves. Bring to a gentle boil, then reduce the heat and simmer uncovered for 35 minutes until the vegetables are tender and the broth is fragrant.

STRAIN THE VEG
Remove the vegetables, bay leaves and peppercorns with a slotted spoon or strain the broth through a fine-mesh sieve for a clearer soup.

ADJUST THE SEASONING
Taste the broth and season with salt as needed.

COOK THE NOODLES
In a separate pot, bring some water to the boil and add the egg noodles. Cook according to the packet instructions until just tender.

WARM THE SHREDDED CHICKEN
Stir the shredded chicken into the broth to warm through for 2–3 minutes.

TO SERVE
Add some warmed shredded chicken and a few cooked carrots from the sieve into each bowl. Add the cooked noodles and spoon over the broth. Sprinkle over the parsley and tuck in.

SOTO AYAM
(INDONESIAN CHICKEN NOODLE SOUP)

This dish is a fragrant, spiced chicken soup from Indonesia that is brightened with fresh herbs and lime. It's often served with rice or noodles and topped with crunchy shallots, boiled eggs and fresh lime wedges. Perfect for a warming lunch or light dinner; this is spoon food at its finest.

SERVES 4
PREP TIME: 15 MINUTES
COOK TIME: 45 MINUTES

1 tablespoon vegetable oil
1 onion, chopped
3 garlic cloves, crushed
2cm (¾ inch) piece of fresh ginger, peeled and sliced
1 teaspoon ground turmeric
1 teaspoon ground coriander
1 cinnamon stick
2 star anise
1 litre (35fl oz) chicken bone broth
300g (10½oz) cooked shredded chicken
100g (3½oz) glass noodles or vermicelli, soaked if dried
Sea salt and freshly ground black pepper

TO SERVE
2 eggs
2 spring onions, sliced
Chopped coriander
Fried shallots
Lime wedges

BOIL YOUR EGGS
Place the eggs in a small saucepan and cover with cold water. Bring to a gentle boil, then reduce the heat and simmer for 9–10 minutes. Transfer to a bowl of cold water to cool, then peel, halve and set aside.

MAKE THE SOUP BASE
Heat the oil in a large pot over medium heat. Add the onion, garlic, ginger, turmeric and coriander. Cook for 5–7 minutes until softened and fragrant.

ADD THE AROMATICS
Add the cinnamon stick, star anise and bone broth. Bring to a simmer and cook gently for 20 minutes to let the flavours infuse and develop.

COOK THE NOODLES
Remove the cinnamon and star anise. Add the shredded chicken and glass noodles to the pot. Simmer for 3–4 minutes until the noodles are soft and the chicken is heated through. Season the soup with salt and pepper to taste.

TO SERVE
Ladle the soup into bowls and top with the halved eggs, spring onions, fresh coriander and fried shallots. Serve with lime wedges on the side to squeeze over.

MALAYSIAN MONKFISH LAKSA

This is a rich, spicy noodle soup with bold, punchy flavours – creamy from coconut milk and deeply savoury from fish bone broth. Traditionally made with prawns or chicken, this version uses monkfish for its meaty texture, which holds up well in the broth.

SERVES 4
PREP TIME: 25 MINUTES
COOK TIME: 40 MINUTES

1 tablespoon neutral oil (groundnut or vegetable)
1 onion, chopped
2 garlic cloves, crushed
1 thumb-sized piece of fresh ginger, grated
2 red chillies, chopped (deseed for less heat)
1 lemongrass stalk, bashed
1 teaspoon ground turmeric
1 tablespoon laksa paste or Thai red curry paste
500ml (17fl oz) fish bone broth
1 x 400ml (14oz) tin coconut milk
150g (5½oz) fine egg noodles
200g (7oz) monkfish fillet, cut into large chunks
1 tablespoon fish sauce
Juice of ½ lime

TO SERVE
100g (3½oz) beansprouts
Mint
Coriander
Fried shallots
Sliced red chilli (optional)
Lime wedges

COOK THE AROMATIC BASE
Heat the oil in a saucepan over medium heat. Add the onion, garlic, ginger, chillies and lemongrass. Cook for 6–8 minutes until softened and fragrant.

COOK OFF THE SPICES AND PASTE
Stir in the turmeric and laksa paste. Cook for 2–3 minutes until aromatic and slightly darkened.

ADD THE BONE BROTH AND COCONUT MILK
Pour in the bone broth and coconut milk. Bring to a simmer and let it gently bubble for 20 minutes.

COOK THE NOODLES
While the broth simmers, cook the fine egg noodles according to the packet instructions. Drain and rinse with cold water to stop them from sticking, and set aside.

POACH YOUR MONKFISH
Carefully lower the monkfish pieces into the broth. Simmer gently for 6–8 minutes until just cooked through – the fish should be opaque and firm.

SEASON
Add the fish sauce and lime juice to balance the broth. Taste and adjust the seasoning.

TO SERVE
Divide the cooked noodles among the bowls. Ladle the hot laksa broth and monkfish over the top. Top each bowl with beansprouts, fresh herbs, fried shallots and extra chilli, if you like. Serve with lime wedges on the side for an extra squeeze of freshness.

SICHUAN SPICY BEEF NOODLES

This fiery bowl of noodles has a little bit of everything: tender chunks of braised beef, slippery noodles and a dollop of crunchy, spicy chilli oil. Using beef bone broth as the base adds depth and richness, while a slow cook makes sure the meat melts apart beautifully.

SERVES 4
PREP TIME: 30 MINUTES
COOK TIME: 2 HOURS 30 MINUTES

1 tablespoon vegetable oil
500g (1lb 2oz) stewing beef (shin or chuck), cut into 4–5cm (1½–2 inch) chunks
1 onion, quartered
4 garlic cloves, crushed
1 thumb-sized piece of fresh ginger, sliced
2 star anise
1 cinnamon stick
1 tablespoon Sichuan peppercorns
1 tablespoon light soy sauce
1 tablespoon dark soy sauce
1 tablespoon Shaoxing wine or dry sherry
1 litre (35fl oz) beef bone broth
200g (7oz) thick flat noodles (look for ho fun or biang biang on the packet)
1 pak choi, halved
Sea salt and freshly ground black pepper

FOR THE CRISPY CHILLI OIL
100ml (3½fl oz) vegetable oil
2 garlic cloves, finely sliced
1 small shallot, finely sliced
3 tablespoons chilli flakes
1 teaspoon Sichuan peppercorns
Pinch of salt

TO SERVE
Sliced spring onions
Coriander
Red chilli
Lime wedges (optional)

BROWN THE BEEF
Heat the oil in a large, heavy-based pan. Sear the beef in batches for 3–4 minutes until browned on all sides. Remove and set aside.

FRY OFF THE BASE INGREDIENTS
To the same pan, add the onion, garlic, ginger, star anise, cinnamon stick and Sichuan peppercorns. Fry for 5 minutes until fragrant.

BRAISE THE BEEF
Return the beef to the pan and add both the soy sauces and the Shaoxing wine. Stir to coat, then pour in the beef bone broth. Bring to the boil, then reduce the heat, cover and simmer gently for 2 hours, or until the beef is fork-tender.

MAKE THE CHILLI OIL
Heat the oil in a small pan over low heat. Add the garlic and shallot and cook gently for 6–8 minutes until golden and crisp. Remove from the heat and stir in the chilli flakes, Sichuan peppercorns and a pinch of salt. Leave to infuse and cool.

COOK THE NOODLES AND PAK CHOI
Once the beef is done, cook the noodles according to the packet instructions. In the final 2–3 minutes, add the pak choi to the pot to wilt slightly, then drain both.

PREPARE THE BROTH
Remove the aromatics from the broth (star anise, cinnamon, ginger) and season to taste with salt and pepper. Pull the beef slightly with two forks.

TO SERVE
Divide the noodles and pak choi among the bowls. Ladle over the hot broth and generous chunks of beef. Spoon over the crispy chilli oil and finish with spring onions, coriander and fresh chilli with lime wedges on the side, if you want.

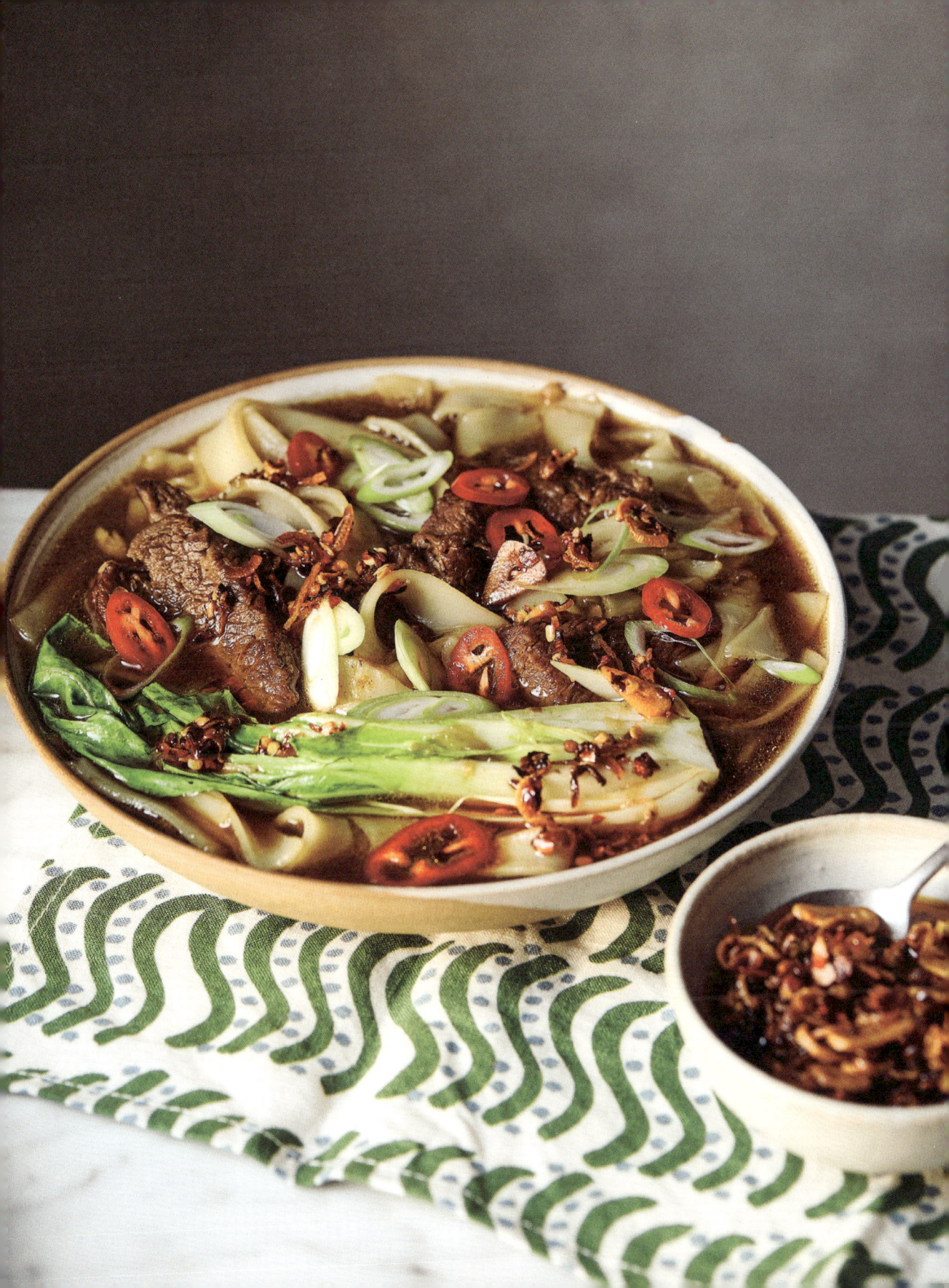

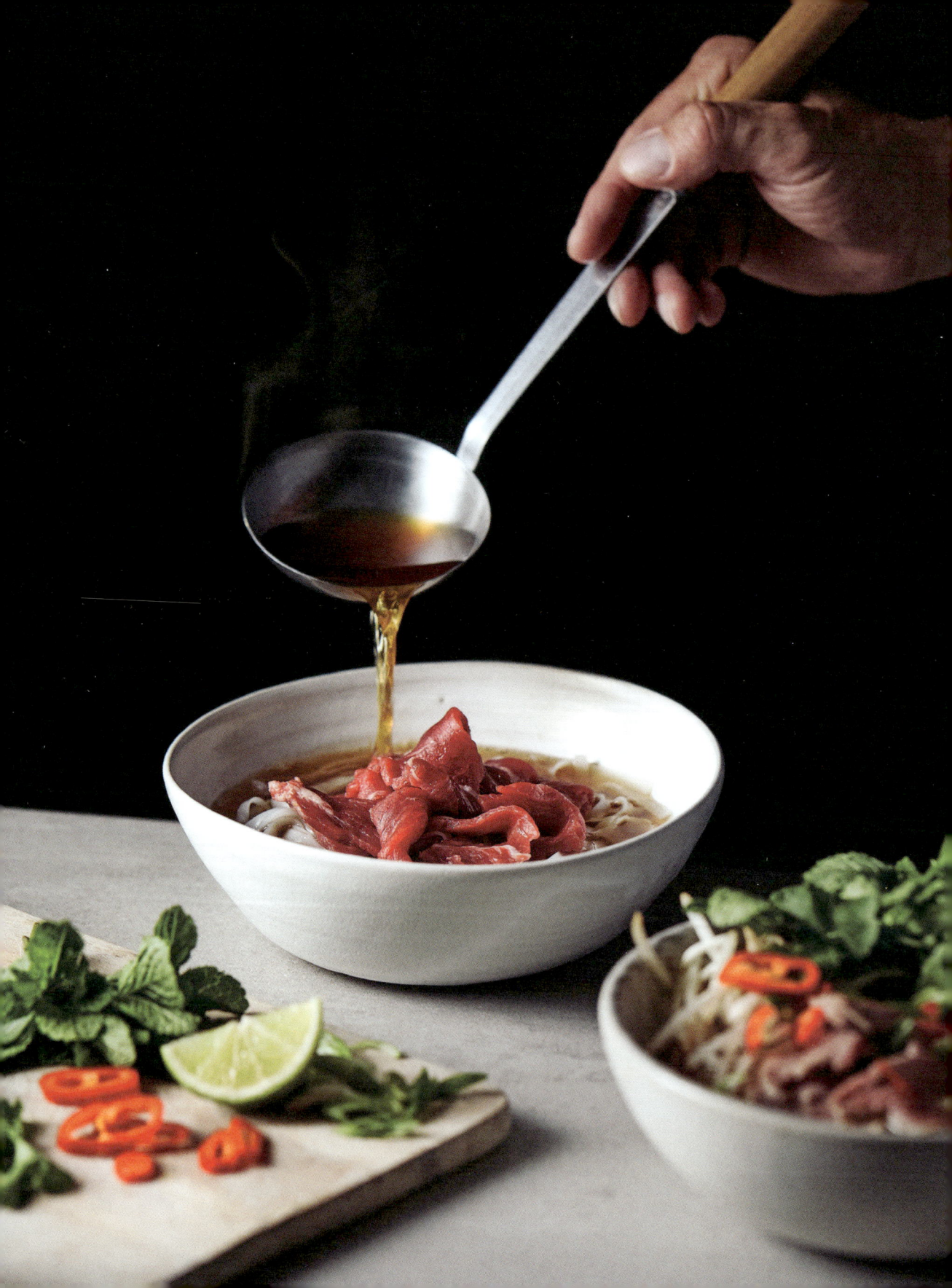

VIETNAMESE BEEF PHO

Pho is Vietnam's most iconic noodle soup. Traditionally simmered for hours, this version uses ready-made beef bone broth as a shortcut without compromising on depth. The broth is perfumed with spices, the noodles are silky and the raw beef is flash-poached in the bowl from the heat of the broth.

SERVES 4
PREP TIME: 20 MINUTES
COOK TIME: 45 MINUTES

- 1 onion, halved
- 1 thumb-sized piece of fresh ginger, halved
- 1.5 litres (52fl oz) beef bone broth
- 2 star anise
- 1 cinnamon stick
- 3 cloves
- 300g (10½oz) flat rice noodles
- 1 tablespoon fish sauce, plus more to taste
- 1 teaspoon sugar
- 300g (10½oz) sirloin or rump steak, very thinly sliced (freeze the beef first to make it easier)

TO SERVE

- 2 spring onions, thinly sliced
- 1 small red chilli, sliced
- Handful of beansprouts
- Lime wedges
- Generous handful of mixed herbs (Thai basil, coriander and mint work well)
- Hoisin sauce (optional)
- Sriracha (optional)

CHAR YOUR VEG
Place the onion and ginger halves directly over a gas flame or under a hot grill. Char for 5–7 minutes until blackened and fragrant.

SIMMER
In a large saucepan, bring the beef bone broth to a simmer. Add the charred onion and ginger, star anise, cinnamon stick and cloves. Simmer gently for 30–40 minutes, uncovered, to infuse the flavours.

COOK YOUR NOODLES
Meanwhile, cook the rice noodles according to the packet instructions. Drain, rinse under cold water and set aside.

FINISH THE BROTH
Strain the broth to remove the aromatics. Stir in the fish sauce and sugar, and taste – adjust the seasoning with more fish sauce or a pinch of salt if needed.

COOK THE BEEF
Arrange the raw beef slices over the noodles in serving bowls. Bring the broth to a fast boil and pour into the bowls – the beef will cook in the heat of the liquid.

TO SERVE
Top with spring onions, chilli and beansprouts. Serve with lime wedges and a generous handful of fresh herbs. Add hoisin or Sriracha to taste at the table, grab your chopsticks and tuck in.

COMFORT COOKING

Comfort cooking is where flavour meets familiarity, where slow-simmered bone broth brings a depth to dishes you know and love, plus some new favourites yet to be discovered. This section is full of hearty, stomach-filling, soul-warming meals, anchored by the broth's rich, comforting flavour.

These recipes aren't about fancy techniques or fuss. They're about honest, satisfying food that feels as good as it tastes and makes the house smell like home. Whether you're stirring a rich Beef Rendang or filling the perfect One-Pot Chicken & Leek Pie, each dish invites you to slow down, savour the simplicity and nourish yourself with real, honest flavour.

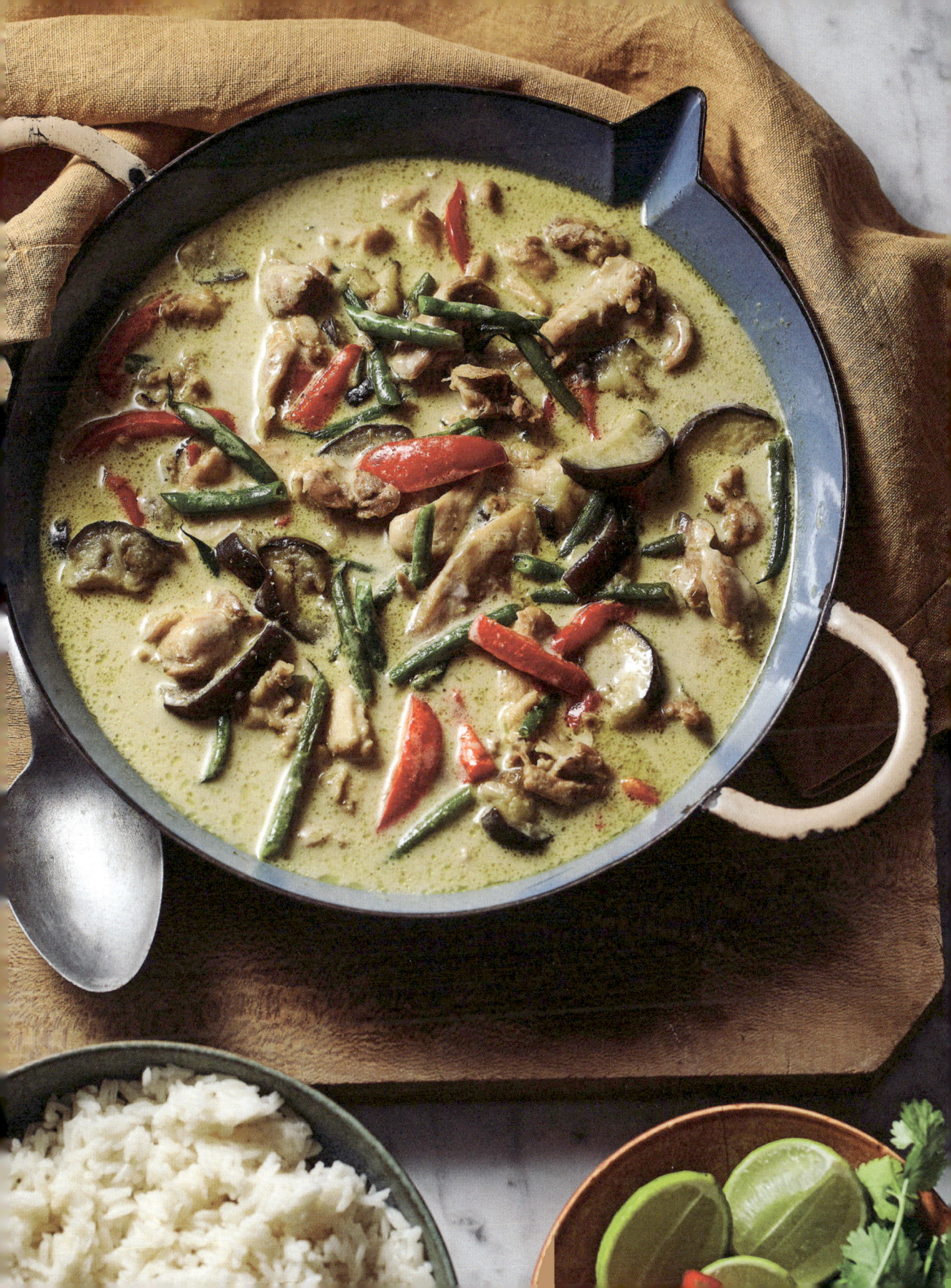

ULTIMATE CHILLI

A family favourite that has evolved over years of tweaking. Using dried chillies rather than fresh adds a complexity of flavour that delivers an unmatchable layered, smoky finish. The flavours only get better with time, so make it a day ahead if you can. We always make twice as much as we need so there's some for the freezer – just double up the quantities for extra.

SERVES 4
PREP TIME: 30 MINUTES
COOK TIME: 3 HOURS

FOR THE SPICE BASE
1 teaspoon cumin seeds
1 teaspoon coriander seeds
1 dried ancho chilli
1 dried chipotle chilli
100ml (3½fl oz) beef bone broth

FOR THE MEAT, VEGETABLES AND BEANS
1 tablespoon olive oil
75g (2½oz) cooking chorizo, diced
250g (9oz) diced stewing beef (chuck or shin), patted dry
100g (3½oz) pork mince
1 large onion, finely chopped
3 garlic cloves, minced
1 red pepper, diced
1 carrot, finely grated
1 tablespoon tomato purée
1 teaspoon dried oregano
1 teaspoon smoked paprika
400ml (14fl oz) beef bone broth
1 x 400g (14oz) tin chopped tomatoes
1 x 400g (14oz) tin black-eyed beans, drained
1 x 400g (14oz) tin kidney beans, drained
Sea salt and freshly ground black pepper

BUILD THE SPICE BASE
This optional step will add an extra layer of complexity to the dish. If it's too much of a faff, the chilli will forgive you for using ground spices and whole dried chillies instead.

Toast the cumin and coriander seeds in a dry pan over medium heat for 1–2 minutes until fragrant. Grind them using a spice grinder or pestle and mortar and set aside.

Rehydrate the dried chillies in the bone broth for 15 minutes. Then blend the chillies and their soaking liquid to a smooth paste. This forms the flavour-packed base for the dish.

BROWN THE MEATS
In a large casserole dish, heat the olive oil. Add the chorizo and cook until it begins to crisp and release its oil. Remove and set aside.

Working in batches, brown the stewing beef until well seared on all sides. Do not crowd the pan. Remove and set aside.

Add the pork mince and cook until browned and caramelised. Push to one side of the pan.

SWEAT THE VEG AND ADD THE SPICES
Add the onion, garlic, red pepper and carrot to the pan. Cook gently for 5–7 minutes until softened.

Stir in the tomato purée, toasted cumin and coriander, oregano and smoked paprika. Cook for another 2–3 minutes until darkened and fragrant.

UMAMI
15g (½oz) dark chocolate
1 tablespoon dark soy sauce

TO FINISH
Chipotle flakes or paste (for smoke) or a small amount of habanero (for heat) (optional)
Splash of red wine vinegar

TO SERVE (OPTIONAL)
Dollop of natural yoghurt
Sprinkle of coriander
Steamed rice or bread

SIMMER THE CHILLI

Return all the browned meats and chorizo to the pan. Add the blended chilli bone broth mix, the bone broth and the chopped tomatoes.

Stir in the dark chocolate and soy sauce. Season lightly with salt and pepper.

Bring to a gentle simmer, cover loosely and cook over low heat for 1 hour 30 minutes, stirring occasionally. Add a splash of water if it gets too thick.

ADD BEANS AND COOK UNCOVERED

Stir in the black-eyed and kidney beans. Simmer uncovered for another 20–30 minutes until thickened and rich.

FINAL ADJUSTMENTS

Taste and adjust the seasoning. Add the chipotle flakes or paste for more smokiness or a touch of habanero for heat, if desired. Be very sparing with these, and simmer for a few minutes to allow the flavour and spice to develop before adding more!

Finally, add a splash of red wine vinegar to lift the flavour.

TO SERVE

Delicious on its own with a dollop of natural yoghurt and a sprinkle of fresh coriander, or piled on top of steamy rice or alongside bread for scooping.

ONE-POT CHICKEN & LEEK PIE

This dish brings together the comfort of a classic chicken pie with the ease of a one-pot method. Make sure to choose a suitable pan that works on the hob, in the oven and at the table (we use a trusty old cast-iron casserole dish). The chicken is braised in marjoram and bay-infused bone broth until tender, then shredded and folded back into a thickened, creamy stew.

SERVES 4
PREP TIME: 30 MINUTES
COOK TIME: 1 HOUR 30 MINUTES

1 litre (35fl oz) chicken bone broth
Zest of ½ lemon (use the other half for the parsley and lemon oil, see below)
4 thyme sprigs
2 bay leaves
2 tablespoons olive oil
8 bone-in, skin-on chicken thighs
2 leeks (white and light green parts), halved lengthways and sliced
2 carrots, diced
2 celery sticks, diced
4 garlic cloves, minced
2 teaspoons Dijon mustard
2 tablespoons plain flour
4 tablespoons crème fraîche
4 tablespoons grated Parmesan cheese
Sea salt and freshly ground black pepper

FOR THE PASTRY TOP
1 sheet ready-rolled all-butter puff pastry
1 egg, beaten

FOR THE PARSLEY AND LEMON OIL (OPTIONAL)
Small handful of flat-leaf parsley
Zest of ½ lemon
2 tablespoons olive oil

INFUSE THE BONE BROTH
Warm the bone broth in a small saucepan with the lemon zest, thyme and bay leaves. Let it infuse gently over low heat for about 5–10 minutes while you prepare the rest of the dish. Strain before using.

SEAR THE CHICKEN
Preheat the oven to 200°C (180°C fan)/400°F/gas 6. In a wide, ovenproof sauté pan or cast-iron skillet, heat the olive oil over medium-high heat. Season the chicken thighs with salt and pepper, then sear, skin-side down, for about 5–6 minutes until golden. Turn and cook for a further 2 minutes. Remove the chicken and set aside.

BUILD THE BASE
Reduce the heat to medium. Add the leeks, carrots, celery and garlic to the same pan. Cook for 5–6 minutes until softened. Pour in the infused broth and return the chicken to the pan. Simmer uncovered for 30–35 minutes, or until the chicken is tender and the liquid has reduced slightly.

SHRED AND ENRICH
Remove the chicken to a plate. Shred the meat into chunky pieces, discarding the bones, and return the meat to the pan. Stir in the Dijon mustard, then sprinkle over the flour, stir to mix and cook for 2–3 minutes to thicken the sauce. Stir in the crème fraîche and season to taste with salt and pepper. Scatter the grated Parmesan over the surface of the filling.

(continues overleaf)

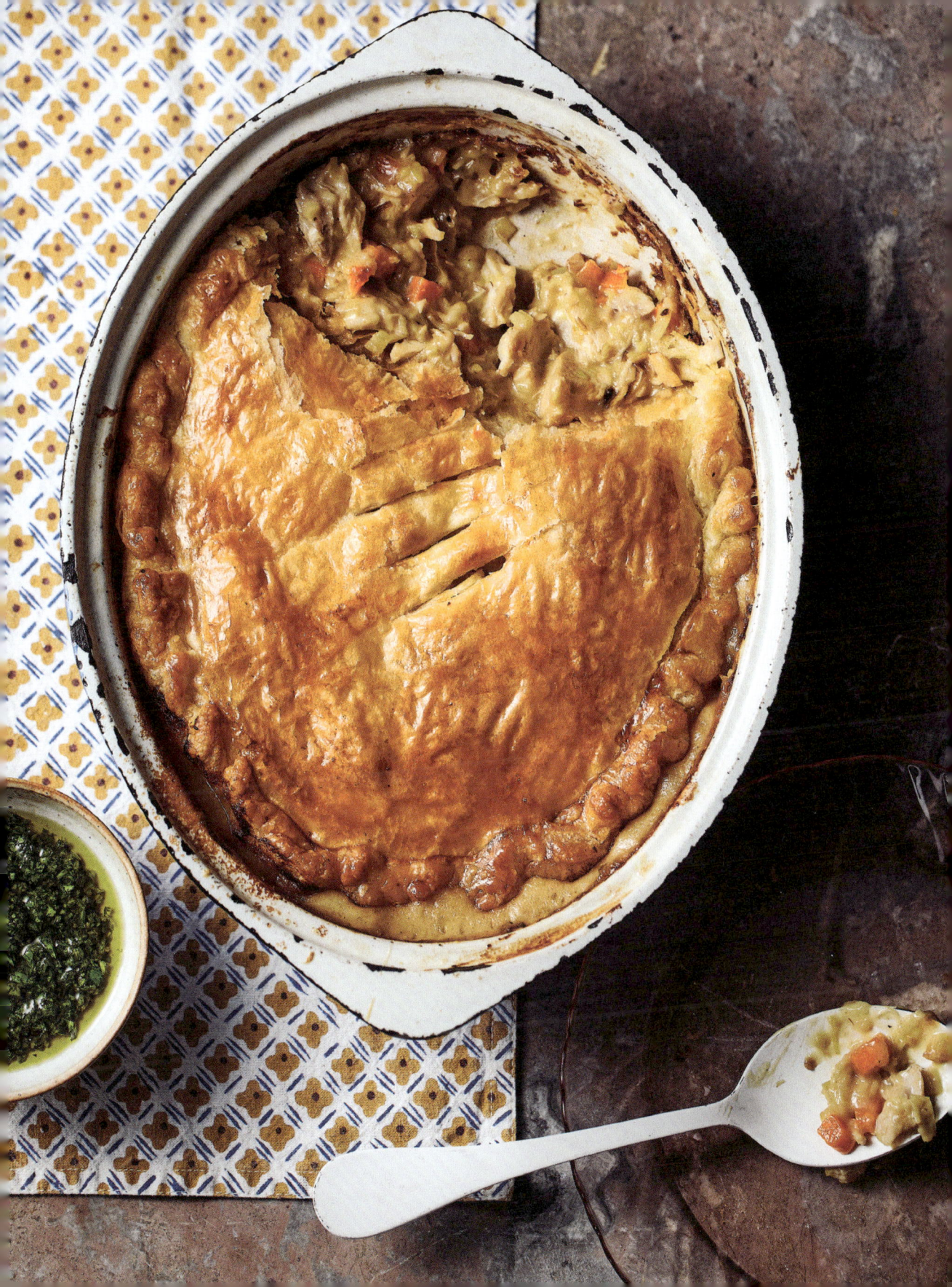

ONE-POT CHICKEN & LEEK PIE (CONTINUED)

ADD THE PASTRY
Remove the pan from the heat. Lay the puff pastry over the top, trimming the edges if needed and pressing down gently to seal. Brush the pastry with the beaten egg, then cut a small slit in the centre to allow steam to escape.

BAKE
Transfer the pan to the oven and bake for 25–30 minutes, or until the pastry is puffed, golden and crisp.

MAKE THE HERB OIL
While the pie bakes, finely chop the parsley and combine with the lemon zest and olive oil. Set aside.

TO SERVE
Let the pie rest for 5 minutes before serving. Drizzle the herb oil over the pastry just before taking it to the table.

> **VARIATION: CHICKEN & MUSHROOM PIE WITH TARRAGON**
> To give the dish a more savoury, earthy flavour, you can substitute the leek with 400–500g (14–17½oz) sliced chestnut or mixed mushrooms. Sauté the mushrooms until browned and their moisture has evaporated before continuing with the braise. Replace the thyme with 2 tablespoons finely chopped fresh tarragon or 1 teaspoon dried. Add half to the broth and stir the rest through at the end.

CLASSIC CHICKEN & APRICOT TAGINE

This sweet and savoury tagine is a Moroccan classic, subtly enhanced with the umami depth of chicken bone broth. If you're feeling adventurous, try swapping out the apricots for dried figs or dates for a deeper, more luxurious twist.

SERVES 4
PREP TIME: 20 MINUTES
COOK TIME: 1 HOUR 10 MINUTES

1 tablespoon olive oil
4 bone-in chicken thighs (skin-on or skinless)
2 onions, finely sliced
3 garlic cloves, minced
1 teaspoon ground ginger
½ teaspoon ground cinnamon
Pinch of saffron threads (or ¼ teaspoon ground turmeric)
250ml (9fl oz) chicken bone broth
12 dried apricots, halved
1 tablespoon runny honey
Squeeze of lemon juice (optional)
Sea salt and freshly ground black pepper

TO SERVE
40g (1½oz) toasted almonds (whole, slivered or chopped)
Handful of chopped coriander or flat-leaf parsley
Couscous, flatbreads or a fresh green salad

BROWN THE CHICKEN
Heat the olive oil in a heavy-based pot or tagine over medium heat. Brown the chicken thighs on both sides for about 5–7 minutes until golden. Remove and set aside.

BUILD THE BASE
Lower the heat and add the sliced onions. Cook for 10 minutes, stirring often, until soft and golden. Add the garlic, ginger, cinnamon and saffron (or turmeric) and stir for 1 minute to release their aroma.

DEGLAZE AND BRAISE
Return the chicken to the pot and pour in the chicken bone broth. Add the apricots and honey, season lightly with salt and pepper and bring to a gentle simmer. Cover and cook for 45–60 minutes until the chicken is tender and the sauce has thickened slightly. For a richer, thicker sauce, remove the lid during the final 10 minutes to allow the liquid to reduce.

FINISH AND GARNISH
Taste and adjust the seasoning, adding a squeeze of lemon juice if needed to balance the sweetness. Just before serving, scatter over the toasted almonds and fresh herbs. For a deeper flavour, toast the almonds in a dry frying pan until golden before using.

TO SERVE
Serve with couscous, flatbreads or a fresh green salad.

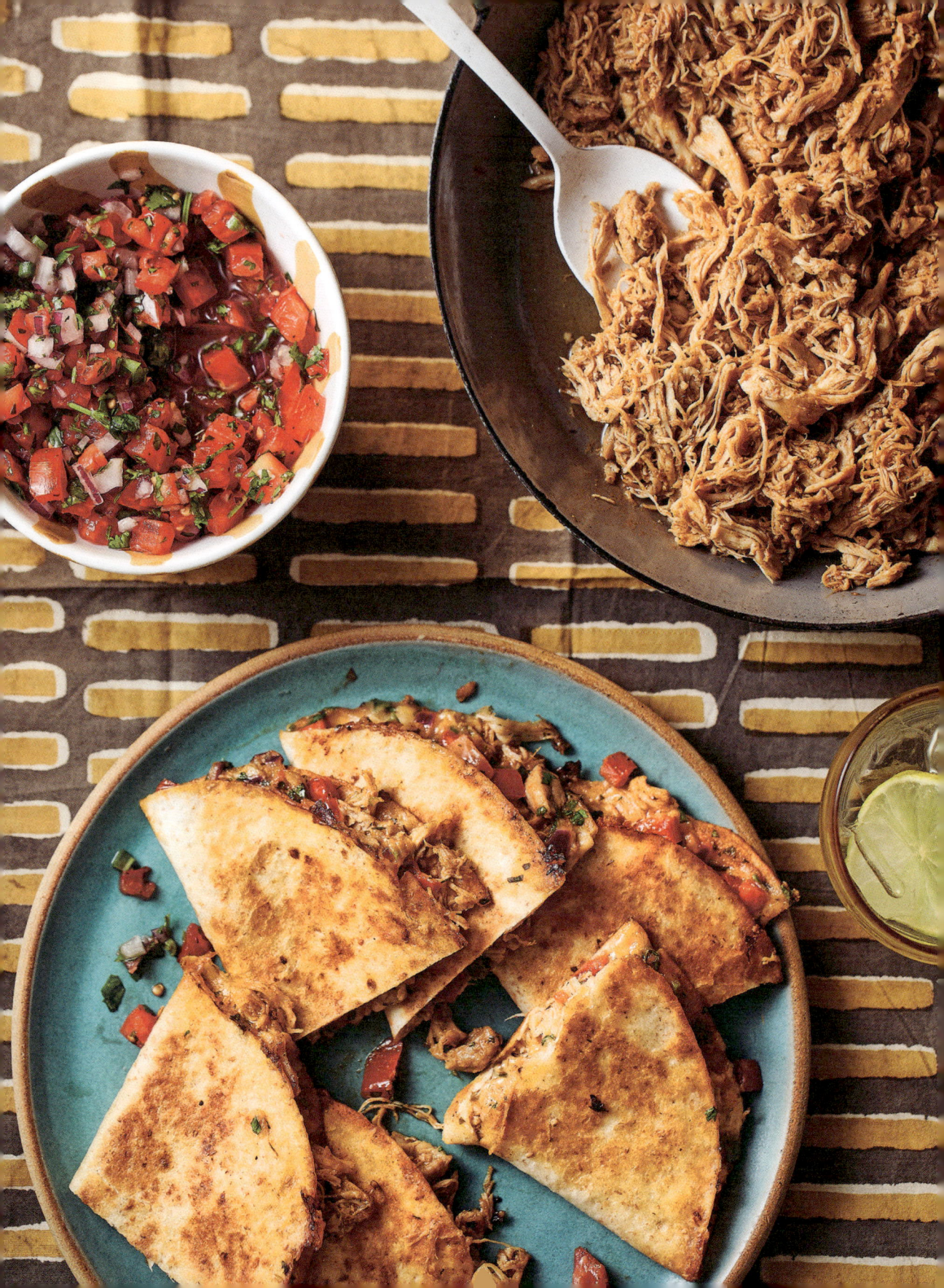

MEXICAN CHICKEN WITH FRESH TOMATO SALSA

As a family, we love batch cooking on the weekend so we can eat well all week. This dish improves with time, becoming more juicy and tasty as the week goes on. We serve it first with rice or tacos, the next day as a quesadilla or burrito, and any leftovers we whizz into a soup with more bone broth, perhaps with added black beans or sweetcorn.

SERVES 4+
PREP TIME: 15 MINUTES
COOK TIME: 55 MINUTES (HOB METHOD)

FOR THE CHICKEN
1 tablespoon olive oil
800g (1lb 12oz) boneless, skinless chicken thighs
1 onion, thinly sliced
2 garlic cloves, finely chopped
1 tablespoon chipotle paste (or 2 teaspoons chipotles in adobo)
2 teaspoons dried oregano
1 teaspoon ground cumin
1 teaspoon smoked paprika, plus more to finish
250ml (9fl oz) chicken bone broth
Juice of 1 lime
Sea salt and freshly ground black pepper

SEAR THE CHICKEN
Heat the olive oil in a deep sauté pan or pressure cooker base. Sear the chicken thighs on both sides until lightly browned. Remove and set aside.

SAUTÉ THE BASE
In the same pan, soften the sliced onion for 2–3 minutes. Add the garlic, chipotle paste, oregano, cumin and paprika. Cook for another 1 minute until aromatic.

DEGLAZE AND COMBINE
Pour in a splash of broth to loosen any brown bits. Return the chicken to the pan with the remaining broth, salt and pepper.

COOK
Pressure cooker: Seal and cook on high pressure for 15 minutes, then natural release for 10 minutes.

On the hob: Cover and simmer gently for 35–40 minutes, turning the chicken halfway, until tender.

Slow cooked: Set it on high and cook for 4 hours until cooked through and tender.

SHRED AND FINISH
Remove the chicken and shred with two forks. Return to the pan and mix with the cooking juices. Add the juice of 1 lime and a final pinch of smoked paprika.

(continues overleaf)

MEXICAN CHICKEN WITH FRESH TOMATO SALSA (CONTINUED)

FOR THE FRESH SALSA
4 ripe tomatoes, finely diced
½ red onion, very finely chopped
1 green chilli, finely chopped (optional)
Small handful of coriander, chopped
Juice of 1 lime
Pinch of sugar and drizzle of extra virgin olive oil to balance acidity (optional)

MAKE THE SALSA

Combine all the salsa ingredients in a bowl. Let it sit for at least 10 minutes to allow the flavours to come together. If your tomatoes are a little sharp, add a pinch of sugar and a drizzle of olive oil to round things out.

TO SERVE

Quesadillas: Fold the chicken and salsa with grated cheese into a tortilla. Pan-fry until crisp and golden.

Tacos or rice bowls: Pile the chicken into warm tortillas or over rice with salsa, black beans, avocado and coriander.

Soup: Simmer leftovers in more broth with sweetcorn and beans for a quick tortilla soup.

STIFADO (GREEK BEEF STEW) WITH FETA MASH

This classic Greek stew is all about warmth and depth – mouthwateringly melty beef, sweet shallots and aromatic spices in a rich tomato and bone broth base. Using bone broth gives the sauce its silky texture and umami flavour, while a creamy, salty feta mash cuts through the richness.

SERVES 4
PREP TIME: 30 MINUTES
COOK TIME: 3 HOURS

- 2 tablespoons olive oil
- 600g (1lb 5oz) stewing beef (chuck or shin), cut into large chunks
- 300g (10½oz) shallots, peeled and left whole
- 2 garlic cloves, crushed
- 1 cinnamon stick
- 2 bay leaves
- 3–4 cloves
- 1 tablespoon tomato purée
- 150ml (5fl oz) red wine
- 1 x 400g (14oz) tin chopped tomatoes
- 250ml (9fl oz) beef bone broth
- 1 teaspoon sugar or honey
- Splash of red wine vinegar or lemon juice
- Sea salt and freshly ground black pepper

FOR THE FETA MASH
- 800g (1lb 12oz) floury potatoes (e.g. Maris Piper), peeled and chopped
- 30g (1oz) butter
- 75ml (2½fl oz) warm milk
- 50g (1¾oz) feta, crumbled

TO SERVE (OPTIONAL)
Green salad or lemony steamed greens

BROWN THE BEEF FOR THE STIFADO
Heat 1 tablespoon of the olive oil in a large, heavy-based pot. Pat the beef dry and brown in batches until well seared. Remove and set aside.

CARAMELISE THE SHALLOTS
Add the remaining oil and cook the shallots over low heat for 10–15 minutes until soft and golden. Add the garlic and cook for 1 minute more.

TOAST THE SPICES
Push the shallots aside and toast the cinnamon, bay leaves and cloves for 30 seconds until fragrant.

DEGLAZE AND DEEPEN
Stir in the tomato purée and cook for 1–2 minutes. Add the red wine and deglaze the pot, scraping up any browned bits.

SIMMER
Return the beef to the pot with the tomatoes, bone broth, sugar, salt and pepper. Stir well. Bring to a simmer, cover and cook on low for 2 hours 30 minutes–3 hours. Uncover for the final 30 minutes if needed to thicken.

SEASON
Taste and adjust the seasoning. Add a splash of red wine vinegar or lemon juice to lift the dish before serving.

BOIL THE POTATOES FOR THE FETA MASH
While the stew simmers, cook the potatoes in salted water for about 15–20 minutes until soft. Drain well and return to the pan to steam dry for 1 minute.

MASH AND MIX
Mash with the butter, warm milk and crumbled feta. Season to taste – the feta brings salt and tang, so go easy.

TO SERVE
Ladle the stifado over generous spoonfuls of feta mash. Add a green salad or lemony steamed greens if you like.

Comfort Cooking

ONE-POT BUTTER CHICKEN CURRY

Butter chicken always feels like a guilty pleasure. Our version uses a quick yoghurt marinade for freshness and to tenderise, and a warm brown butter masala drizzle to finish it off perfectly.

SERVES 4
PREP TIME: 30 MINUTES, PLUS UP TO 2 HOURS TO MARINATE
COOK TIME: 40 MINUTES

FOR THE CHICKEN MARINADE
3 tablespoons full-fat plain yoghurt
1 teaspoon garam masala
1 garlic clove, grated
Juice of ½ lemon
½ teaspoon salt
4 small chicken breasts (or 2 large, halved horizontally)

FOR THE CURRY
2 tablespoons butter or ghee
1 large onion, finely chopped
3 garlic cloves, minced
1 tablespoon grated fresh ginger
2 tablespoons tomato purée
2 teaspoons garam masala
1 teaspoon ground cumin
1 teaspoon ground coriander
½ teaspoon ground turmeric
½ teaspoon smoked paprika (optional)
½ teaspoon chilli powder (adjust to taste)
500ml (17fl oz) chicken bone broth
100ml (3½fl oz) double cream
Juice of ½ lemon
2 tablespoons chopped toasted cashews (or flaked almonds)
Sea salt and freshly ground black pepper

FOR THE GARNISH
1 tablespoon butter
¼ teaspoon garam masala

TO SERVE
Steamed basmati rice or flatbreads

MARINATE THE CHICKEN
In a bowl, mix the yoghurt, garam masala, garlic, lemon juice and salt. Add the chicken breasts and coat well. Marinate for at least 30 minutes (or up to 2 hours chilled). Before cooking, lightly scrape off any excess marinade.

START THE SAUCE
In a deep sauté pan or shallow casserole dish, melt the butter and add the chopped onion. Cook for 6–8 minutes until soft. Stir in the garlic and ginger and cook for another 1–2 minutes.

TOAST THE SPICES AND TOMATO PASTE
Add the tomato purée, garam masala, cumin, coriander, turmeric, paprika and chilli powder. Stir well and cook for 2–3 minutes to deepen the colour and aroma.

REDUCE
Pour in the chicken bone broth. Simmer uncovered for 10–12 minutes until the liquid reduces and the sauce thickens slightly.

ADD CREAM AND POACH THE CHICKEN
Stir in the cream and season. Nestle the chicken breasts in the sauce. Reduce the heat to low, cover and poach gently for 15–18 minutes, turning once, until cooked through.

REST AND SLICE
Transfer the chicken to a board and rest for 5 minutes before slicing. Meanwhile, reduce the sauce uncovered for a few minutes if needed. Add the lemon juice to lift the flavour.

MAKE THE BROWN BUTTER DRIZZLE
In a small pan, melt the butter over medium heat until golden and nutty. Remove from the heat and stir in the garam masala.

TO FINISH
Return the sliced chicken to the pan. Top with toasted cashews and spoon over the brown butter masala drizzle.

TO SERVE
Serve hot with basmati rice or warm flatbreads.

RED WINE, PORCINI & BEEF CHEEK RAGU

This wonderfully rich, savoury ragu is a luxurious alternative to a traditional bolognese. Bone broth adds some 'oomph' and extra depth to the sauce, giving it that glossy, slow-cooked texture without needing hours of reduction.

SERVES 4
PREP TIME: 30 MINUTES, PLUS SOAKING THE MUSHROOMS
COOK TIME: 3 HOURS 30 MINUTES

30g (1oz) dried porcini mushrooms
800g (1lb 12oz) beef cheeks, trimmed and cut into 4–6 large pieces
2 tablespoons olive oil
1 onion, finely chopped
2 carrots, finely diced
2 celery sticks, finely diced
3 garlic cloves, minced
1 tablespoon tomato purée
200ml (7fl oz) dry red wine
250ml (9fl oz) beef bone broth
1 tablespoon balsamic vinegar
1 teaspoon white or red miso paste (optional but recommended)
2 rosemary sprigs
2 thyme sprigs
1 bay leaf
1 Parmesan rind (optional)
Knob of cold butter
Sea salt and freshly ground black pepper

TO SERVE
Fresh pappardelle or polenta

SOAK THE MUSHROOMS
Cover the dried porcini with 150ml (5fl oz) just-boiled water. Leave to soak for 20 minutes, then lift out the mushrooms, finely chop them and strain the soaking liquid through a coffee filter or muslin. Reserve both the mushrooms and liquid.

BROWN THE BEEF CHEEKS
Season the beef cheeks generously with salt and pepper. Heat the olive oil in a heavy casserole or Dutch oven. Sear the cheeks in batches until dark brown on all sides. Remove and set aside.

BUILD THE SOFFRITTO
Lower the heat. Add the onion, carrot and celery with a pinch of salt. Cook slowly for 10–15 minutes, stirring often, until soft and translucent. Add the garlic and cook for 1 minute more.

DEGLAZE AND REDUCE
Stir in the tomato purée and cook for 2 minutes. Pour in the red wine and scrape the base of the pan to release any caramelised bits. Let the wine reduce by half.

ASSEMBLE THE BRAISE
Return the beef cheeks to the pan. Add the chopped porcini, reserved mushroom liquid, bone broth, balsamic vinegar, miso paste (if using), herbs and Parmesan rind. Bring to a gentle simmer, cover and cook on the lowest heat (or in a 170°C (150°C fan)/350°F/gas 4 oven) for 2½–3 hours until the cheeks are fork-tender and falling apart.

FINISH THE RAGU
Remove the beef cheeks and discard the herbs and Parmesan rind. Shred the meat using two forks. Return the meat to the pan and simmer uncovered for 15 minutes to reduce and thicken the sauce. Adjust the seasoning to taste. For a glossy finish, whisk in a knob of cold butter before serving.

TO SERVE
Spoon the ragu over fresh pappardelle, tossing with a splash of pasta water. Alternatively, serve over cheesy polenta (see page 142)

COTTAGE PIE WITH HERBY LEMON MASH

We've taken a proper British classic and dialled up the flavour and freshness to create this new family favourite. We like to create a deep, beefy base by carefully reducing the bone broth, and contrast this with a zesty herb mash. A sure-fire crowd pleaser for even the fussiest eaters!

SERVES 4
PREP TIME: 20 MINUTES, PLUS 5 MINUTES REST TIME
COOK TIME: 1 HOUR 55 MINUTES

1 tablespoon olive oil
1 onion, finely chopped
2 carrots, finely diced
2 celery sticks, finely diced
2 garlic cloves, crushed
500g (1lb 2oz) beef mince
2 tablespoons tomato purée
1 tablespoon Worcestershire sauce
100ml (3½fl oz) red wine (or use extra broth)
250ml (9fl oz) beef bone broth
1 teaspoon fresh thyme leaves or ½ teaspoon dried
1 teaspoon finely chopped fresh rosemary or ½ teaspoon dried
Sea salt and freshly ground black pepper

FOR THE MASH TOPPING
900g (2lb) floury potatoes (such as Maris Piper or King Edward), peeled and chopped
50g (1¾oz) butter
75ml (2½fl oz) whole milk (more if needed)
Zest of 1 lemon
2 tablespoons chopped parsley
1 tablespoon chopped chives or spring onions

TO SERVE
Extra chives
Freshly steamed greens

START THE BASE
Heat the olive oil in a large sauté pan over medium heat. Add the onion, carrots and celery with a pinch of salt. Cook gently for 8–10 minutes until soft and slightly golden. Stir in the garlic and cook for 1 minute more.

BROWN THE BEEF
Increase the heat and add the mince. Break it up with a wooden spoon and fry for about 6–8 minutes until well browned. You want some colour here for flavour, so do not rush this step.

BUILD THE FLAVOUR
Stir in the tomato purée and Worcestershire sauce. Cook for 2 minutes to remove any raw taste. Add the wine (if using) and let it reduce by half, scraping the bottom of the pan to lift any sticky bits.

SIMMER
Pour in the beef bone broth and add the thyme and rosemary. Season with salt and pepper. Reduce the heat and simmer gently, uncovered, for 25–30 minutes until the sauce is thick and glossy. It should look spoonable, not soupy – take your time to reduce properly. If it's still loose, turn up the heat for the final few minutes and stir often.

MAKE THE MASH
While the filling simmers, cook the potatoes in a large pan of salted boiling water for 15–20 minutes until completely tender. Drain well, then return them to the hot pan for 1 minute to steam dry. This helps the mash stay fluffy and firm, not wet.

MASH AND SEASON
Add the butter, milk, lemon zest, parsley and chives to the potatoes. Mash until smooth, adding more milk only if needed. Season generously. The lemon zest should brighten the flavour without overpowering.

ASSEMBLE AND BAKE

Preheat the oven to 200°C (180°C fan)/400°F/gas 6. Spoon the beef mixture into a baking dish. Let it cool slightly before topping – this helps the mash sit on top, rather than sink. Spoon the mash over gently, starting from the edges and working inwards to seal. Use a fork to rough up the surface, which helps it crisp.

FINISH IN THE OVEN

Bake for 20–25 minutes until golden and bubbling. For a deeper crust, place under the grill for 2–3 minutes at the end. Let the pie rest for 5 minutes before serving – this makes slicing much easier.

TO SERVE

Sprinkle some extra chives on top and serve with a side of freshly steamed greens like Tenderstem broccoli or asparagus.

BONE BROTH BOLOGNESE

Bone broth brings natural collagen and slow-cooked depth to this bolognese. Definitely not your average mince.

SERVES 4
PREP TIME: 25 MINUTES
COOK TIME: 2–3 HOURS

250g (9oz) beef mince (15–20% fat)
250g (9oz) pork mince
½ teaspoon fine sea salt
½ teaspoon freshly ground black pepper
1 teaspoon finely chopped fresh sage or ½ teaspoon dried

FOR THE SAUCE
1 tablespoon olive oil
50g (1¾ oz) smoked pancetta or lardons
1 large onion, finely diced
1 carrot, finely diced
1 celery stick, finely diced
3 garlic cloves, minced
3 anchovy fillets in oil
½ teaspoon ground nutmeg
1 tablespoon tomato purée
150ml (5fl oz) dry white wine
1 x 400g (14oz) tin plum tomatoes, crushed by hand
500ml (17fl oz) beef bone broth
1 small piece of Parmesan rind (optional)
1 bay leaf
1 teaspoon red wine vinegar or balsamic vinegar
1 teaspoon sugar (if needed, to balance acidity)
Sea salt and freshly ground black pepper

TO FINISH
100ml (3½fl oz) whole milk or 50ml (1¾fl oz) double cream
25g (1oz) unsalted butter
25g (1oz) Parmesan cheese, grated

TO SERVE
400g (14oz) tagliatelle or pappardelle
Extra grated Parmesan cheese

FORM THE MEAT PATTY
In a large bowl, mix the beef and pork mince with the salt, pepper and sage. Gently shape into one large, thick patty.

BROWN THE MEAT
Heat the olive oil in a large, heavy-based pan over medium-high heat. Sear the patty on both sides until well browned, about 3 minutes per side. Do not stir. Once browned, break into small chunks with a wooden spoon and set aside.

RENDER PANCETTA AND BUILD AROMATICS
In the same pan, cook the pancetta for 3 minutes until the fat melts away. Add the onion, carrot and celery. Sauté over medium heat for 8–10 minutes until soft and lightly golden.

ADD THE GARLIC AND ANCHOVY
Stir in the garlic, anchovy and nutmeg. Cook for 2–3 minutes until the anchovies melt.

TOMATO PURÉE AND WINE
Stir in the tomato purée and cook for 1 minute. Add the white wine and scrape up any bits stuck to the bottom of the pan. Let it reduce by half.

BUILD THE SAUCE
Return the browned meat to the pan. Add the crushed tomatoes, bone broth, Parmesan rind, bay leaf and vinegar. Simmer gently, uncovered or partially covered, for 2–3 hours, stirring occasionally. Add water if it reduces too far.

FINISH THE SAUCE
Remove the Parmesan rind and bay leaf. Stir in the milk or cream, butter and grated Parmesan. Season to taste and add sugar if needed. The sauce should be rich, thick and glossy.

COOK THE PASTA
Cook the pasta in salted boiling water. Reserve 100ml (3½fl oz) pasta water before draining. Toss the pasta with the sauce and a splash of pasta water over a low heat to bind.

TO SERVE
Pile into a deep pasta bowl, then cover with more grated Parmesan.

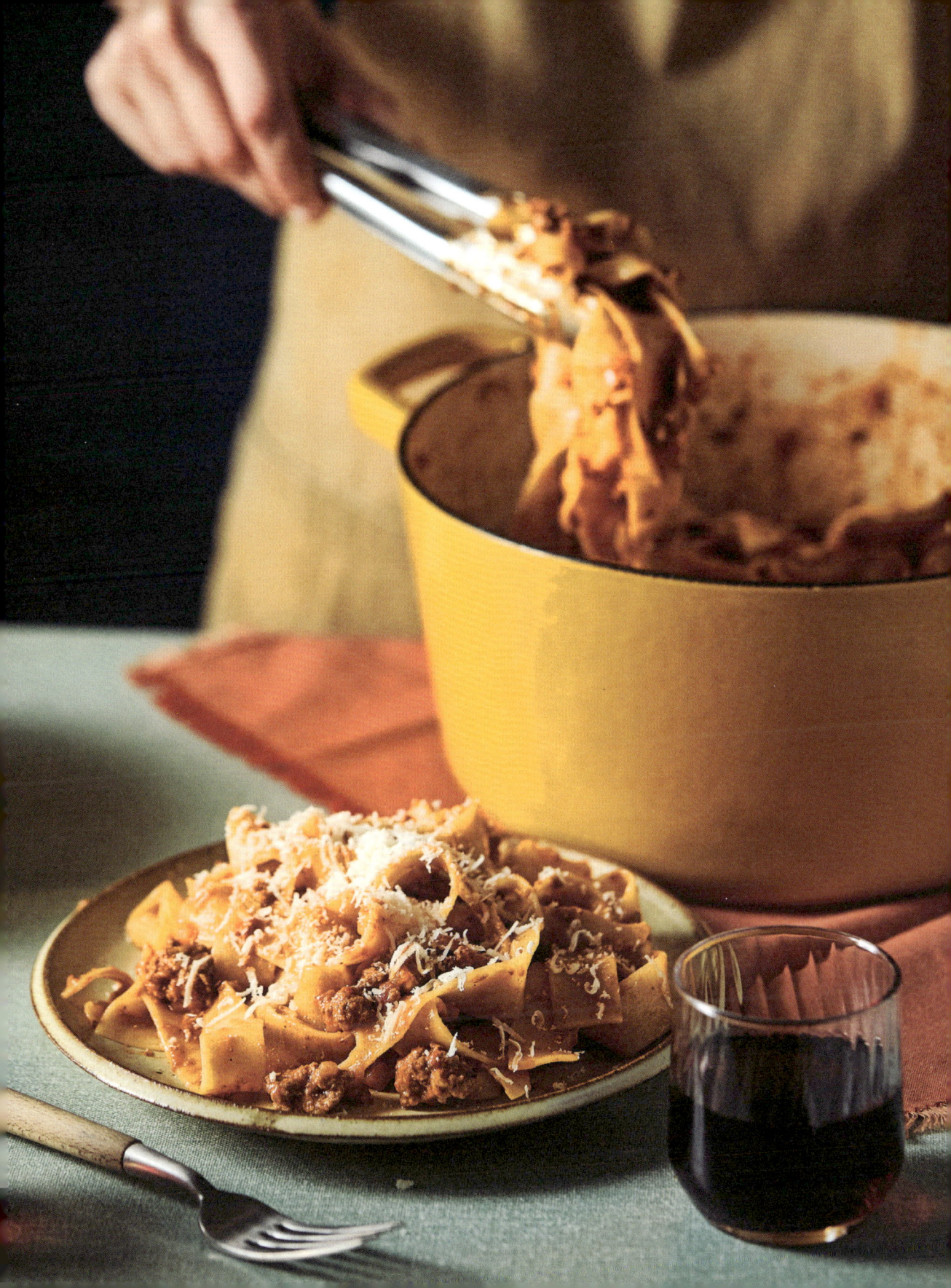

CHICKEN VINDALOO WITH A COOLING RAITA

Bone broth adds both nutrition and complexity to this vindaloo's heat, acidity and sweetness. Its natural gelatine gives the dish a rich, glossy finish, while also deepening the flavour. Warning, this is a hot one – we added a cooling raita out of necessity!

SERVES 4
PREP TIME: 30 MINUTES, PLUS 30 MINUTES (UP TO 12 HOURS) TO MARINATE
COOK TIME: 45 MINUTES

600g (1lb 5oz) boneless, skinless chicken thighs, cut into bite-size chunks
2 teaspoons ground cumin
2 teaspoons ground coriander
1 teaspoon ground turmeric
1 tablespoon white wine or apple cider vinegar
2 tablespoons ghee or neutral oil (such as sunflower)
1 large onion, finely sliced
1 teaspoon smoked paprika
1–2 teaspoons chilli powder (adjust to taste)
1 teaspoon ground cinnamon
4 garlic cloves, minced
2.5cm (1 inch) piece of fresh ginger, grated
1 tablespoon tomato purée
250ml (9fl oz) chicken bone broth
1 teaspoon sugar or honey
1 small red chilli, finely chopped
1 tablespoon cold butter
Squeeze of lemon or lime juice (optional)
Sea salt and freshly ground black pepper

MARINATE
Combine the chicken with half the cumin, coriander and turmeric, along with the vinegar and a pinch of salt. Set aside for at least 30 minutes, or up to 12 hours.

CARAMELISE THE ONIONS
Heat the ghee or oil in a heavy-based pan. Add the onion and cook slowly over medium heat for 10–15 minutes until deeply golden brown. This step builds sweetness and depth.

TOAST THE SPICES
Push the onions to one side of the pan. In the cleared space, add a splash of oil if needed, then toast the remaining ground spices for 30 seconds to release their aroma.

BUILD THE BASE
Add the garlic and ginger and stir through the spices for 1–2 minutes. Stir in the tomato purée and cook for another minute.

DEGLAZE AND SIMMER
Pour in a splash of bone broth to deglaze the pan, scraping up any browned bits. Add the rest of the broth, sugar, fresh chilli and the chicken. Bring to a simmer.

COOK DOWN
Cover and cook gently for 20 minutes. Remove the lid and simmer for a further 10–15 minutes, allowing the sauce to reduce and thicken. The bone broth will concentrate naturally to a rich, glossy finish.

SEASON
Taste and adjust the seasoning. Just before serving, swirl in the cold butter to enrich and smooth the sauce. Add a squeeze of lemon or lime if desired.

FOR THE RAITA
½ cucumber, grated or finely diced
Pinch of salt
250g (9oz) Greek or natural yoghurt
¼ teaspoon ground cumin
Small handful of mint or coriander, finely chopped
Pinch of ground chilli or sumac

TO SERVE
Chopped coriander
Steamed rice or naan

START THE RAITA
Sprinkle the grated or diced cucumber with a little salt and let it sit for 10 minutes. Squeeze out the moisture using a clean tea towel or kitchen paper.

ADD THE YOGHURT TO THE RAITA
Combine the yoghurt, cucumber, cumin and herbs in a bowl and season with salt. Finish with extra chopped herbs and a pinch of ground chilli or sumac for colour.

TO SERVE
Garnish the chicken vindaloo with a scattering of chopped coriander. Serve hot with rice or naan, and raita on the side.

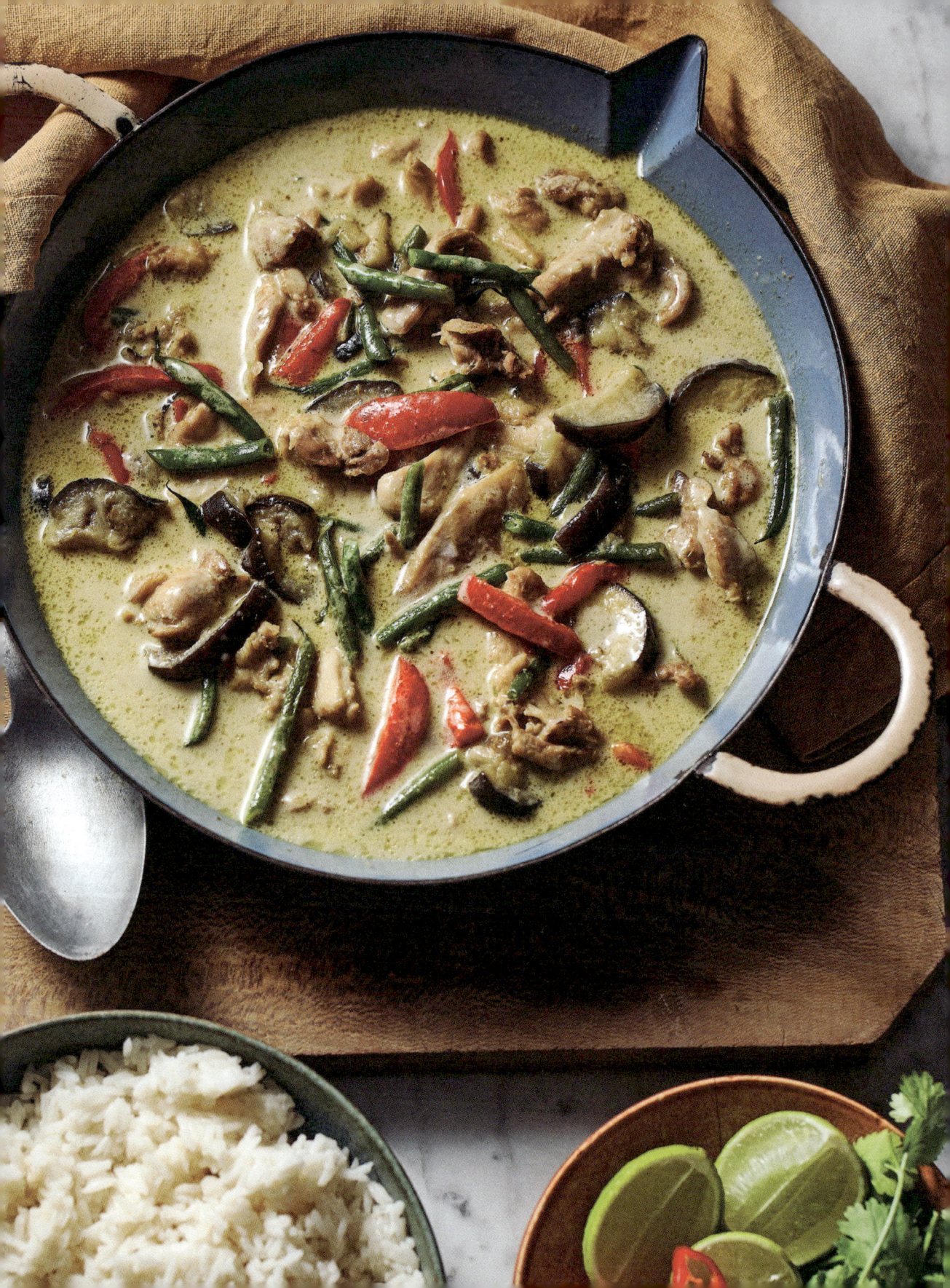

THAI GREEN CHICKEN CURRY

Thai green curry is one of our favourite ways to use bone broth! A homemade curry paste adds extra zing and freshness to the flavour, but store bought paste is totally fine too. Most curry pastes freeze well once opened.

SERVES 4
PREP TIME: 25 MINUTES
COOK TIME: 30 MINUTES

FOR THE GREEN CURRY PASTE
- 4–5 medium green chillies, deseeded for less heat
- 1 shallot, roughly chopped
- 2 garlic cloves, peeled
- 1 thumb-sized piece of fresh galangal (or ginger), peeled and chopped
- 1 lemongrass stalk, tender inner part only, finely sliced
- 1 teaspoon makrut lime zest or 2 lime leaves (central vein removed)
- Small bunch of coriander stems (roots if you have them)
- 1 teaspoon ground coriander
- 1 teaspoon ground cumin
- 1 tablespoon fish sauce or ½ teaspoon salt
- ½ teaspoon shrimp paste (optional, but authentic)
- Juice of ½ lime

FOR THE CURRY
- 1 tablespoon coconut oil
- 2–3 tablespoons green curry paste (see above, or use a good ready made one)
- 1 x 400ml (14oz) tin full-fat coconut milk
- 250ml (9fl oz) chicken bone broth
- 500g (1lb 2oz) boneless, skinless chicken thighs, sliced into strips
- 1 small aubergine, cut into chunks
- 100g (3½oz) green beans, trimmed
- 1 red pepper, thinly sliced
- 1 tablespoon fish sauce, or to taste
- 1 teaspoon palm sugar or light brown sugar
- Zest of 1 lime

TO SERVE
- Steamed jasmine rice
- Coriander
- 1 red chilli, finely sliced
- Lime wedges

MAKE THE CURRY PASTE
Blend everything in a small food processor with a splash of water or neutral oil to loosen. Scrape down and blend again until smooth. You can make it ahead and freeze in portions.

COOK THE CURRY PASTE
Heat the coconut oil in a wide pan over medium heat. Add the green curry paste and fry for 2–3 minutes until fragrant. The paste should sizzle and darken slightly to build flavour.

ADD THE COCONUT MILK AND BONE BROTH
Stir in the coconut milk and bone broth. Bring to a gentle simmer, but avoid boiling hard – this can reduce the sauce too quickly.

POACH THE CHICKEN
Add the chicken strips and simmer gently for 10–12 minutes until just cooked. Don't stir too often, let the broth gently do its work.

ADD THE VEG IN STAGES
Add the aubergine first and simmer for about 8 minutes until starting to soften. Add the green beans and red pepper and cook for a final 3–4 minutes. This layering adds texture and colour.

SEASON
Stir in the fish sauce, sugar and lime zest. Taste and adjust. Add more fish sauce for salt, sugar for roundness or lime juice for acidity.

TO SERVE
Spoon over fragrant jasmine rice and finish with fresh coriander, red chilli and lime wedges.

BEEF KOFTA CURRY

A rich, spiced curry built on a classic rogan josh base. The koftas are lightly browned, then gently poached to stay tender and full of flavour. Serve with rice or flatbreads to soak up the bold, aromatic sauce.

SERVES 4
PREP TIME: 25 MINUTES, PLUS CHILLING
COOK TIME: 45 MINUTES

FOR THE KOFTAS
1 small onion
500g (1lb 2oz) beef mince (15–20% fat)
2 garlic cloves, minced
1 teaspoon grated fresh ginger
2 tablespoons chopped coriander stalks
1 teaspoon ground cumin
1 teaspoon garam masala
½ teaspoon Kashmiri chilli powder
1 teaspoon salt
1 egg yolk
2 tablespoons breadcrumbs or chickpea flour

FOR THE ROGAN JOSH BASE
2 tablespoons ghee or neutral oil (vegetable or sunflower)
2 onions, thinly sliced
4 garlic cloves, minced
1 tablespoon grated fresh ginger
3 green cardamom pods, lightly crushed
1½ teaspoons ground coriander
1½ teaspoons paprika
1 teaspoon Kashmiri chilli powder
1 teaspoon ground turmeric
1 teaspoon ground cumin
½ teaspoon ground cinnamon
2 tablespoons tomato purée
200ml (7fl oz) passata or finely chopped tomatoes
250ml (9fl oz) beef bone broth
Sea salt

TO FINISH
1 teaspoon garam masala
Juice of ½ lemon

TO SERVE
Handful of chopped coriander and mint
Drizzle of yoghurt or cream (optional)
Steamed basmati rice, naan or jeera rice

PREP THE ONION FOR THE KOFTAS
Grate the onion into a fine sieve, sprinkle over a little salt and leave to drain for 10 minutes. This removes excess water, helping your koftas hold together better.

MAKE THE KOFTAS
In a large bowl, mix the beef, drained grated onion, garlic, ginger, coriander stalks, spices, salt, egg yolk and breadcrumbs. Mix gently with your hands until just combined. Do not overwork. Roll into 16 golf ball-sized meatballs and chill for 15–30 minutes to firm up.

START THE SAUCE
Heat the ghee in a wide, deep pan over medium heat. Add the onions and cook slowly for 10–15 minutes until deep golden brown. Add the garlic, ginger and cardamom pods and cook for 1 minute. Stir in all the ground spices and toast them for 30 seconds until fragrant.

BUILD FLAVOUR
Add the tomato purée and cook for 2–3 minutes until it darkens and starts to caramelise. Stir in the passata, bring to a simmer and cook for 5 minutes to reduce slightly.

ADD THE BONE BROTH
Pour in the beef bone broth and season with salt. Simmer gently while you brown the koftas.

BROWN AND POACH THE KOFTAS
In a non-stick frying pan, brown the koftas lightly on all sides. They should take on some colour but remain raw in the centre. Once browned, gently lower them into the curry base. Simmer over low heat, covered, for 12–15 minutes until fully cooked.

FINISH
Stir in the final teaspoon of garam masala and a good squeeze of lemon juice to lift the dish.

TO SERVE
Scatter the curry with chopped herbs and a drizzle of yoghurt then serve with basmati or jeera rice, or naan.

COMFORTING CHICKEN & DUMPLINGS

Almost every culture has its own version of dumplings, and it's no wonder. The familiar, satisfying comfort of a rich stew topped with plump dumplings never gets old. This recipe is a British classic, ideal for using up leftover roast chicken.

SERVES 4
PREP TIME: 25 MINUTES
COOK TIME: 1 HOUR 5 MINUTES

- 1 tablespoon olive oil or reserved chicken fat
- 1 leek, white and pale green only, finely sliced
- 2 carrots, diced
- 2 celery sticks, diced
- 2 garlic cloves, minced
- 2 teaspoons fresh thyme or 1 teaspoon dried
- 150ml (5fl oz) dry white wine or vermouth (optional)
- 500ml (17fl oz) chicken bone broth
- 1 bay leaf
- 1 tablespoon Dijon mustard
- 250–300g (9–10½oz) shredded cooked chicken
- 1 tablespoon crème fraîche or double cream (optional)
- Dash of lemon juice or sherry vinegar (optional)
- Sea salt and freshly ground black pepper

FOR THE DUMPLINGS
- 125g (4½oz) self-raising flour
- 1 teaspoon baking powder
- ½ teaspoon fine sea salt
- 1 tablespoon finely chopped herbs (parsley or chives work well)
- 50g (1¾oz) cold butter, diced (or lard or suet if available – see note)
- 75ml (2½fl oz) cold milk

TO SERVE
Chopped parsley

BUILD YOUR BASE
Heat the olive oil or chicken fat in a large, heavy-based pan. Add the leek, carrots and celery with a generous pinch of salt. Sweat over low heat for 8–10 minutes until soft but not browned. Stir in the garlic and thyme, cooking for 1 minute more.

ADD DEPTH
Pour in the wine or vermouth and allow it to bubble for about 2–3 minutes. Add the bone broth, 250ml (9fl oz) water, the bay leaf and mustard. Bring to a simmer and cook uncovered for about 10–15 minutes until the veg are tender and the broth slightly reduced.

ENRICH AND LAYER
Stir in the shredded chicken and crème fraîche, if using. Simmer for another 5 minutes to let the flavours combine. Taste and adjust the seasoning. A dash of lemon juice or sherry vinegar at this stage can help lift the broth and balance the richness.

MAKE THE DUMPLINGS
In a bowl, combine the flour, baking powder, salt and herbs. Rub in the cold butter (or lard or suet) using your fingertips until it resembles coarse breadcrumbs. Stir in the milk gradually to form a soft dough. Divide and shape into eight dumplings.

STEAM THE DUMPLINGS
Place the dumplings on the surface of the stew, leaving space between them to expand. Cover with a tight-fitting lid and simmer gently for 15 minutes. Do not lift the lid during this time. For a golden crust, uncover after 15 minutes and cook for a further 5 minutes with the heat turned up slightly.

TO SERVE
Scatter with fresh parsley and serve it simply in warm bowls.

Note: Traditionally, British dumplings are made with suet – a firm beef or lamb fat prized for creating light, fluffy textures. It is less commonly stocked in supermarkets today, but lard is a great substitute for richness, while cold butter works reliably too.

BEEF RENDANG WITH CARROT & CABBAGE SALAD

This rich, slow-cooked Indonesian beef dish is taken to the next level with bone broth, adding a nourishing depth to the sauce as it reduces. The crisp, fresh salad contrasts delightfully with the hearty beef and creamy coconut flavour.

SERVES 4
PREP TIME: 30 MINUTES
COOK TIME: 3 HOURS, PLUS RESTING TIME

800g (1lb 12oz) beef chuck or shin, cut into 4–5 cm (1½–2 inch) cubes
2 tablespoons coconut oil or neutral oil (vegetable or sunflower)
200ml (7fl oz) coconut cream
2 tablespoons coconut paste or grated creamed coconut
2 teaspoons fish sauce
500ml (17fl oz) beef bone broth
2 lime leaves (optional)
1 cinnamon stick
1 star anise
Sea salt

FOR THE SPICE PASTE
4 shallots, peeled
4 garlic cloves, peeled
2 red chillies (adjust to taste)
1 thumb-sized piece of fresh ginger
1 thumb-sized piece of fresh galangal (or use more ginger)
1 lemongrass stalk, white part only, chopped
1 teaspoon ground coriander
1 teaspoon ground cumin
1 teaspoon ground turmeric
1 teaspoon palm sugar or light brown sugar

PREPARE THE BEEF
Pat the beef dry with kitchen paper. Brown in batches in a heavy pot over medium-high heat with a little oil to build deep flavour. Remove and set aside.

COOK THE SPICE PASTE
Blend all the spice paste ingredients. Lower the heat to medium and cook the blended spice paste in the same pan for 7–10 minutes until fragrant, darkened slightly and the oil begins to separate.

BUILD THE SAUCE
Add the coconut cream, coconut paste, fish sauce and bone broth. Stir well, scraping up any browned bits from the base. Return the beef to the pot along with the lime leaves, cinnamon and star anise.

SLOW SIMMER
Simmer uncovered for 2 hours 30 minutes–3 hours, stirring occasionally. The sauce should reduce to a thick, rich coating. Stir more frequently near the end. Season to taste.

REST (IF YOU CAN)
The flavour improves if made a day ahead and reheated gently before serving.

(continues overleaf)

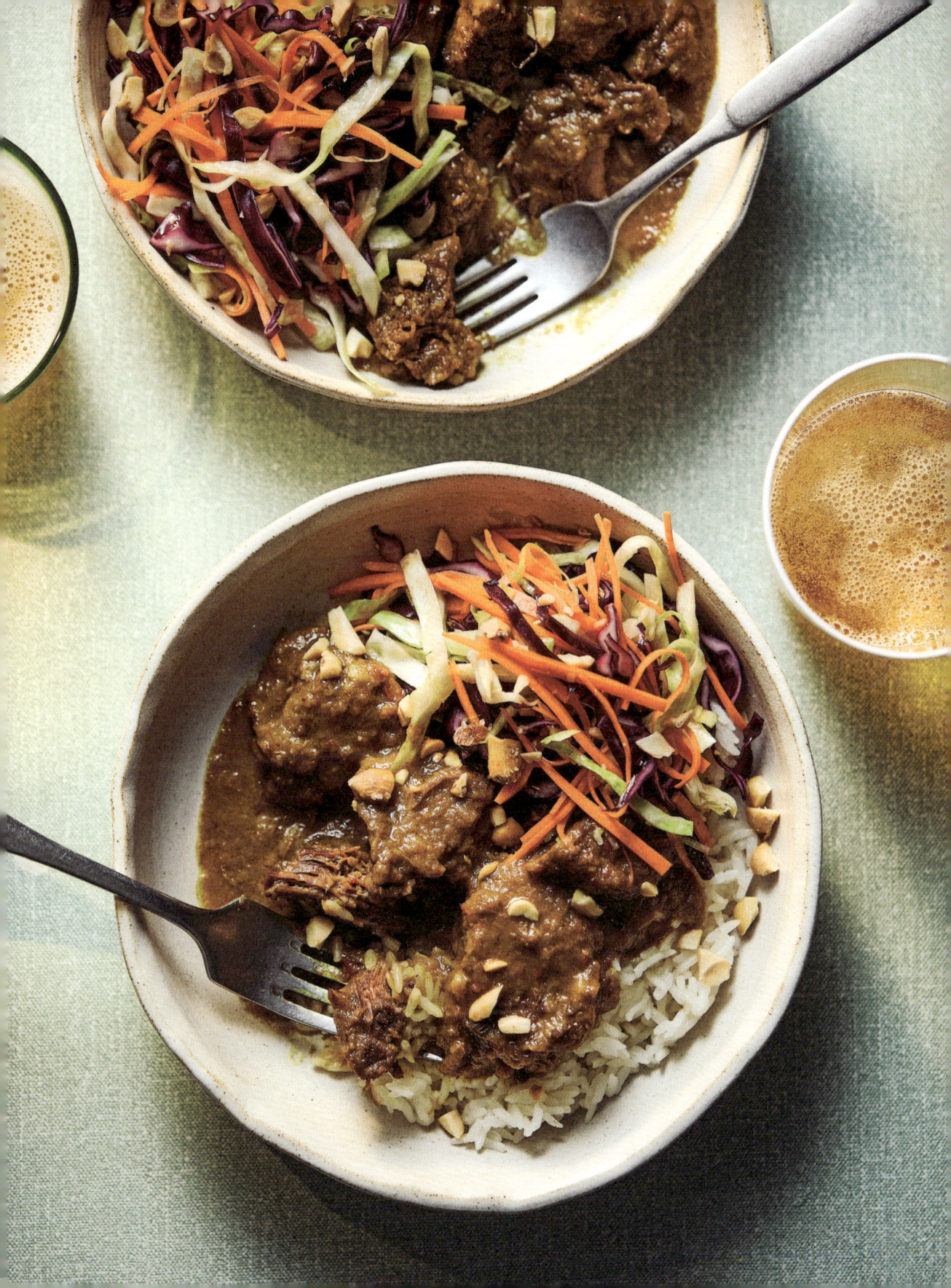

BEEF RENDANG WITH CARROT & CABBAGE SALAD (CONTINUED)

FOR THE CARROT AND CABBAGE SALAD
¼ green cabbage, finely sliced
¼ red cabbage, finely sliced (optional, for colour)
2 carrots, julienned or coarsely grated
2 spring onions, thinly sliced
Small handful of coriander leaves
2 tablespoons roasted peanuts or cashews, chopped
Sea salt

FOR THE DRESSING
2 tablespoons lime juice
1 tablespoon fish sauce or light soy sauce
1 teaspoon rice vinegar
1 teaspoon honey or maple syrup
1 teaspoon sesame oil
1 small red chilli, finely chopped (optional)

TO SERVE
Steamed rice

MAKE THE SALAD
If time allows, sprinkle a little salt over the shredded cabbage and leave it to sit for 10 minutes while you prep the other veg. This softens the texture without making it soggy.

FINISH THE SALAD
Whisk the dressing ingredients together. Just before serving, toss all the salad ingredients together with the dressing, finishing with chopped nuts for added texture and crunch.

TO SERVE
Spoon the warming rendang into a bowl atop steamed rice, then finish with the fresh salad on the side.

BO KHO (VIETNAMESE BEEF STEW)

This classic Vietnamese stew is deliciously fragrant, rich with warming spices and lifted by the fresh brightness of lemongrass and herbs. It's all the more satisfying with bone broth as its base.

SERVES 4
PREP TIME: 30 MINUTES, PLUS 1 HOUR (OR OVERNIGHT) TO MARINATE
COOK TIME: 3 HOURS

700g (1lb 9oz) boneless beef shin or brisket, cut into large 6–7.5cm (2½–3 inch) chunks
2 teaspoons fish sauce
¾ teaspoon Chinese five-spice powder
3 lemongrass stalks, 1 smashed (for marinating), 2 bruised and cut into thirds
1 tablespoon neutral oil (vegetable or sunflower)
1 small onion, finely diced
2 garlic cloves, minced
1 small thumb-sized piece of fresh ginger, peeled and minced
2 star anise
½ teaspoon freshly ground black pepper

FOR THE SAUCE
1½ tablespoons tomato purée
2 teaspoons light brown sugar
1½ tablespoons fish sauce
2 teaspoons soy sauce
¼ teaspoon chilli flakes or ½ dried chilli (optional)
500ml (17fl oz) beef bone broth
2 carrots, thickly sliced

TO FINISH
Extra fish sauce
Extra palm sugar or light brown sugar
Lime juice

TO SERVE
Thai basil or coriander
Lime wedges
Crusty baguette, rice noodles or jasmine rice

MARINATE THE BEEF
Combine the beef with the fish sauce, five-spice and 1 smashed lemongrass stalk. Marinate for at least 1 hour, ideally overnight.

SEAR THE BEEF
Dry the beef thoroughly. Heat the oil in a heavy-based pot and brown in batches until golden. Remove and set aside.

SWEAT THE AROMATICS
In the same pot, sauté the onion, garlic, ginger, remaining lemongrass, star anise and pepper over medium heat for 5–7 minutes until soft and fragrant.

CARAMELISE THE PASTE
Stir in the tomato purée and sugar. Cook for 2–3 minutes until deepened in colour and sticking slightly to the base of the pot.

DEGLAZE AND SEASON
Return the beef to the pot. Add the fish sauce, soy sauce and optional chilli. Stir, then pour in the beef bone broth and just enough water to cover.

SIMMER LOW AND SLOW
Bring to a boil, skim any foam, then reduce to a low simmer. Cover and cook for 2 hours, checking occasionally.

ADD CARROTS AND REDUCE
Uncover, add the carrots and simmer for 25–30 minutes until tender and the broth thickens slightly.

TASTE AND FINISH
Adjust with more fish sauce, sugar or lime juice to balance savoury, sweet and bright.

TO SERVE
Spoon into bowls, top with the herbs and lime wedges. Ideal with a warm, crusty baguette for scooping up the sauce or stirred through with rice noodles.

Comfort Cooking

LIGHT KERALAN FISH CURRY WITH KACHUMBER
(INDIAN SALAD)

This dish is a perfect showcase for fish broth. It adds savoury depth without overpowering the light, freshness of the curry. Coconut, curry leaves and zingy lime keep things bright, and a final drizzle of spiced oil gives the dish a warm, fragrant lift.

SERVES 4
PREP TIME: 15 MINUTES
COOK TIME: 35 MINUTES

- 500ml (17fl oz) fish broth (or use vegetable or chicken broth with a splash of fish sauce)
- 8–10 fresh curry leaves
- 1 tablespoon coconut oil,
- 1 teaspoon black mustard seeds
- 1 small onion, finely sliced
- 1 green chilli, slit lengthways
- 1 teaspoon grated fresh ginger or ginger paste
- 1 teaspoon grated garlic or garlic paste
- ½ teaspoon ground turmeric
- ½ teaspoon Kashmiri chilli powder or mild paprika
- 1 tomato, chopped
- 100ml (3½fl oz) coconut milk
- 500g (1lb 2oz) firm white fish (cod, pollock, hake), cut into large chunks
- Juice of ½ lime
- Handful of coriander, chopped

FOR THE KACHUMBER
- ½ cucumber, finely diced
- 1 small red onion, finely diced
- 1 tomato, finely diced or 6 cherry tomatoes, chopped
- Juice of ½ lime
- Small handful of coriander or mint, chopped
- Sea salt

TO FINISH
- 1 teaspoon coconut oil
- Pinch of black mustard seeds
- Pinch of Kashmiri chilli powder

TO SERVE
Steamed rice

PREPARE THE KACHUMBER
Mix the cucumber, onion, tomato, lime juice, herbs and salt in a bowl. Chill until ready to serve. For a milder onion flavour, soak the diced onion in cold water for 10 minutes, then drain before mixing with the other ingredients.

INFUSE THE BONE BROTH
Gently simmer the fish broth with a few curry leaves or a slice of fresh ginger for 5 minutes, then strain before using.

BEGIN THE CURRY BASE
Heat the coconut oil in a wide pan. Add the mustard seeds. Once they pop, add the remaining curry leaves. Stir for about 30 seconds.

BUILD THE FLAVOUR
Add the onion and cook gently for 5–6 minutes until soft and lightly golden. Add the green chilli, ginger, garlic, turmeric and chilli powder. Stir for 30 seconds until fragrant.

ADD LIQUID AND SIMMER
Stir in the chopped tomato and cook for 2 minutes. Pour in the broth and simmer for 5 minutes. Add the coconut milk, season with salt and simmer for another 2–3 minutes.

ADD THE FISH AND FINISH WITH LIME
Place the fish pieces into the curry. Cover and cook over low heat for 5–6 minutes until just cooked through. Stir in the lime juice and chopped coriander.

MAKE THE SPICED OIL
In a small pan, warm the remaining teaspoon of coconut oil with a pinch of mustard seeds and a little chilli powder. Once aromatic, drizzle over the curry before serving.

TO SERVE
Spoon the curry over warm rice, with the kachumber served on the side for freshness.

BEST-EVER BEEF BONE BROTH GRAVY

This is a proper grown-up gravy. The black garlic packs a rich, sweet punch that blends into the beef bone broth for real depth. It's brilliant with roast beef, venison or any red meat and makes everything on your plate taste that little bit more indulgent.

SERVES 4
PREP TIME: 10 MINUTES
COOK TIME: 25 MINUTES

30g (1oz) unsalted butter
1 banana shallot or ½ small onion, finely chopped
1 teaspoon tomato purée
1 tablespoon black garlic paste (or 3 garlic cloves, mashed)
½ teaspoon white miso paste (optional, boosts savoury depth)
1 tablespoon plain flour
100ml (3½fl oz) red wine (Cabernet Sauvignon or similar)
500ml (17fl oz) beef bone broth
Sea salt and freshly ground black pepper

SWEAT THE SHALLOT
In a saucepan, melt the butter over medium-low heat. Add the chopped shallot and cook gently for 5–7 minutes until soft and just beginning to colour.

BUILD THE FLAVOUR BASE
Add the tomato purée and black garlic paste to the shallot and stir for 1–2 minutes. The paste should darken slightly and begin to smell sweet and savoury. Stir in the miso, if using.

MAKE THE ROUX
Sprinkle over the flour and stir to form a loose paste. Cook for a further 1–2 minutes to get rid of the raw flour taste.

DEGLAZE AND SIMMER
Pour in the red wine and stir well, scraping the bottom of the pan. Let it bubble for a minute or two. Slowly whisk in the bone broth until the mixture is smooth.

SIMMER AND SEASON
Simmer gently for 10 minutes, stirring occasionally, until the gravy has thickened and the flavours have come together. Taste and season with salt and black pepper.

STRAIN FOR SMOOTHNESS
Pour the finished gravy through a fine-mesh sieve into a warm jug or saucepan. This makes it silky and removes any pieces of shallot or black garlic.

SERVE OR STORE
Serve hot over roast beef or mash. Cool and store in the fridge for up to 3 days. Reheat gently with a splash of water or broth to loosen, whisking until smooth again.

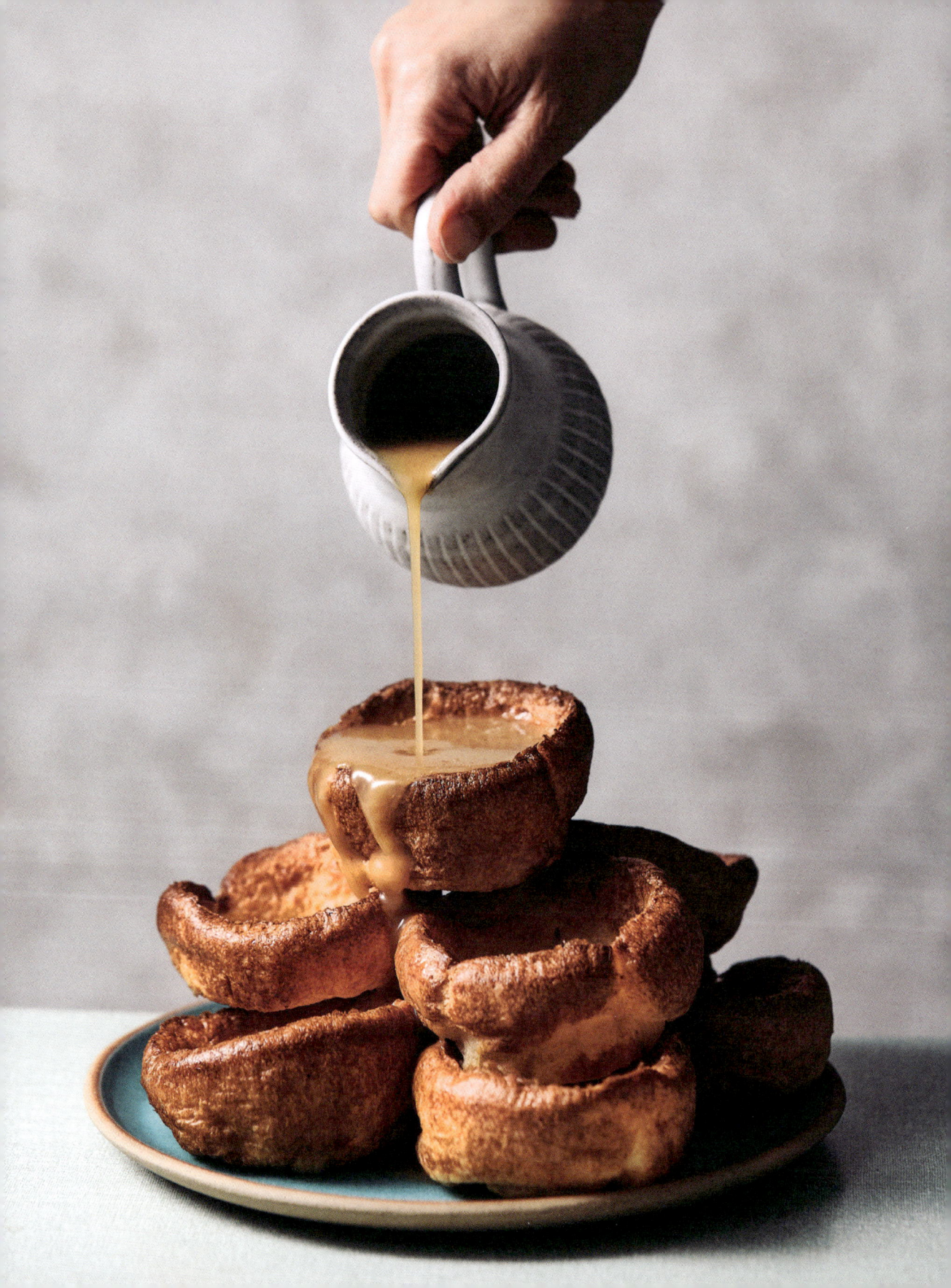

BEST-EVER CHICKEN BONE BROTH GRAVY

This is the kind of gravy that takes a roast dinner from delicious to extraordinary. Brown butter brings a nutty richness, and the chicken bone broth gives it depth without needing to simmer for hours. It's worth making extra – it keeps well and reheats beautifully.

SERVES 4
PREP TIME: 10 MINUTES
COOK TIME: 25 MINUTES

60g (2¼oz) unsalted butter
3 thyme sprigs
1 banana shallot or ½ small onion, finely chopped
1 tablespoon plain flour
75ml (2½fl oz) dry white wine (or dry vermouth)
500ml (17fl oz) chicken bone broth
1 teaspoon white miso paste (optional, for umami)
Squeeze of lemon juice (optional)
Sea salt and freshly ground black pepper

MAKE THE BROWN BUTTER
In a saucepan, melt the butter over medium heat. Add the thyme sprigs and let it bubble gently, swirling occasionally. Cook for about 4–5 minutes until the butter turns golden brown and smells nutty. Remove the thyme with tongs and discard.

SWEAT THE SHALLOT
Turn the heat to low, then add the chopped shallot to the brown butter. Cook for 5–7 minutes, stirring often, until soft and translucent.

BUILD THE ROUX
Sprinkle the flour over the butter and shallots. Cook, stirring, for 1–2 minutes to cook out the raw taste and form a loose paste.

DEGLAZE AND COMBINE
Pour in the wine and whisk well to smooth out any lumps. Let it simmer for 1–2 minutes. Gradually whisk in the bone broth, a little at a time. Keep whisking until the gravy is smooth and begins to thicken.

FINISH AND SEASON
Let the gravy simmer gently for another 5–10 minutes, stirring now and then. Stir in the miso paste, if using, and season with salt and pepper. Add a squeeze of lemon juice to lift the flavour, if needed.

STRAIN FOR SILKINESS
Pass the gravy through a fine-mesh sieve into a warm jug or serving bowl. This removes the shallot and any thyme bits, giving it a smooth, glossy finish.

SERVE OR STORE
Serve straight away, or cool and store in the fridge for up to 3 days. Reheat gently and whisk to bring it back together, adding a splash of water or broth if needed.

BONE-IN DISHES

Throughout this book, we've explored many different ways broth can be used to make everyday recipes and ingredients richer, deeper, more nutritious and, ultimately, tastier.

This chapter takes things up a notch. It's packed with delicious bone-in recipes, designed to be simmered low and slow, drawing out the best of the flavour and nutrients directly from the bones and meat.

You'll notice there's no added bone broth here, because you're making it as you go! From Coq au Vin to Ossobuco alla Milanese, these are meals that take time – some three hours or more – but repay you with incredibly rich, deep and satisfying flavour. This is slow food at its absolute best.

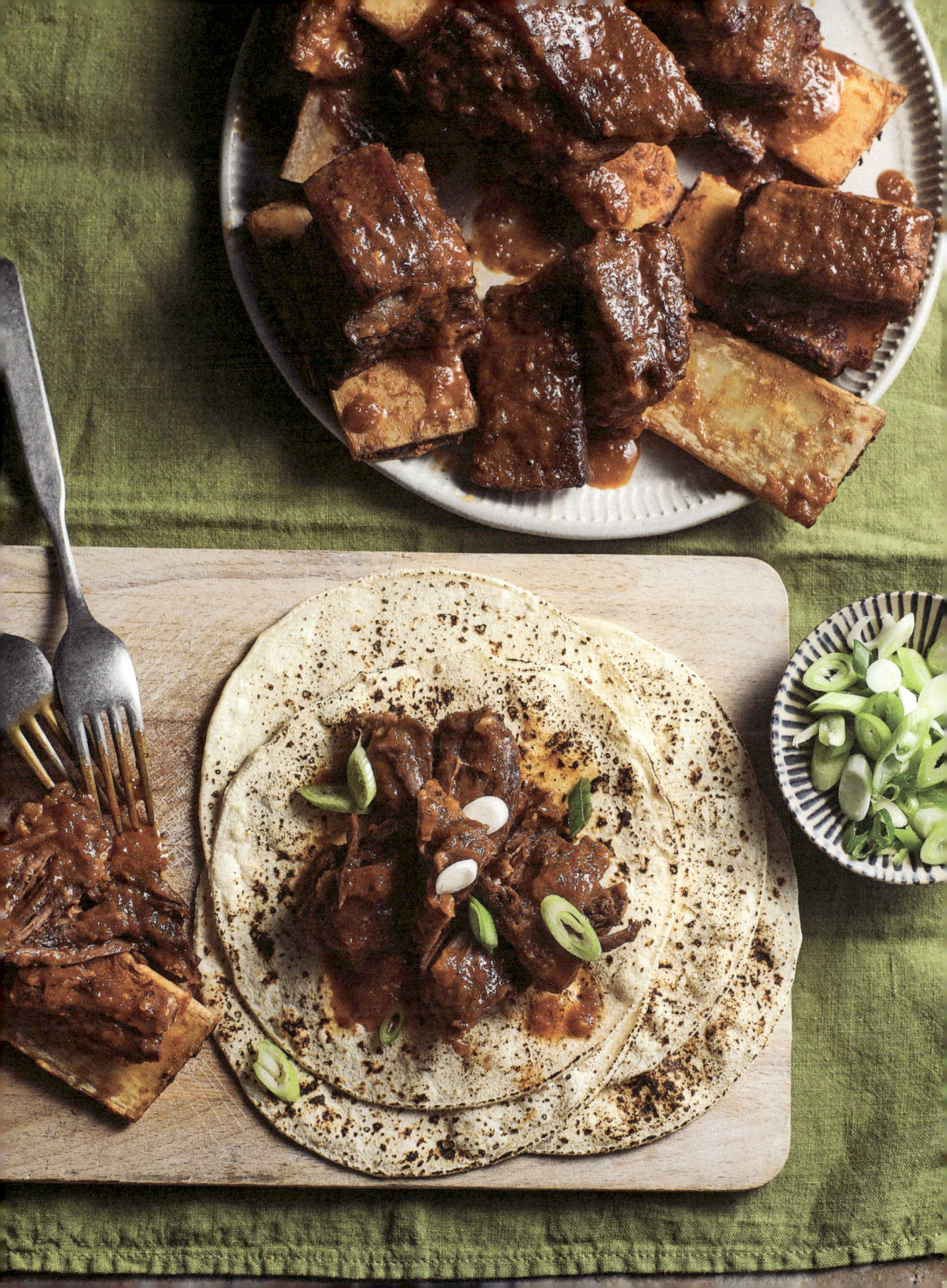

JAMAICAN OXTAIL BEANS

Slow-cooked oxtail on the bone creates a glossy sauce for this classic. You get heat from the Scotch bonnet (it can be milder if removed during cooking), warmth from the pimento and earthiness from the thyme and garlic.

SERVES 4
PREP TIME: 20 MINUTES, PLUS 2 HOURS OR OVERNIGHT MARINATING
COOK TIME: 4 HOURS

FOR THE MARINADE (CAN BE DONE THE NIGHT BEFORE)
4 garlic cloves, peeled
4 spring onions
1 small onion, peeled
6 fresh thyme sprigs or 1 teaspoon dried
1 teaspoon allspice (pimento)
1 teaspoon salt
½ teaspoon freshly ground black pepper
1.2–1.5kg (2lb 10oz–3lb 5oz) oxtail
1 tablespoon browning sauce (or 2 teaspoons dark soy sauce plus 1 teaspoon molasses)
1 tablespoon apple cider vinegar

FOR COOKING
1 tablespoon neutral oil (such as vegetable or rapeseed)
1 Scotch bonnet (left whole)
1 x 400g (14oz) tin butter beans, drained and rinsed

TO SERVE
Extra chopped spring onions
Few thyme leaves
1 lime
Steamed rice and peas

MAKE YOUR GREEN SEASONING PASTE
Put the garlic, spring onions, onion, thyme, allspice, salt and pepper in a food processor or blender. Blitz to a thick paste.

MARINATE THE OXTAIL
Place the oxtail in a large bowl. Pour over the green paste, browning sauce (or soy/molasses mix) and vinegar. Mix well to coat. Cover and leave in the fridge overnight, or for at least 2 hours if short on time.

BROWN THE MEAT
Heat the oil in a large, heavy pot (like a Dutch oven) over medium heat. Remove the oxtail from the marinade, letting most of the paste stay stuck to the meat. Working in batches, brown the oxtail on all sides until well coloured. Set the browned pieces aside.

BUILD THE STEW
Once all the meat is browned, return it to the pot. Add the reserved marinade, the whole Scotch bonnet (do not cut it) and 500ml (17fl oz) water. Bring to a simmer, then cover and reduce the heat to low.

SLOW COOK
Let it simmer gently for 3–3 hours 30 minutes, stirring occasionally, until the meat is tender and the sauce is rich and glossy. Top up with a splash of hot water if it starts to dry out too early.

ADD THE BEANS
Stir in the butter beans and simmer uncovered for another 15–20 minutes until the beans are warmed through and the sauce thickens a little more.

FINISH AND SERVE
Remove the Scotch bonnet. Taste and adjust the salt if needed.

TO SERVE
Just before serving, stir through some chopped spring onions, a few thyme leaves and a good squeeze of lime juice. Add to a warm, deep bowl with plain rice or rice and peas.

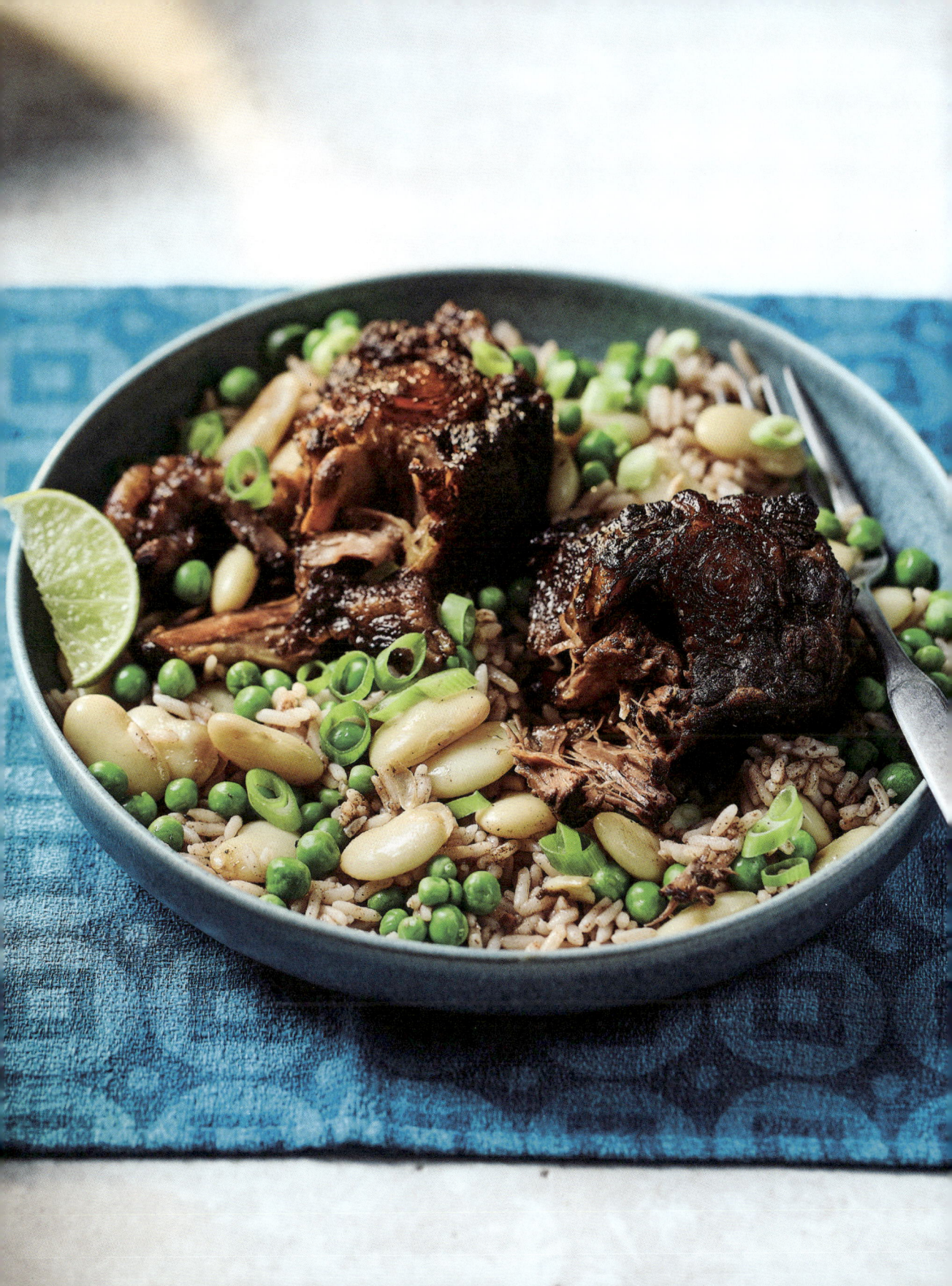

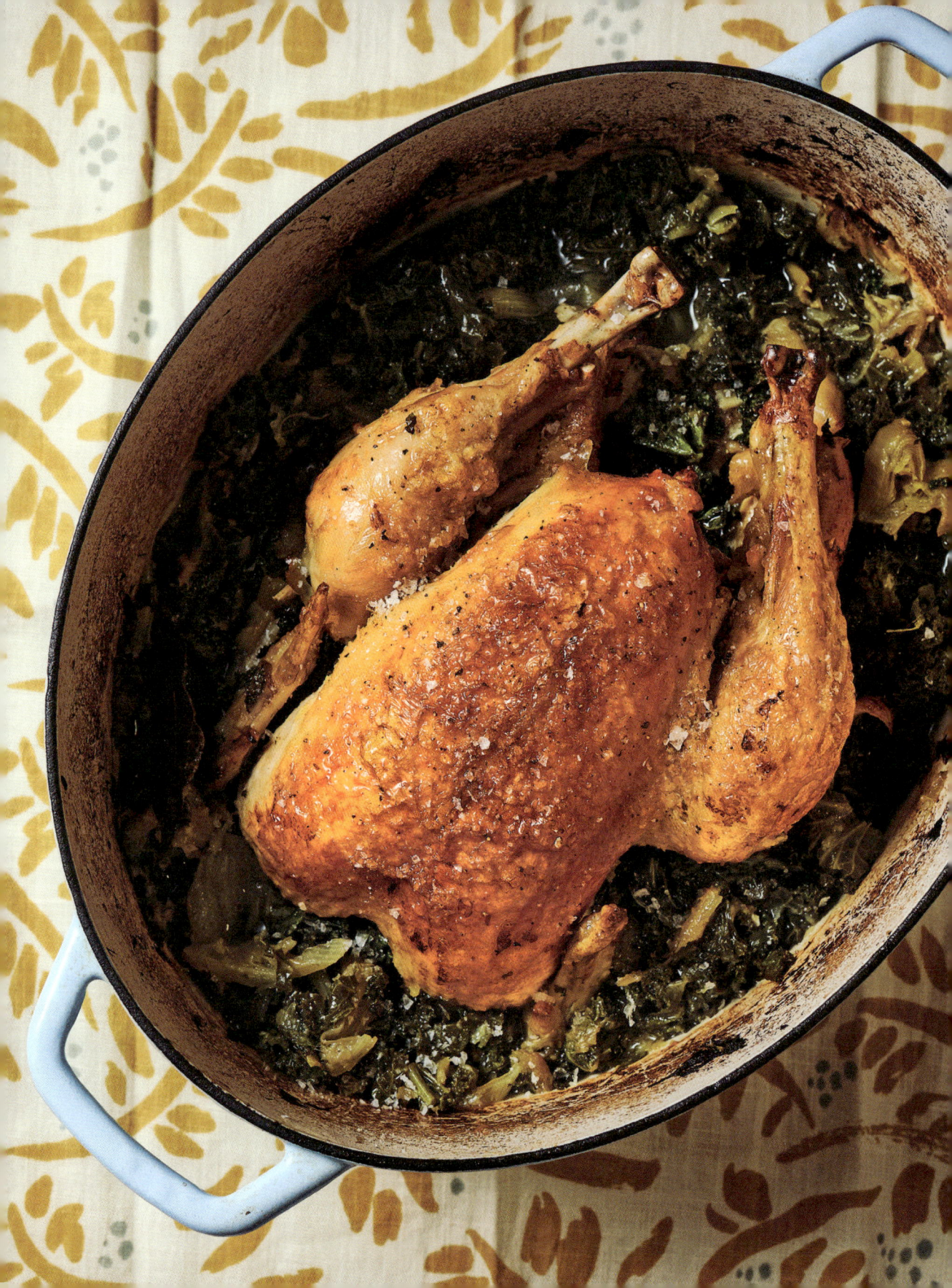

POT ROAST CHICKEN WITH GREENS & LEMON

A comforting way to cook a whole chicken without the faff of a roast. The chicken stays juicy and tender, making its own broth. It's simple enough for a weekday but still feels like something you've put effort into – plus far less washing up. Leftovers are brilliant in soup or shredded over rice.

SERVES: 4
PREP TIME: 15 MINUTES, PLUS OPTIONAL 12–24 HOURS FOR SALTING
COOK TIME: 2 HOURS, PLUS RESTING TIME

- 1 medium whole chicken (1.5–1.8kg/3lb 5oz–4lb), ideally pre-salted for 12–24 hours
- 2 tablespoons olive oil
- 2 large leeks, cleaned and thickly sliced
- 1 bulb fennel, cored and sliced
- 4 garlic cloves, crushed (no need to peel)
- 2 bay leaves
- ½ preserved lemon, finely chopped (or zest of 1 fresh lemon)
- 200g (7oz) kale or spring greens, roughly chopped
- Sea salt and freshly ground black pepper

PRE-SALT THE CHICKEN (OPTIONAL BUT WORTH IT)
The day before cooking, rub 2 teaspoons of sea salt all over the chicken, including under the legs and wings. Leave uncovered in the fridge overnight. This helps it stay juicy and seasons the meat all the way through.

PREP YOUR VEG BASE
Heat 1 tablespoon of the olive oil in a large lidded casserole dish over medium heat. Add the leeks, fennel and garlic. Cook for 5–7 minutes, stirring occasionally, until they soften slightly.

BROWN THE CHICKEN
Push the veg to the sides and add the chicken, breast-side down. Brown for 3–4 minutes, then turn and brown the other side. This gives great flavour even though it will mostly cook covered with a lid.

ADD WATER AND AROMATICS
Scatter in the bay leaves and preserved lemon (or lemon zest). Pour in 500ml (17fl oz) water. You want the liquid to come about 2–3cm (1 inch) up the sides of the bird.

COVER AND ROAST
Preheat the oven to 180°C (160°C fan)/350°F/gas 4. Put the lid on and cook for 1 hour 15 minutes.

CRISP THE SKIN AND FINISH THE GREENS
Remove the lid and turn the oven up to 220°C (200°C fan)/425°F/gas 7. Add the chopped greens to the pot, tucking them around the bird. Drizzle the remaining tablespoon of oil over the top. Roast uncovered for a final 25–30 minutes, until the skin is golden and the greens are tender.

REST BEFORE SERVING
Take the dish out of the oven and let the chicken rest in the broth for 10 minutes before carving.

TO SERVE
Carve the chicken and serve with the greens, covered with spoonfuls of the lemony broth and softened veg.

SLOW-COOKED NIHARI (PAKISTANI BEEF STEW)

A slow-cooked spiced beef stew, traditionally eaten at breakfast in South Asia, but perfect for a cold evening in Northern Europe. It's made with bone-in beef, so the broth makes itself as it cooks. The result is rich, warming and full of flavour.

SERVES 4
PREP TIME: 20 MINUTES, PLUS SOAKING TIME (OPTIONAL)
COOK TIME: 4 HOURS (MOSTLY HANDS-OFF)

- 800g (1lb 12oz) bone-in chunks of beef shin or oxtail (ask your butcher for marrow bones if possible)
- 1 tablespoon plain flour or wholewheat flour (atta)
- 3 tablespoons neutral oil (vegetable or sunflower) or ghee
- 1 large piece (7.5cm/3 inches) of fresh ginger, half grated, half finely sliced into matchsticks
- 3 garlic cloves, finely grated
- 1 teaspoon sea salt

FOR THE SPICES
- 1 heaped tablespoon nihari masala (store-bought is fine, like Shan or Laziza)

Or use:
- 1 teaspoon ground coriander
- 1 teaspoon ground cumin
- ½ teaspoon paprika
- ½ teaspoon ground cinnamon
- ¼ teaspoon ground cloves
- ¼ teaspoon fennel seeds
- Pinch of ground nutmeg or mace (optional)

TO FINISH
- Juice of ½ lime or lemon
- Small handful of coriander, roughly chopped
- 1 green chilli, finely sliced (optional)

TO SERVE
Warm naan, chapatti or crusty bread

OPTIONAL PREP
If you're using marrow bones or oxtail, soak them in cold water for 30–60 minutes to draw out any excess blood. Drain and pat dry.

TOAST THE FLOUR
In a dry pan over medium heat, toast the flour for about 3–4 minutes until it turns golden and smells nutty. Set aside.

BROWN THE MEAT
In a large heavy-based pot or Dutch oven, heat 2 tablespoons of the oil or ghee over medium-high heat. Add the beef pieces and brown on all sides for 6–8 minutes. Remove and set aside.

TOAST THE AROMATICS
Lower the heat to medium. Add another tablespoon of oil or ghee, the grated ginger and garlic. Stir for 30 seconds, then add your spice mix. Toast for 1 minute until fragrant, being careful not to burn.

DEGLAZE
Add a splash of water to loosen any stuck bits from the bottom of the pan.

SIMMER
Return the meat to the pot, along with any juices. Pour in 1 litre (35fl oz) cold water and add the salt. Bring to the boil, then skim off any scum from the surface. Lower the heat to the gentlest simmer, cover with the lid slightly ajar and cook for 3 hours, stirring occasionally.

THICKEN
After 3 hours, whisk the toasted flour with a few spoonfuls of hot liquid from the pot to make a slurry. Pour into the stew and stir well. Simmer uncovered for another 30 minutes, until the sauce thickens and the meat is tender. Taste and adjust the salt.

TO SERVE
Stir in the lime juice. Ladle into bowls and top with the ginger matchsticks, coriander and green chilli, if using. Serve with warm naan, chapatti or crusty bread.

CANJA DE GALINHA
(BRAZILIAN CHICKEN & RICE SOUP)

This is Brazilian comfort food at its best – the kind of soup you'd want someone to make for you when you're feeling run down. The rice thickens the soup naturally, and the flavours come from time and care, not shortcuts. Some versions may include fresh tomatoes or potatoes, but we've kept this version beautifully simple.

SERVES 4
PREP TIME: 15 MINUTES
COOK TIME: 1 HOUR

1 tablespoon olive oil
1 onion, finely chopped
2 garlic cloves, crushed
2 carrots, diced
1 celery stick, finely chopped
4 bone-in, skin-on chicken thighs
1 bay leaf
Small handful of parsley stalks (save leaves for garnish)
100g (3½oz) long-grain rice
Sea salt and freshly ground black pepper

TO SERVE
Lemon wedges

FRY THE AROMATICS
Heat the olive oil in a large saucepan over medium heat. Add the onion, garlic, carrots and celery and cook for 8–10 minutes until soft but not coloured.

ADD THE CHICKEN AND HERBS
Add the chicken pieces, bay leaf, parsley stalks and 1.5 litres (52fl oz) water. Bring to a gentle boil, skimming off any foam that rises to the top.

SIMMER THE CHICKEN
Lower the heat and simmer for 30 minutes, partially covered. Remove the chicken and set aside to cool slightly. Discard the bay leaf and parsley stalks.

COOK THE RICE
Add the rice to the pan and cook for 15–20 minutes until tender and the soup has thickened slightly.

FINISH THE SOUP
While the rice is cooking, shred the chicken off the bone and return it to the pan. Simmer for a further 5 minutes to warm through. Season well with salt and black pepper.

TO SERVE
Serve hot, scattered with chopped parsley and a wedge of lemon on the side.

STICKY SHORT RIB BIRRIA (MEXICAN STYLE STEW)

Here, short ribs are cooked on the bone, then finished in a rich, sticky sauce with Mexican flavours. Quick to prep, slow to simmer, this dish is a low-effort showstopper.

SERVES 4
PREP TIME: 30 MINUTES
COOK TIME: 3 HOURS 30 MINUTES, PLUS RESTING

1.2–1.5kg (2lb 10oz–3lb 5oz) bone-in beef short ribs
1 teaspoon sea salt
1 tablespoon neutral oil (such as rapeseed or vegetable)
Freshly ground black pepper

FOR THE SAUCE
4 dried guajillo chillies, deseeded
2 dried ancho chillies, deseeded (or use 1 tablespoon chipotle paste as a shortcut)
1 large tomato, halved
1 large onion, peeled and quartered
4 garlic cloves, unpeeled
1 tablespoon tomato purée
1 tablespoon red wine vinegar
1 teaspoon sugar
1 teaspoon ground cumin
1 teaspoon dried oregano
1 teaspoon smoked paprika
Pinch of sea salt

TO SERVE
Rice or corn tortillas
Sliced spring onions

TOAST AND PREP THE SAUCE BASE
Place the dried chillies, tomato, onion and garlic in a dry frying pan over medium heat. Toast for 3–4 minutes, turning occasionally, until slightly charred. Tip into a saucepan, cover with water and simmer for 10 minutes until softened, then drain.

If using chipotle paste skip the above and roast the tomato, onion and garlic in the oven or grill until slightly blackened.

BLEND THE SAUCE
Peel the garlic, then blend all the softened ingredients with the tomato purée, vinegar, sugar, cumin, oregano, smoked paprika and a pinch of salt. Add a splash of water to help it blend. You want a thick, smooth paste.

BROWN THE BEEF
Season the short ribs all over. In a large oven-safe pot, heat the oil over medium-high heat. Brown the ribs for 3–4 minutes per side in batches. Set aside.

BUILD THE BRAISE
Pour off any excess fat, then return the beef to the pot. Pour the sauce over, add 400ml (14fl oz) water and stir to coat. The liquid should come about two-thirds of the way up the meat.

SLOW COOK
Preheat the oven to 150°C (130°C fan)/300°F/gas 2. Cover the pot with a tight-fitting lid and cook for 3 hours. Check once halfway and turn the ribs.

REDUCE UNTIL STICKY
After 3 hours, carefully remove the ribs and set aside in a warm place. Skim off some fat (or leave it in for richness). Put the pot back on the hob over medium heat and simmer uncovered for 15–20 minutes until the sauce thickens slightly. You want it sticky enough to coat the meat, but still spoonable.

FINISH AND SERVE
Return the ribs to the pot and gently turn to coat in the sticky sauce. Rest for 10–15 minutes, then serve with rice or tortillas and sliced spring onions.

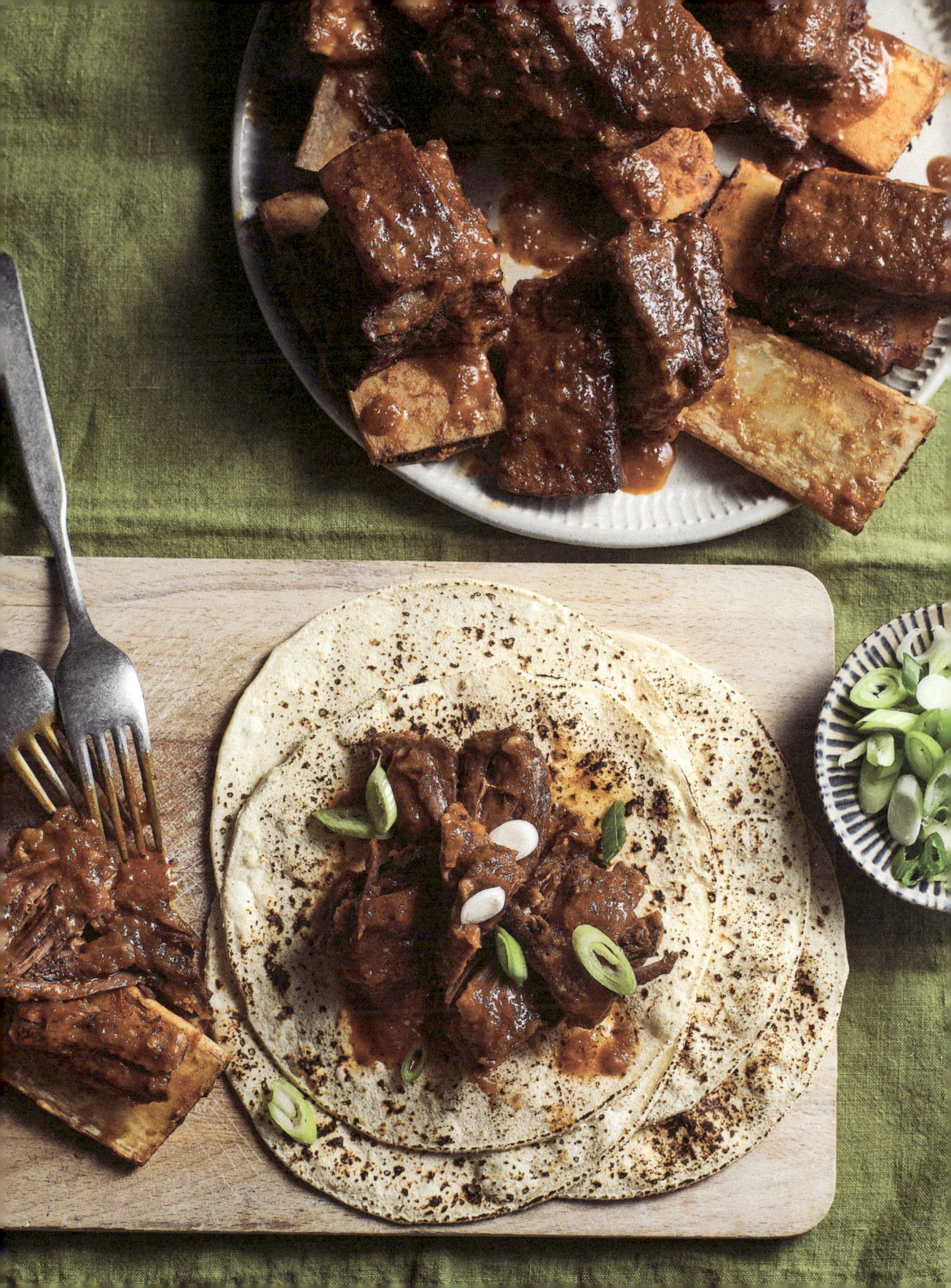

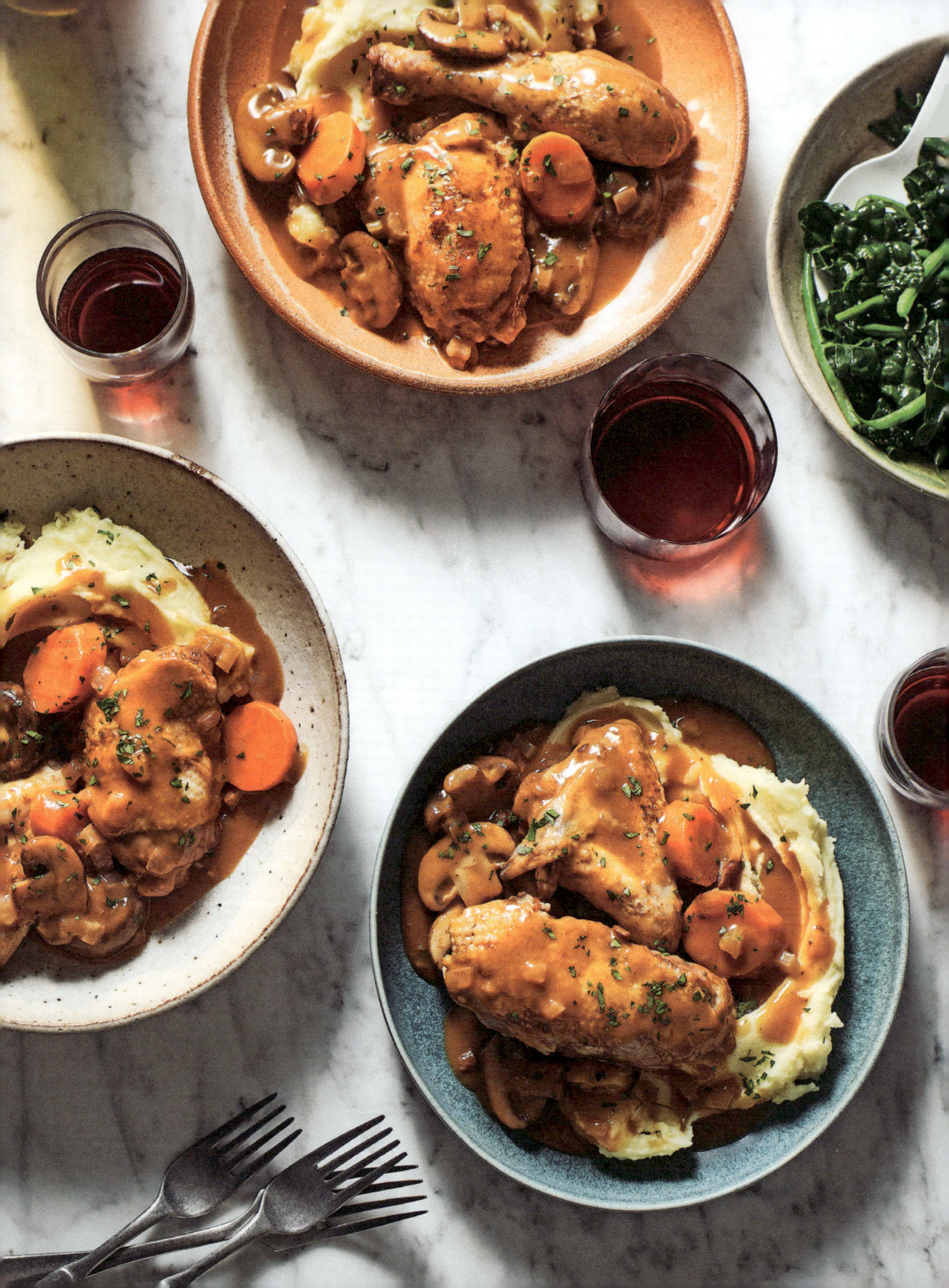

COQ AU VIN

This is one of those classic French dishes that sounds fancy but is deliciously simple home cooking at its finest. It's rich, hearty and perfect for slow Sunday cooking. It also reheats brilliantly the next day.

SERVES 4
PREP TIME: 25 MINUTES
COOK TIME: 2 HOURS

FOR THE MEAT AND BROTH
1 whole chicken, jointed into 8 pieces (or 8 bone-in, skin-on thighs)
Splash of neutral oil (vegetable or sunflower)
100g (3½oz) pancetta or streaky bacon, diced
1 large onion, chopped
2 carrots, sliced into thick rounds
2 celery sticks, chopped
3 garlic cloves, crushed
2 tablespoons tomato purée
2 bay leaves
4 sprigs thyme sprigs
Small bunch of parsley stalks (save the leaves for garnish)
400ml (14fl oz) red wine (Burgundy or similar, not too heavy)
Sea salt and freshly ground black pepper

TO FINISH
2 tablespoons butter
200g (7oz) chestnut mushrooms, halved if large
Pinch of salt
1 tablespoon plain flour

TO SERVE
Mashed potatoes, crusty bread or buttered greens

BROWN THE CHICKEN
Pat the chicken dry and season with salt and pepper. In a large casserole dish, heat a splash of oil over medium-high heat. Brown the chicken pieces in batches, skin-side down first, for 5–6 minutes until golden. Remove and set aside.

COOK THE PANCETTA AND VEG
Lower the heat and add the pancetta to the same pan. Fry for 4–5 minutes until just crisp. Add the onion, carrots, celery and garlic. Cook gently for 8–10 minutes until softened and golden. Stir in the tomato purée and cook for 1–2 minutes. Return the chicken to the pan along with any resting juices.

ADD THE AROMATICS
Tie the bay, thyme and parsley stalks together with kitchen string and add to the pot. Pour in the wine and simmer for 5 minutes to reduce slightly, scraping the base of the pan.

ADD THE WATER AND BRAISE
Add 500ml (17fl oz) water. Bring to a gentle simmer, cover loosely with a lid and cook over low heat for 1 hour 15 minutes. The chicken should be very tender but not falling apart.

COOK THE MUSHROOMS
Meanwhile, in a frying pan, heat 1 tablespoon of the butter and sauté the mushrooms with a pinch of salt for 6–8 minutes until golden and just cooked through. Set aside.

THICKEN THE SAUCE
Once the chicken is cooked, remove and set aside. Discard the herb bundle. In a small bowl, mash 1 tablespoon of the butter with the flour to form a paste. Whisk this into the sauce and cook for 8–10 minutes until slightly thickened.

FINISH AND SERVE
Return the chicken and mushrooms to the dish and warm through for 5–10 minutes. Season to taste. Scatter over chopped parsley leaves before serving.

TO SERVE
Serve with mashed potatoes, crusty bread or buttered greens.

OSSOBUCO ALLA MILANESE (BRAISED VEAL SHANKS)

This dish shows exactly what happens when you cook with the bone instead of just adding broth. You get depth, richness and that unmistakably silky texture that comes from letting time and heat work their magic. Ossobuco means 'bone with a hole'; you'll see why when you serve it!

SERVES 4
PREP TIME: 20 MINUTES
COOKING TIME: 3 HOURS

4 bone-in veal shanks (about 300g/10½oz) each (or use bone-in beef shin if easier to find, just cook slightly longer)
2 tablespoons plain flour
2 tablespoons olive oil
1 onion, finely chopped
1 carrot, finely chopped
1 celery stick, finely chopped
2 garlic cloves, sliced
150ml (5fl oz) dry white wine or white vermouth
1 tablespoon tomato purée
1 bay leaf
1 fresh rosemary sprig or a pinch of dried
Sea salt and freshly ground black pepper

FOR THE GREMOLATA (OPTIONAL BUT RECOMMENDED)
Zest of 1 lemon
1 garlic clove, very finely chopped or grated
Small handful of parsley, finely chopped

TO SERVE
Risotto (ideally with saffron), mashed potato, polenta or crusty bread
Wilted greens or roasted veg

PREP THE MEAT
Pat the shanks dry. Season generously, then dust lightly with flour. This helps them brown and thickens the sauce.

BROWN IN BATCHES
Heat the oil in a large, heavy-based pan or casserole dish. Sear the shanks until golden brown (about 3–4 minutes per side). Don't crowd the pan – do this in batches if needed. Set aside.

BUILD THE BASE
Turn the heat down a little. Add the onion, carrot, celery and a pinch of salt. Cook gently for 6–8 minutes until soft and starting to colour. Stir in the garlic and cook for another minute.

DEGLAZE WITH WINE
Pour in the wine or vermouth and let it bubble for a minute, scraping up any browned bits from the pan. Stir in 400ml (14fl oz) water, the tomato purée, bay leaf and rosemary.

RETURN THE MEAT
Nestle the shanks back into the pan. The liquid should come halfway up the sides of the meat – top up with a splash more water if needed. Bring to a gentle simmer.

SLOW COOK
Preheat the oven to 180°C (160°C fan)/350°F/gas 4. Cover tightly and cook for 2½–3 hours, turning the shanks once or twice. The meat is done when it pulls away from the bone with a fork and the marrow has mostly melted into the sauce.

MAKE THE GREMOLATA
Mix together the lemon zest, garlic and parsley.

FINAL TOUCHES
If the sauce seems thin, remove the lid and simmer for about 10–15 minutes to reduce slightly. Taste and adjust the seasoning.

TO SERVE
Serve the shanks with the sauce spooned over and sprinkle with gremolata.

CANTONESE BRAISED DUCK LEGS

This dish is all about the balance of savoury, sweet and warming, aromatic flavours. Braising the duck legs slowly in soy and Shaoxing wine gives the meat that fall-off-the-bone tenderness, steeped in a deep, sticky sauce. This also works beautifully with skin-on chicken thighs if you'd prefer.

SERVES 4
PREP TIME: 20 MINUTES
COOK TIME: 2 HOURS 30 MINUTES

4 duck legs
4 garlic cloves, crushed
5cm (2 inch) piece of fresh ginger, sliced
2 spring onions, cut into 5cm (2 inch) lengths
1 star anise
1 cinnamon stick
1 strip of dried orange peel or 2 strips of fresh orange zest
3 tablespoons dark soy sauce
3 tablespoons light soy sauce
3 tablespoons Shaoxing wine or dry sherry
1 tablespoon oyster sauce
1 tablespoon soft brown sugar

TO FINISH
1 teaspoon cornflour mixed with 1 tablespoon cold water (optional, to thicken)

TO SERVE
Steamed rice or steamed greens

BROWN THE DUCK
Pat the duck legs dry with kitchen paper. Place them skin-side down in a cold, wide pan and turn the heat to medium. Let the fat render out slowly and cook for 8–10 minutes until the skin is deep golden. Turn and cook the other side for 2–3 minutes. Remove and set aside. Pour off most of the fat, leaving about 1 tablespoon in the pan.

FRY THE AROMATICS
Add the garlic, ginger, spring onions, star anise, cinnamon and orange peel or zest to the pan. Fry for 2–3 minutes until fragrant but not charred.

ADD THE BRAISING LIQUID
Pour in 500ml (17fl oz) water, both soy sauces, Shaoxing wine, oyster sauce and the brown sugar. Stir well to combine and bring to a gentle simmer.

BRAISE THE DUCK
Return the duck legs to the pan, skin-side up. The liquid should come about halfway up the sides of the legs. Cover with a lid or foil and simmer over low heat for 2 hours, turning the legs once halfway through. The meat should be tender but still holding together.

REDUCE AND THICKEN
Remove the duck legs and keep warm. Turn the heat up and reduce the sauce for 10–15 minutes until slightly thickened. If you want a glossier finish, stir in the cornflour slurry and cook for 2–3 minutes until thickened and shiny.

FINISH AND SERVE
Return the duck to the pan to coat in the sauce or spoon the sauce over the top.

TO SERVE
Serve with rice or steamed greens, with plenty of sauce. Leftovers can be shredded and added to noodles or fried rice the next day. The flavour only gets better overnight!

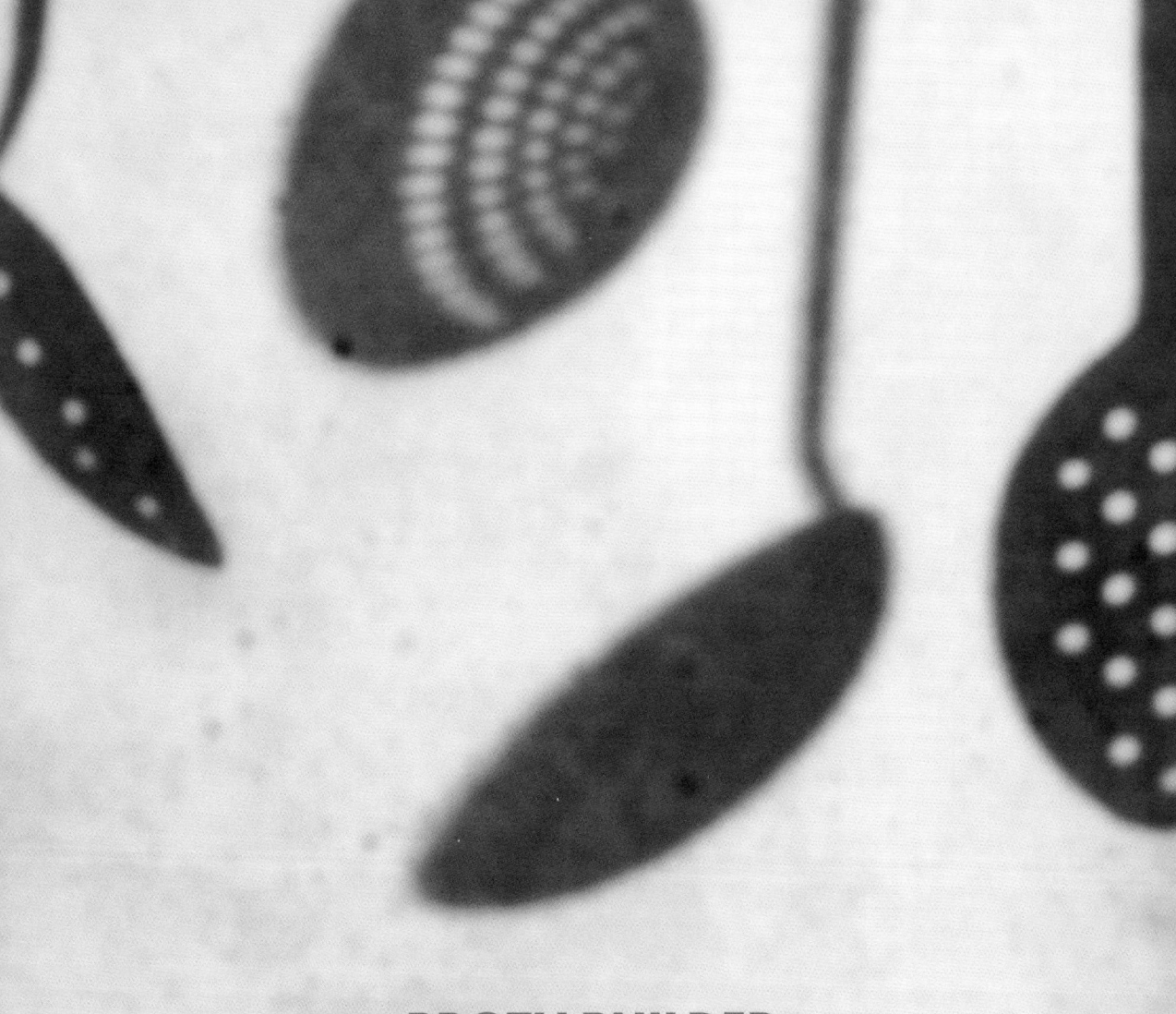

BROTH BUILDER

There's something really satisfying about making a good old broth bowl from scratch with whatever you've got in your fridge. This Broth Builder is your go-to for mix and matching your way to a quick and deliciously nourishing meal. Whether you're craving something light and simple or rich and comforting, there are plenty of ideas here for you to pick and choose from!

Just start at the left with your brothy base and work your way across, picking one or two things from each column. Use what's in season, what's in your kitchen and what tastes good to you. Quantities are for one person, but you can easily scale them up if needed.

START WITH A BASE BROTH	CHOOSE A PROTEIN	ADD YOUR VEGETABLES (2+)	CHOOSE A CARB	FLAVOUR AND SEASONING	ADDITION
300ML (10½FL OZ) PER PERSON	A SMALL HANDFUL (75–100G/ 2½–3½OZ)	2 HANDFULS TOTAL (150G/5½OZ)	80–100G (2¾–3½OZ) COOKED	1–2 TSP (PASTE, SAUCE) 1 TBSP (CREAM)	1 TBSP (OR WHOLE EGG)
CHICKEN	SHREDDED CHICKEN THIGH	LEEKS, FINELY SLICED	PEARL BARLEY	CREAM	JAMMY BOILED EGG
BEEF	MEXICAN-SPICED CHICKEN	CARROTS, JULIENNED	GNOCCHI	PESTO	CRISPY CHILLI OIL
FISH	CHORIZO	CELERY, DICED	NOODLES (EGG, UDON, GLASS)	MISO PASTE	CHOPPED PEANUTS
	PULLED BEEF	CAVOLO NERO OR SPINACH, TORN	RICE (JASMINE, SUSHI, WILD, BROWN)	GOCHUJANG	SPRING ONIONS
	MEATBALLS (PORK OR BEEF)	OYSTER MUSHROOMS	BEANS (BLACK OR CANNELLINI)	PEANUT BUTTER	CHOPPED FRESH HERBS
	SHAVED STEAK	CHINESE CABBAGE, SHREDDED	DUMPLINGS OR GYOZA	HARISSA	FRESH RED CHILLI
	TEMPEH	COURGETTE RIBBONS	NEW POTATOES	CHIPOTLE PASTE	GRATED CHEESE
	FIRM TOFU	ROASTED BEETROOT OR BUTTERNUT SQUASH	FREEKEH	SOY SAUCE	ROASTED CHICKPEAS
	WHITE FISH (COD, HADDOCK)	CHARGRILLED PEPPERS	PASTA (BROKEN LINGUINE, STELLINE, ORZO)	SRIRACHA	KIMCHI
	MUSSELS	EDAMAME BEANS	TORTELLINI	COCONUT MILK	SOURDOUGH CROUTONS
	SALMON	BROCCOLI FLORETS OR TENDERSTEM		TAHINI	CRISPY PANCETTA
Warm your broth in a pan to a gentle simmer	Cook separately in a pan (grilled, pan-fried, roasted, etc.) then add to broth	Prep to taste: slice thinly, roast, sauté, steam or add directly to broth	Cook carbs separately if needed (e.g. rice, pasta), or directly in broth	Add a dollop of flavour and stir into the broth. Start small, taste and adjust	Add just before serving for texture, crunch or creaminess

REFERENCES

GUT HEALTH

Bone broth is rich in glutamine and glycine, which support gut lining repair, reduce inflammation and improve digestion.

Chen J, Yang Y, Yang Y, Dai Z, Kim IH, Wu G, Wu Z. 'Dietary Supplementation with Glycine Enhances Intestinal Mucosal Integrity and Ameliorates Inflammation in C57BL/6J Mice with High-Fat Diet-Induced Obesity', J Nutr. 2021 Jul 1;151(7):1769-1778. doi: 10.1093/jn/nxab058. PMID: 33830211.

Genton L, Pruijm M, Teta D, Bassi I, Cani PD, Gaïa N, Herrmann FR, Marangon N, Mareschal J, Muccioli GG, Stoermann C, Suriano F, Wurzner-Ghajarzadeh A, Lazarevic V, Schrenzel J. 'Gut barrier and microbiota changes with glycine and branched-chain amino acid supplementation in chronic haemodialysis patients', J Cachexia Sarcopenia Muscle. 2021 Dec;12(6):1527-1539. doi: 10.1002/jcsm.12781. Epub 2021 Sep 18. PMID: 34535959; PMCID: PMC8718035.

Wang B, Wu G, Zhou Z, Dai Z, Sun Y, Ji Y, Li W, Wang W, Liu C, Han F, Wu Z. 'Glutamine and intestinal barrier function', Amino Acids. 2015 Oct;47(10):2143-54. doi: 10.1007/s00726-014-1773-4. Epub 2014 Jun 26. PMID: 24965526.

Zhong Z, Wheeler MD, Li X, Froh M, Schemmer P, Yin M, Bunzendaul H, Bradford B, Lemasters JJ. 'L-Glycine: a novel antiinflammatory, immunomodulatory, and cytoprotective agent', Curr Opin Clin Nutr Metab Care. 2003 Mar;6(2):229-40. doi: 10.1097/00075197-200303000-00013. PMID: 12589194.

IMMUNE HEALTH

Glycine, glutamine and zinc in bone broth reduce inflammation, support immune cell function and boost antioxidant production (via glutathione), helping fight infections and maintain immune balance.

Newsholme P. 'Why is L-glutamine metabolism important to cells of the immune system in health, postinjury, surgery or infection?' J Nutr. 2001 Sep;131(9 Suppl):2515S-22S; discussion 2523S-4S. doi: 10.1093/jn/131.9.2515S. PMID: 11533304.

Prasad AS. 'Zinc in human health: effect of zinc on immune cells', Mol Med. 2008 May-Jun;14(5-6):353-7. doi: 10.2119/2008-00033.Prasad. PMID: 18385818; PMCID: PMC2277319.

Wheeler MD, Ikejema K, Enomoto N, Stacklewitz RF, Seabra V, Zhong Z, Yin M, Schemmer P, Rose ML, Rusyn I, Bradford B, Thurman RG. 'Glycine: a new anti-inflammatory immunonutrient', Cell Mol Life Sci. 1999 Nov 30;56(9-10):843-56. doi: 10.1007/s000180050030. PMID: 11212343; PMCID: PMC11147092.

SKIN HEALTH

Collagen/gelatine and glycine support skin repair, hydration and elasticity. The gut-skin axis means improved gut health can reduce inflammation-driven skin issues.

Al-Atif H. 'Collagen Supplements for Aging and Wrinkles: A Paradigm Shift in the Fields of Dermatology and Cosmetics', Dermatol Pract Concept. 2022 Jan 1;12(1):e2022018. doi: 10.5826/dpc.1201a18. PMID: 35223163; PMCID: PMC8824545.

Bolke L, Schlippe G, Gerß J, Voss W. 'A Collagen Supplement Improves Skin Hydration, Elasticity, Roughness, and Density: Results of a Randomized, Placebo-Controlled, Blind Study', Nutrients. 2019 Oct 17;11(10):2494. doi: 10.3390/nu11102494. PMID: 31627309; PMCID: PMC6835901.

Takaoka M, Okumura S, Seki T, Ohtani M. 'Effect of amino-acid intake on physical conditions and skin state: a randomized, double-blind, placebo-controlled, crossover trial', J Clin Biochem Nutr. 2019 Jul;65(1):52-58. doi: 10.3164/jcbn.18-108. Epub 2019 May 24. PMID: 31379414; PMCID: PMC6667387.

HEALTHY HAIR

Zinc and collagen in bone broth support hair follicle health, keratin synthesis and scalp repair.

Guo EL, Katta R. 'Diet and hair loss: effects of nutrient deficiency and supplement use', Dermatol Pract Concept. 2017 Jan 31;7(1):1-10. doi: 10.5826/dpc.0701a01. PMID: 28243487; PMCID: PMC5315033.

Kil MS, Kim CW, Kim SS. 'Analysis of serum zinc and copper concentrations in hair loss', Ann Dermatol. 2013 Nov;25(4):405-9. doi: 10.5021/ad.2013.25.4.405. Epub 2013 Nov 30. PMID: 24371385; PMCID: PMC3870206.

FURTHER READING

BONE HEALTH

Collagen/gelatine and glucosamine in bone broth support joint cartilage and reduce inflammation, potentially easing arthritis or joint pain. Minerals aid bone health.

Benito-Ruiz, P., Camacho-Zambrano, M., Carrillo-Arcentales, J., Mestanza-Peralta, M., Vallejo-Flores, C., Vargas-López, S., Villacís-Tamayo, R., and Zurita-Gavilanes, L. (2009). 'A randomized controlled trial on the efficacy and safety of a food ingredient, collagen hydrolysate, for improving joint comfort', International Journal of Food Sciences and Nutrition, 60, 113 - 99. https://doi.org/10.1080/09637480802498820.

Campos LD, Santos Junior VA, Pimentel JD, Carregã GLF, Cazarin CBB. 'Collagen supplementation in skin and orthopedic diseases: A review of the literature', Heliyon. 2023 Mar 28;9(4):e14961. doi: 10.1016/j.heliyon.2023.e14961. PMID: 37064452; PMCID: PMC10102402.

WEIGHT MANAGEMENT

Gelatine in bone broth promotes satiety, helping control appetite and supporting weight management.

Hochstenbach-Waelen A, Westerterp-Plantenga MS, Veldhorst MA, Westerterp KR. 'Single-protein casein and gelatin diets affect energy expenditure similarly but substrate balance and appetite differently in adults', J Nutr. 2009 Dec;139(12):2285-92. doi: 10.3945/jn.109.110403. Epub 2009 Oct 28. PMID: 19864402.

Rubio IG, Castro G, Zanini AC, Medeiros-Neto G. 'Oral ingestion of a hydrolyzed gelatin meal in subjects with normal weight and in obese patients: Postprandial effect on circulating gut peptides, glucose and insulin', Eat Weight Disord. 2008 Mar;13(1):48-53. doi: 10.1007/BF03327784. PMID: 18319637.

Want to dive deeper into the world of bone broth, its benefits and creative ways to use it? Here's a curated list of books to expand your knowledge and inspire your cooking.

Nourishing Broth: An Old-Fashioned Remedy for the Modern World by Sally Fallon Morell and Kaayla T. Daniel (Grand Central Publishing, 2014)

Nourishing Diets: How Paleo, Ancestral and Traditional Peoples Really Ate by Sally Fallon Morell (Life and Style, 2018)

Better Broths & Healing Tonics: 75 Bone Broth and Vegetarian Broth-Based Recipes for Everyone by Jill Shepphard Davenport and Kara N Fitzgerald (Hachette Go, 2022)

The Bone Broth Secret: Recipes and Wisdom for Health, Beauty, and Strength by Louise Hay and Heather Dane (Hay House Inc., 2016)

Broth and Stock from the Nourished Kitchen by Jennifer McGruther (Ten Speed Press, 2016)

The Bare Bones Broth Cookbook: 125 Gut-Friendly Recipes by Katherine and Ryan Harvey (Harper Wave, 2016)

Ramen Forever: Recipes for Ramen Success by Tim Anderson (Hardie Grant Books UK, 2023)

Catching Fire: How Cooking Made Us Human by Richard Wrangham (Profile Books, 2010)

Soup Through the Ages: A Culinary History with Period Recipes by Victoria Rumble (MacFarland, 2009)

ENDNOTES

1 Reilly DM, Lozano J. 'Skin collagen through the lifestages: importance for skin health and beauty', *Plastic and Aesthetic Research*. 2021;8:2. http://dx.doi.org/10.20517/2347-9264.2020.153

2 Zhong Z, Wheeler MD, Li X, Froh M, Schemmer P, Yin M, Bunzendaul H, Bradford B, Lemasters JJ. 'L-Glycine: a novel antiinflammatory, immunomodulatory, and cytoprotective agent', *Current Opinion in Clinical Nutrition & Metabolic Care*. 2003 Mar;6(2):229-40. doi: 10.1097/00075197-200303000-00013.

3 Proksch E, Segger D, Degwert J, Schunck M, Zague V, Oesser S. 'Oral supplementation of specific collagen peptides has beneficial effects on human skin physiology: a double-blind, placebo-controlled study', *Skin Pharmacology and Physiology*. 2014;27(1):47–55. https://pubmed.ncbi.nlm.nih.gov/23949208/

4 Guo EL, Katta R. 'Diet and hair loss: effects of nutrient deficiency and supplement use', *Dermatology Practical & Conceptual*. 2017 Jan 31;7(1):1-10. doi: 10.5826/dpc.0701a01.

5 Peng HY, Man CF, Xu J, Fan Y. 'Elevated homocysteine levels and risk of cardiovascular and all-cause mortality: a meta-analysis of prospective studies', *Journal of Zhejiang University Science B*. 2015 Jan;16(1):78-86. doi: 10.1631/jzus.B1400183

6 Feng X. 'Chemical and Biochemical Basis of Cell-Bone Matrix Interaction in Health and Disease', *Current Chemical Biology*. 2009 May 1;3(2):189-196. doi: 10.2174/187231309788166398.

7 Razak MA, Begum PS, Viswanath B, Rajagopal S. 'Multifarious Beneficial Effect of Nonessential Amino Acid, Glycine: A Review', *Oxidative Medicine and Cellular Longevity*. 2017;2017:1716701. doi: 10.1155/2022/9857645.

8 Donald A. Vessey 'The biochemical basis for the conjugation of bile acids with either glycine or taurine', *Biochemical Journal* 15 August 1978; 174 (2): 621–626. https://doi.org/10.1042/bj1740621

9 Gundersen RY, Vaagenes P, Breivik T, Fonnum F, Opstad PK. 'Glycine – an important neurotransmitter and cytoprotective agent', *Acta Anaesthesiologica Scandinavica*. 2005 Sep;49(8):1108-16. doi: 10.1111/j.1399-6576.2005.00786.x.

10 Morrione TG, Seifter S. 'Alteration in the collagen content of the human uterus during pregnancy and post partum involution', *Journal of Experimental Medicine*. 1962 Feb 1;115(2):357-65. doi: 10.1084/jem.115.2.357.

11 Paddon-Jones, Douglas; Rasmussen, Blake B. 'Dietary protein recommendations and the prevention of sarcopenia', *Current Opinion in Clinical Nutrition and Metabolic Care* 12(1):p 86-90, January 2009. | doi: 10.1097/MCO.0b013e32831cef8b

12 Gallicchio L, Miller SR, Kiefer J, Greene T, Zacur HA, Flaws JA. 'Change in body mass index, weight, and hot flashes: a longitudinal analysis from the midlife women's health study', *Journal of Women's Health (Larchmont)*. 2014 Mar;23(3):231-7. doi: 10.1089/jwh.2013.4526.

13 Rubio IG, Castro G, Zanini AC, Medeiros-Neto G. 'Oral ingestion of a hydrolyzed gelatinemeal in subjects with normal weight and in obese patients: Postprandial effect on circulating gut peptides, glucose and insulin', *Eating and Weight Disorders*. 2008 Mar;13(1):48-53. doi: 10.1007/BF03327784.

14 https://frejafoods.com/pages/nhs-trial
 *Trialled in an NHS menopause & gut health surgery with 28 women experiencing menopausal symptons

15 McAfee AJ, McSorley EM, Cuskelly GJ, Fearon AM, Moss BW, Beattie JA, Wallace JM, Bonham MP, Strain JJ. 'Red meat from animals offered a grass diet increases plasma and platelet n-3 PUFA in healthy consumers', *British Journal of Nutrition*. 2011 Jan;105(1):80-9. doi: 10.1017/S0007114510003090.

ACKNOWLEDGEMENTS

This book has no single author. It's a collective effort from the Freja team, a group of bone broth evangelists who care deeply about simple, nourishing food and the benefits it can bring. Every member of the team helped bring it to life; with special thanks to Rosie Wildgoose, Lara Southwell-Moore, Tamsin Exley, Lily Convey and Jordan Moore for their creativity, skill and persistence along the way.

A big thanks goes to Tom Asker, Simeon Greenway, Georgina Atsiaris and to the whole team at HarperCollins for their guidance, enthusiasm and belief in this project. And also to the fantastic photography team Andrew Burton, Pippa Leon, Georgia Rudd and Faye Wears for capturing our recipes so beautifully.

Finally, thank you to our customers – the people who inspire everything we do. You've shared your stories of how bone broth has supported your health, recovery and wellbeing, and shown us countless ways to use it, many of which have found their way into this book.

INDEX

A
Africa 23
ageing 26
amino acids 14–15
anchovies
    bone broth bolognese 194
    one-pot puttanesca 163
apples: oven-braised red cabbage with horseradish cream 127
apricots: classic chicken & apricot tagine 185
aromatics: bone broth ingredients 42–47
arroz caldoso (brothy rice with wild mushrooms) 146
Asia 21–22, 153, 216
asparagus: creamy asparagus soup with lemon & pancetta pangrattato 95
aubergines
    baked rigatoni with aubergine 162
    braised aubergine with spring 132
    cheat's ratatouille 122
    Thai green chicken curry 199
avgolemono (Greek egg & lemon chicken soup) 78
avocado: sopa de lima (Mexican lime & chicken soup) 81

B
bacon
    baked potato soup with sour cream & chives 91
    coq au vin 221
    feijoada (Brazilian black bean stew) 148
barley: Scotch beef & barley broth 109
basil:
    baked rigatoni with aubergine 162
    bo kho (Vietnamese beef stew) 205
    cheat's ratatouille 122
    Italian pesto & gnocchi soup 116
    gazpacho 96
    Vietnamese beef pho 177
bay leaves: bone broth use and method 45

beans
    braised aubergine with spring onion 132
    Bristol baked beans with crispy pork belly 154
    fasolia (lamb & white bean stew) 141
    feijoada (Brazilian black bean stew) 148
    Italian pesto & gnocchi soup 116
    Jamaican oxtail beans 212
    rustic French cassoulet 147
    Sri Lankan vegetable & coconut soup 101
    sumac-spiced tomatoes & green beans 120
    Thai green chicken curry 199
    Tuscan ribollita-style minestrone 104
    ultimate chilli 180–181
beansprouts
    Malaysian monkfish laksa 173
    Vietnamese beef pho 177
    yukgaejang (Korean spicy beef soup) 84
beef
    beef kofta curry 200
    beef rendang with carrot & cabbage salad 202–204
    bo kho (Vietnamese beef stew) 205
    bone broth bolognese 194
    bone broth cuts 36
    cottage pie with herby lemon mash 192–193
    Hungarian smoky beef goulash 113
    Italian wedding soup 75
    Jamaican oxtail beans 212
    Liverpudlian beef scouse broth 77
    miyeok-guk (Korean seaweed soup) 86
    red wine, porcini & beef cheek ragu 191
    Scotch beef & barley broth 109
    Sichuan spicy beef noodles 174

    slow-cooked nihari (Pakistani beef stew) 216
    sticky short rib birria (Mexican style stew) 218
    stifado (Greek beef stew) with feta mash 189
    ultimate chilli 180–181
    Vietnamese beef pho 177
    yukgaejang (Korean spicy beef soup) 84
beef bone broth
    arroz caldoso (brothy rice with wild mushrooms) 146
    baked rigatoni with aubergine 162
    beef kofta curry 200
    beef rendang with carrot & cabbage salad 202–204
    beef tomato soup 94
    best-ever beef bone broth gravy 207
    bloody bullshot 67
    bo kho (Vietnamese beef stew) 205
    bone broth bolognese 194
    bone broth hot chocolate 67
    boozy beef mushrooms on toast 128
    'boulangoise' (boulangère meets dauphinoise) 125
    braised aubergine with spring 132
    Bristol baked beans with crispy pork belly 154
    bulletproof coffee bone broth 66
    chunky beetroot borscht 107
    cottage pie with herby lemon mash 192–193
    eggs Florentine soup 90
    feijoada (Brazilian black bean stew) 148
    fondant potatoes 130
    Hungarian smoky beef goulash 113
    Liverpudlian beef scouse broth 77
    miyeok-guk (Korean seaweed soup) 86

    one-pot puttanesca 163
    oven-braised red cabbage with horseradish cream 127
    proper beef tea 60
    red wine, porcini & beef cheek ragu 191
    Scotch beef & barley broth 109
    Sichuan spicy beef noodles 174
    spring greens with garlic & lemon 126
    stifado (Greek beef stew) with feta mash 189
    tortellini in brodo 158
    Tuscan ribollita-style minestrone 104
    ultimate chilli 180–181
    ultimate French onion soup 110
    umami Marmite tea 65
    Vietnamese beef pho 177
    youvetsi (Greek orzo with lamb) 166
    yukgaejang (Korean spicy beef soup) 84
beetroot: chunky beetroot borscht 107
bile salts 14–15
bisque, fennel & crab 98
black beans: feijoada (Brazilian black bean stew) 148
bloody bullshot 67
bo kho (Vietnamese beef stew) 205
bolognese, bone broth 194
bone broth
    broth builder 224–225
    buying 55
    compared to stock 16
    composition 13–15
    culture 13, 21–23
    ingredients 34–47
    method 48–49
    pork bone broth 50
    problem solving 53–55
    roasting bones 40–41
    storage 50
bone health 26
borscht, chunky beetroot 107
bouillabaisse, cheat's 82
'boulangoise' (boulangère meets dauphinoise) 125

brandy: fennel & crab bisque 98
Brazilian black bean stew 148
Brazilian chicken & rice soup 217
bread
  boozy beef mushrooms on toast 128
  leek & mussel chowder in a sourdough bowl 114
  ultimate French onion soup 110
breadcrumbs
  creamed shallots & garlic with pangrattato 121
  creamy asparagus soup with lemon & pancetta pangrattato 95
  Italian wedding soup 75
  rustic French cassoulet 147
Bristol baked beans with crispy pork belly 154
broth builder 224–225
bulletproof coffee bone broth 66
butter beans: Jamaican oxtail beans 212
butter
  bulletproof coffee bone broth 66
  one-pot butter chicken curry 190
butternut squash: harissa butternut squash soup 100

C
cabbage
  beef rendang with carrot & cabbage salad 202–204
  chunky beetroot borscht 107
  oven-braised red cabbage with horseradish cream 127
  rustic cabbage & smoked sausage broth 85
calcium 15, 26
canja de galinha (Brazilian chicken & rice soup) 217
cannellini beans: Tuscan ribollita-style minestrone 104
Cantonese braised duck legs 223

capers: one-pot puttanesca 163
cardamom:
  beef kofta curry 200
  spiced chai bone broth 66
carrots
  beef rendang with carrot & cabbage salad 202–204
  bo kho (Vietnamese beef stew) 205
  bone broth bolognese 194
  bone broth use and method 44
  canja de galinha (Brazilian chicken & rice soup) 217
  chunky beetroot borscht 107
  comforting chicken & dumplings 201
  coq au vin 221
  cottage pie with herby lemon mash 192–193
  fennel & crab bisque 98
  instant ramen upgrade 168
  Italian penicillin soup 161
  Italian wedding soup 75
  Liverpudlian beef scouse broth 77
  Nordic salmon & dill chowder 108
  one-pot chicken & leek pie 182–184
  ossobuco alla Milanese (braised veal shanks) 222
  perfect Puy lentils 138
  red wine, porcini & beef cheek ragu 191
  rosół (classic Polish noodle soup) 171
  rustic cabbage & smoked sausage broth 85
  rustic French cassoulet 147
  Scotch beef & barley broth 109
  Sri Lankan vegetable & coconut soup 101
  Tuscan ribollita-style minestrone 104
  ultimate chilli 180–181
cashews: beef rendang with carrot & cabbage salad 202–204

cavolo nero
  Italian wedding soup 75
  Tuscan ribollita-style minestrone 104
celery
  bone broth bolognese 194
  bone broth use and method 44
  canja de galinha (Brazilian chicken & rice soup) 217
  cheat's bouillabaisse (classic French fish soup) 82
  comforting chicken & dumplings 201
  coq au vin 221
  cottage pie with herby lemon mash 192–193
  Italian penicillin soup 161
  Italian wedding soup 75
  Liverpudlian beef scouse broth 77
  one-pan prawn jambalaya 145
  one-pot chicken & leek pie 182–184
  ossobuco alla Milanese (braised veal shanks) 222
  perfect Puy lentils 138
  red wine, porcini & beef cheek ragu 191
  rosół (classic Polish noodle soup) 171
  rustic cabbage & smoked sausage broth 85
  rustic French cassoulet 147
  Scotch beef & barley broth 109
  Tuscan ribollita-style minestrone 104
celery salt: bloody bullshot 67
Central America 23
chai bone broth, spiced 66
chard: spring greens with garlic & lemon 126
cheat's bouillabaisse (classic French fish soup) 82
cheat's ratatouille 122
cheese
  baked potato soup with sour cream & chives 91

  baked rigatoni with aubergine 162
  'boulangoise' (boulangère meets dauphinoise) 125
  eggs Florentine soup 90
  Italian penicillin soup 161
  Italian wedding soup 75
  one-pot chicken & leek pie 182–184
  polenta quattro formaggi (four cheese polenta) 142
  risotto blanco 152
  stifado (Greek beef stew) with feta mash 189
  tagliolini al tartufo (pasta with white truffle) 167
  tortellini in brodo 158
  Tuscan ribollita-style minestrone 104
  ultimate French onion soup 110
chicken
  avgolemono (Greek egg & lemon chicken soup) 78
  bone broth cuts 35
  canja de galinha (Brazilian chicken & rice soup) 217
  chicken vindaloo with a cooling raita 196–197
  Chinese chicken & sweetcorn soup 76
  classic chicken & apricot tagine 185
  comforting chicken & dumplings 201
  coq au vin 221
  instant ramen upgrade 168
  Italian penicillin soup 161
  Mexican chicken with fresh tomato salsa 187–188
  one-pot butter chicken curry 190
  one-pot chicken & leek pie 182–184
  pot roast chicken with greens & lemon 215
  rosół (classic Polish noodle soup) 171
  sopa de lima (Mexican lime & chicken soup) 81

soto ayam (Indonesian chicken noodle soup) 172
Thai green chicken curry 199
chicken bone broth
  avgolemono (Greek egg & lemon chicken soup) 78
  baked potato soup with sour cream & chives 91
  best-ever chicken bone broth gravy 209
  caramelised onion freekeh pilaf 140
  cheat's ratatouille 122
  chicken vindaloo with a cooling raita 196–197
  Chinese chicken & sweetcorn soup 76
  classic chicken & apricot tagine 185
  classic cream of mushroom soup 97
  comforting chicken & dumplings 201
  congee with sliced belly pork 153
  creamed shallots & garlic with pangrattato 121
  creamy asparagus soup with lemon & pancetta pangrattato 95
  creamy mustard-glazed fennel 131
  fasolia (lamb & white bean stew) 141
  fondant potatoes 130
  foolproof couscous 137
  gazpacho 96
  get-well-soon chicken broth 60
  harissa butternut squash soup 100
  hot toddy broth 64
  immune-boosting tonic 61
  instant ramen upgrade 168
  Italian penicillin soup 161
  Italian pesto & gnocchi soup 116
  Italian wedding soup 75
  Mexican chicken with fresh tomato salsa 187–188
  miso bone broth 65
  one-pot butter chicken curry 190
  one-pot chicken & leek pie 182–184

perfect Puy lentils 138
polenta quattro formaggi (four cheese polenta) 142
protein power-up (egg drop broth) 64
Provençal garlic & sage broth 61
red daal with crispy onions 151
risotto blanco 152
rosół (classic Polish noodle soup) 171
rustic cabbage & smoked sausage broth 85
rustic French cassoulet 147
sopa de lima (Mexican lime & chicken soup) 81
soto ayam (Indonesian chicken noodle soup) 172
spiced chai bone broth 66
Sri Lankan vegetable & coconut soup 101
sumac-spiced tomatoes & green beans 120
tagliolini al tartufo (pasta with white truffle) 167
Thai green chicken curry 199
ultimate fluffy rice 136
chilli, ultimate 180–181
chillies
  beef rendang with carrot & cabbage salad 202–204
  braised aubergine with spring 132
  chicken vindaloo with a cooling raita 196–197
  hot & sour prawn tom yum 72
  Jamaican oxtail beans 212
  light Keralan fish curry with kachumber (Indian salad) 206
  linguine alle vongole (pasta with clams) 164
  Malaysian monkfish laksa 173
  Mexican chicken with fresh tomato salsa 187–188
  Sichuan spicy beef noodles 174
  sopa de lima (Mexican lime & chicken soup) 81
  Sri Lankan vegetable & coconut soup 101

sticky short rib birria (Mexican style stew) 218
Thai green chicken curry 199
ultimate chilli 180–181
Vietnamese beef pho 177
Chinese chicken & sweetcorn soup 76
chives
  baked potato soup with sour cream & chives 91
  cottage pie with herby lemon mash 192
  cullen skink (Scottish smoked haddock chowder) 117
  leek & mussel chowder in a sourdough bowl 114
chocolate
  bone broth hot chocolate 67
  ultimate chilli 180–181
chondroitin 15, 26
chorizo
  feijoada (Brazilian black bean stew) 148
  ultimate chilli 180–181
chowder
  cullen skink 117
  leek & mussel in a sourdough bowl 114
  Nordic salmon & dill 108
cider: Bristol baked beans with crispy pork belly 154
cinnamon
  bone broth use and method 46
  spiced chai bone broth 66
clams: linguine alle vongole (pasta with clams) 164
cloudiness 53–54
cloves
  bone broth use and method 46
  stifado (Greek beef stew) with feta mash 189
  Vietnamese beef pho 177
cocoa powder: bone broth hot chocolate 67
coconut cream: beef rendang with carrot & cabbage salad 202–204
coconut milk
  light Keralan fish curry with kachumber (Indian salad) 206
  Malaysian monkfish laksa 173

red daal with crispy onions 151
Sri Lankan vegetable & coconut soup 101
Thai green chicken curry 199
coffee: bulletproof coffee bone broth 66
collagen 13–15, 25–26, 28, 54–55
congee with sliced belly pork 153
coq au vin 221
coriander seeds:
  bone broth use and method 46
  ultimate chilli 180–181
cottage pie with herby lemon mash 192–193
courgettes: cheat's ratatouille 122
couscous, foolproof 137
couscous: classic chicken & apricot tagine 185
crab: fennel & crab bisque 98
cream
  bone broth bolognese 194
  'boulangoise' (boulangère meets dauphinoise) 125
  classic cream of mushroom soup 97
  comforting chicken & dumplings 201
  creamed shallots & garlic with pangrattato 121
  creamy asparagus soup with lemon & pancetta pangrattato 95
  creamy mustard-glazed fennel 131
  cullen skink (Scottish smoked haddock chowder) 117
  fennel & crab bisque 98
  Italian pesto & gnocchi soup 116
  leek & mussel chowder in a sourdough bowl 114
  Nordic salmon & dill chowder 108
  one-pot butter chicken curry 190
creatine 14
crème fraîche
  beef tomato soup 94
  comforting chicken & dumplings 201
  eggs florentine soup 90
  one-pot chicken & leek pie 182–184

oven-braised red cabbage with horseradish cream 127
cucumber
    chicken vindaloo with a cooling raita 196–197
    gazpacho 96
    light Keralan fish curry with kachumber (Indian salad) 206
cullen skink (Scottish smoked haddock chowder) 117
curry
    beef kofta curry 200
    beef rendang with carrot & cabbage salad 202–204
    chicken vindaloo with a cooling raita 196–197
    light Keralan fish curry with kachumber (Indian salad) 206
    Malaysian monkfish laksa 173
    one-pot butter chicken 190
    slow-cooked nihari (Pakistani beef stew) 216
    Thai green chicken curry 199

D

daal, red, with crispy onions 151
digestive health 26, 29
dill:
    chunky beetroot borscht 107
    Nordic salmon & dill chowder 108
duck: Cantonese braised duck legs 223

E

East Asia 21–22
eggs
    avgolemono (Greek egg & lemon chicken soup) 78
    beef kofta curry 200
    Bristol baked beans with crispy pork belly 154
    Chinese chicken & sweetcorn soup 76
    eggs Florentine soup 90
    instant ramen upgrade 168
    Italian wedding soup 75
    one-pot chicken & leek pie 182
    protein power-up (egg drop broth) 64
    soto ayam (Indonesian chicken noodle soup) 172
electrolytes 28
equipment 33–34
essential amino acids (EAAs) 14
Europe 22

F

fasolia (lamb & white bean stew) 141
feijoada (Brazilian black bean stew) 148
fennel
    bone broth use and method 45
    cheat's bouillabaisse (classic French fish soup) 82
    creamy mustard-glazed fennel 131
    fennel & crab bisque 98
    pot roast chicken with greens & lemon 215
feta: stifado (Greek beef stew) with feta mash 189
fish
    bone broth ingredients 38
    cheat's bouillabaisse (classic French fish soup) 82
    light Keralan fish curry with kachumber (Indian salad) 206
    Malaysian monkfish laksa 173
    Nordic salmon & dill chowder 108
    one-pot puttanesca 163
fish bone broth
    cheat's bouillabaisse (classic French fish soup) 82
    cullen skink (Scottish smoked haddock chowder) 117
    fennel & crab bisque 98
    hot & sour prawn tom yum 72
    leek & mussel chowder in a sourdough bowl 114
    light Keralan fish curry with kachumber (Indian salad) 206
    linguine alle vongole (pasta with clams) 164
    Malaysian monkfish laksa 173
    Nordic salmon & dill chowder 108
    one-pan prawn jambalaya 145
fish sauce
    beef rendang with carrot & cabbage salad 202–204
    bo kho (Vietnamese beef stew) 205
    hot & sour prawn tom yum 72
    Malaysian monkfish laksa 173
    miyeok-guk (Korean seaweed soup) 86
    Thai green chicken curry 199
    Vietnamese beef pho 177
    yukgaejang (Korean spicy beef soup) 84
flexitarians 19–20
fondant potatoes 130
freekeh: caramelised onion freekeh pilaf 140
freezer use 50
Freja 7, 238

G

galangal: hot & sour prawn tom yum 72
garlic
    bone broth use and method 44
    creamed shallots & garlic with pangrattato 121
    Provençal garlic & sage broth 61
    spring greens with garlic & lemon 126
gazpacho 96
gelatine 14, 27
get-well-soon chicken broth 60
ginger
    beef kofta curry 200
    beef rendang with carrot & cabbage salad 202–204
    bo kho (Vietnamese beef stew) 205
    bone broth use and method 45
    braised aubergine with spring 132
    Cantonese braised duck legs 223
    chicken vindaloo with a cooling raita 196–197
    Chinese chicken & sweetcorn soup 76
    congee with sliced belly pork 153
    immune-boosting tonic 61
    light Keralan fish curry with kachumber (Indian salad) 206
    Malaysian monkfish laksa 173
    one-pot butter chicken curry 190
    red daal with crispy onions 151
    Sichuan spicy beef noodles 174
    slow-cooked nihari (Pakistani beef stew) 216
    soto ayam (Indonesian chicken noodle soup) 172
    spiced chai bone broth 66
    yukgaejang (Korean spicy beef soup) 84
glucosamine 15, 26
glutamine 15, 26
glutathione 15
glycine 14–15, 25, 26, 27, 28
glycosaminoglycans (GAGs) 15, 25
gnocchi: Italian pesto & gnocchi soup 116
gochugaru: yukgaejang (Korean spicy beef soup) 84
goulash, Hungarian smoky beef 113
gravy
    best-ever beef bone broth 207
    best-ever chicken bone broth 209
green beans
    Italian pesto & gnocchi soup 116
    Sri Lankan vegetable & coconut soup 101
    sumac-spiced tomatoes & green beans 120
    Thai green chicken curry 199
gut health 26

H

haddock, smoked:
　cullen skink (Scottish smoked haddock chowder) 117
haemoglobin 14
hair health 25
haricot beans: Bristol baked beans with crispy pork belly 154
harissa butternut squash soup 100
hazelnuts: oven-braised red cabbage with horseradish cream 127
health benefits 13–15, 25–29
heart health 26
homocysteine 26
honey
　classic chicken & apricot tagine 185
　hot toddy broth 64
　immune-boosting tonic 61
horseradish: oven-braised red cabbage with horseradish cream 127
hot & sour prawn tom yum 72
hot toddy broth 64
Hungarian smoky beef goulash 113
hyaluronic acid 15, 25, 26
hydration 15, 19, 25, 28

I

immune system 25
immune-boosting tonic 61
India 22
Indigenous cultures 22
Indonesian chicken noodle soup 172
instant ramen upgrade 168
iron 15
Italian penicillin soup 161
Italian pesto & gnocchi soup 116
Italian wedding soup 75

J

Jamaican oxtail beans 212
jambalaya, one-pan prawn 145
joint health 26

K

kale
　pot roast chicken with greens & lemon 215
　Tuscan ribollita-style minestrone 104
kombu *see* seaweed

L

laksa, Malaysian monkfish 173
lamb
　fasolia (lamb & white bean stew) 141
　youvetsi (Greek orzo with lamb) 166
leeks
　bone broth use and method 44
　Bristol baked beans with crispy pork belly 154
　cheat's bouillabaisse (classic French fish soup) 82
　comforting chicken & dumplings 201
　creamy asparagus soup with lemon & pancetta pangrattato 95
　cullen skink (Scottish smoked haddock chowder) 117
　leek & mussel chowder in a sourdough bowl 114
　Nordic salmon & dill chowder 108
　one-pot chicken & leek pie 182–184
　pot roast chicken with greens & lemon 215
　rosół (classic Polish noodle soup) 171
　yukgaejang (Korean spicy beef soup) 84
lemongrass
　beef rendang with carrot & cabbage salad 202–204
　bo kho (Vietnamese beef stew) 205
　hot & sour prawn tom yum 72
　Malaysian monkfish laksa 173
　Thai green chicken curry 199
lemons
　avgolemono (Greek egg & lemon chicken soup) 78
　basil pesto 122
　bloody bullshot 67
　classic chicken & apricot tagine 185
　creamy asparagus soup with lemon & pancetta pangrattato 95
　fasolia (lamb & white bean stew) 141
　fennel & crab bisque 98
　foolproof couscous 137
　harissa butternut squash soup 100
　hot toddy broth 64
　immune-boosting tonic 61
　Italian penicillin soup 161
　linguine alle vongole (pasta with clams) 164
　one-pot butter chicken curry 190
　one-pot chicken & leek pie 182–184
　ossobuco alla Milanese (braised veal shanks) 222
　pot roast chicken with greens & lemon 215
　red daal with crispy onions 151
　spring greens with garlic & lemon 126
lentils
　perfect Puy lentils 138
　red daal with crispy onions 151
lime leaves
　bone broth use and method 46
　hot & sour prawn tom yum 72
　Thai green chicken curry 199
limes
　beef rendang with carrot & cabbage salad 202–204
　bo kho (Vietnamese beef stew) 205
　chicken vindaloo with a cooling raita 196–197
　hot & sour prawn tom yum 72
　Jamaican oxtail beans 212
　light Keralan fish curry with kachumber (Indian salad) 206
　Malaysian monkfish laksa 173
　Mexican chicken with fresh tomato salsa 187–188
　Sichuan spicy beef noodles 174
　soto ayam (Indonesian chicken noodle soup) 172
　slow-cooked nihari (Pakistani beef stew) 216
　sopa de lima (Mexican lime & chicken soup) 81
　Sri Lankan vegetable & coconut soup 101
　Thai green chicken curry 199
　Vietnamese beef pho 177
　linguine alle vongole (pasta with clams) 164
Liverpudlian beef scouse broth 77

M

magnesium 15, 27
Malaysian monkfish laksa 173
Marmite
　Liverpudlian beef scouse broth 77
　umami Marmite tea 65
melatonin 27
menopause 28–29
methionine 26
Mexican chicken with fresh tomato salsa 187–188
Mexican lime & chicken soup 81
Middle East 23
milk
　baked potato soup with sour cream & chives 91
　bone broth bolognese 194
　bone broth hot chocolate 67
　comforting chicken & dumplings 201
　cullen skink (Scottish smoked haddock chowder) 117
　spiced chai bone broth 66
minerals 15, 19
miso paste
　best-ever beef bone broth gravy 207
　best-ever chicken bone broth gravy 209
　miso bone broth 65
　red wine, porcini & beef cheek ragu 191
miyeok-guk (Korean seaweed soup) 86
monkfish: Malaysian monkfish laksa 173
mood 27
MSG (monosodium glutamate) 23
mushrooms
　arroz caldoso (brothy rice with wild mushrooms) 146
　bone broth use and method 47

Index

boozy beef mushrooms on toast 128
chicken & mushroom pie with tarragon 184
classic cream of mushroom soup 97
coq au vin 221
hot & sour prawn tom yum 72
red wine, porcini & beef cheek ragu 191
yukgaejang (Korean spicy beef soup) 84

mussels
  cheat's bouillabaisse (classic French fish soup) 82
  leek & mussel chowder in a sourdough bowl 114

mustard
  boozy beef mushrooms on toast 128
  Bristol baked beans with crispy pork belly 154
  comforting chicken & dumplings 201
  creamy mustard-glazed fennel 131
  leek & mussel chowder in a sourdough bowl 114
  one-pot chicken & leek pie 182–184

N
nail health 25
Native American cultures 22
nihari, slow cooked 216
noodles
  bo kho (Vietnamese beef stew) 205
  instant ramen upgrade 168
  Malaysian monkfish laksa 173
  rosół (classic Polish noodle soup) 171
  Sichuan spicy beef noodles 174
  soto ayam (Indonesian chicken noodle soup) 172
  Vietnamese beef pho 177
Nordic salmon & dill chowder 108
nose-to-tail eating 17

O
olives: one-pot puttanesca 163

onions
  arroz caldoso (brothy rice with wild mushrooms) 146
  baked potato soup with sour cream & chives 91
  beef kofta curry 200
  beef tomato soup 94
  best-ever beef bone broth gravy 207
  best-ever chicken bone broth gravy 209
  bo kho (Vietnamese beef stew) 205
  bone broth bolognese 194
  bone broth use and method 44
  'boulangoise' (boulangère meets dauphinoise) 125
  Bristol baked beans with crispy pork belly 154
  canja de galinha (Brazilian chicken & rice soup) 217
  caramelised onion freekeh pilaf 140
  cheat's ratatouille 122
  chicken vindaloo with a cooling raita 196–197
  chunky beetroot borscht 107
  classic chicken & apricot tagine 185
  classic cream of mushroom soup 97
  coq au vin 221
  cottage pie with herby lemon mash 192–193
  creamy asparagus soup with lemon & pancetta pangrattato 95
  cullen skink (Scottish smoked haddock chowder) 117
  eggs Florentine soup 90
  feijoada (Brazilian black bean stew) 148
  gazpacho 96
  harissa butternut squash soup 100
  hot & sour prawn tom yum 72
  Hungarian smoky beef goulash 113
  Italian penicillin soup 161
  Italian pesto & gnocchi soup 116
  Italian wedding soup 75
  Jamaican oxtail beans 212
  light Keralan fish curry with kachumber (Indian salad) 206
  Liverpudlian beef scouse broth 77
  Mexican chicken with fresh tomato salsa 187–188
  one-pan prawn jambalaya 145
  one-pot butter chicken curry 190
  ossobuco alla Milanese (braised veal shanks) 222
  oven-braised red cabbage with horseradish cream 127
  red daal with crispy onions 151
  red wine, porcini & beef cheek ragu 191
  risotto blanco 152
  rosół (classic Polish noodle soup) 171
  rustic cabbage & smoked sausage broth 85
  rustic French cassoulet 147
  Scotch beef & barley broth 109
  Sichuan spicy beef noodles 174
  sopa de lima (Mexican lime & chicken soup) 81
  Sri Lankan vegetable & coconut soup 101
  sticky short rib birria (Mexican style stew) 218
  Tuscan ribollita-style minestrone 104
  ultimate chilli 180–181
  ultimate French onion soup 110
  Vietnamese beef pho 177
  youvetsi (Greek orzo with lamb) 166
  yukgaejang (Korean spicy beef soup) 84
oranges: cheat's bouillabaisse (classic French fish soup) 82
ossobuco alla Milanese (braised veal shanks) 222
oxtail
  Jamaican oxtail beans 212
  slow-cooked nihari (Pakistani beef stew) 216
oyster sauce: braised aubergine with spring 132

P
pak choi: Sichuan spicy beef noodles 174
Pakistani beef stew 216
palm sugar: hot & sour prawn tom yum 72
pancetta
  bone broth bolognese 194
  coq au vin 221
  creamy asparagus soup with lemon & pancetta pangrattato 95
paprika: Hungarian smoky beef goulash 113
parsley: bone broth use and method 45
parsnips
  bone broth use and method 44
  rosół (classic Polish noodle soup) 171
pasta
  baked rigatoni with aubergine 162
  bone broth bolognese 194
  Italian penicillin soup 161
  Italian wedding soup 75
  linguine alle vongole (pasta with clams) 164
  one-pot puttanesca 163
  tagliolini al tartufo (pasta with white truffle) 167
  tortellini in brodo 158
  youvetsi (Greek orzo with lamb) 166
peanuts: beef rendang with carrot & cabbage salad 202–204
peas: Italian pesto & gnocchi soup 116
peppercorns
  bone broth use and method 47
  spiced chai bone broth 66
peppers
  cheat's ratatouille 122
  gazpacho 96
  Hungarian smoky beef goulash 113
  one-pan prawn jambalaya 145
  Thai green chicken curry 199
  ultimate chilli 180–181
pesto
  cheat's ratatouille 122
  Italian pesto & gnocchi soup 116

Index

235

pies
  chicken & mushroom pie with tarragon 184
  cottage pie with herby lemon mash 192–193
  one-pot chicken & leek pie 182–184
pilaf, caramelised onion freekeh 140
pine nuts
  caramelised onion freekeh pilaf 140
  cheat's ratatouille 122
polenta quattro formaggi (four cheese polenta) 142
Polish noodle soup 171
pork
  bone broth bolognese 194
  Bristol baked beans with crispy pork belly 154
  congee with sliced belly pork 153
  feijoada (Brazilian black bean stew) 148
  Italian wedding soup 75
  pork bone broth 50
  rustic French cassoulet 147
  ultimate chilli 180–181
potato gnocchi: Italian pesto & gnocchi soup 116
potatoes
  baked potato soup with sour cream & chives 91
  'boulangoise' (boulangère meets dauphinoise) 125
  chunky beetroot borscht 107
  cottage pie with herby lemon mash 192–193
  cullen skink (Scottish smoked haddock chowder) 117
  eggs Florentine soup 90
  fondant potatoes 130
  Liverpudlian beef scouse broth 77
  Nordic salmon & dill chowder 108
  stifado (Greek beef stew) with feta mash 189
prawns
  cheat's bouillabaisse (classic French fish soup) 82
  hot & sour prawn tom yum 72
  one-pan prawn jambalaya 145
pregnancy 28
pressure cookers 33

problem solving 53–55
proline 14, 15, 26
proper beef tea 60
protein power-up 64
proteoglycans 15
Provençal garlic & sage broth 61
puttanesca, one-pot 163

R
raisins: foolproof couscous 137
ramen upgrade, instant 168
ratatouille, cheat's 122
red cabbage
  beef rendang with carrot & cabbage salad 202–204
  oven-braised red cabbage with horseradish cream 127
red wine, porcini & beef cheek ragu 191
rice
  arroz caldoso (brothy rice with wild mushrooms) 146
  avgolemono (Greek egg & lemon chicken soup) 78
  canja de galinha (Brazilian chicken & rice soup) 217
  congee with sliced belly pork 153
  one-pan prawn jambalaya 145
  risotto blanco 152
  ultimate fluffy rice 136
risotto blanco 152
roasting bones 40–41
rosemary: bone broth use and method 45
rosół (classic Polish noodle soup) 171

S
saffron
  cheat's bouillabaisse (classic French fish soup) 82
  classic chicken & apricot tagine 185
sage: Provençal garlic & sage broth 61
salmon: Nordic salmon & dill chowder 108
sausages
  feijoada (Brazilian black bean stew) 148

  rustic cabbage & smoked sausage broth 85
  rustic French cassoulet 147
Scandinavia 22
Scotch beef & barley broth 109
Scottish smoked haddock chowder 117
scouse broth 77
seaweed
  bone broth use and method 47
  miyeok-guk (Korean seaweed soup) 86
serotonin 27
shallots
  beef rendang with carrot & cabbage salad 202–204
  best-ever chicken bone broth gravy 209
  boozy beef mushrooms on toast 128
  Bristol baked beans with crispy pork belly 154
  creamed shallots & garlic with pangrattato 121
  fennel & crab bisque 98
  Malaysian monkfish laksa 173
  soto ayam (Indonesian chicken noodle soup) 172
  stifado (Greek beef stew) with feta mash 189
shellfish: bone broth ingredients 38
Sichuan spicy beef noodles 174
sipping broths 20, 60–67
skimmers 34
skimming 42, 48, 53
skin health 25
sleep 27
slow cookers 33–34
smoked haddock: cullen skink (Scottish smoked haddock chowder) 117
sopa de lima (Mexican lime & chicken soup) 81
soto ayam (Indonesian chicken noodle soup) 172
soups
  avgolemono (Greek egg & lemon chicken soup) 78
  baked potato soup with sour cream & chives 91
  beef tomato soup 94

canja de galinha (Brazilian chicken & rice soup) 217
cheat's bouillabaisse (classic French fish soup) 82
Chinese chicken & sweetcorn soup 76
chunky beetroot borscht 107
classic cream of mushroom soup 97
creamy asparagus soup with lemon & pancetta pangrattato 95
cullen skink (Scottish smoked haddock chowder) 117
eggs Florentine soup 90
fennel & crab bisque 98
gazpacho 96
harissa butternut squash soup 100
hot & sour prawn tom yum 72
Hungarian smoky beef goulash 113
instant ramen upgrade 168
Italian penicillin soup 161
Italian pesto & gnocchi soup 116
Italian wedding soup 75
leek & mussel chowder in a sourdough bowl 114
Liverpudlian beef scouse broth 77
Malaysian monkfish laksa 173
miyeok-guk (Korean seaweed soup) 86
Nordic salmon & dill chowder 108
rosół (classic Polish noodle soup) 171
rustic cabbage & smoked sausage broth 85
Scotch beef & barley broth 109
sopa de lima (Mexican lime & chicken soup) 81
soto ayam (Indonesian chicken noodle soup) 172
Sri Lankan vegetable & coconut soup 101
tortellini in brodo 158
Tuscan ribollita-style minestrone 104
ultimate French onion soup 110

Vietnamese beef pho 177
yukgaejang (Korean spicy beef soup) 84
sour cream: baked potato soup with sour cream & chives 91
South America 23
soy sauce
  bo kho (Vietnamese beef stew) 205
  braised aubergine with spring 132
  Cantonese braised duck legs 223
  Chinese chicken & sweetcorn soup 76
  congee with sliced belly pork 153
  instant ramen upgrade 168
  Jamaican oxtail beans 212
  miyeok-guk (Korean seaweed soup) 86
  Sichuan spicy beef noodles 174
  ultimate chilli 180–181
  yukgaejang (Korean spicy beef soup) 84
spiced chai bone broth 66
spinach
  eggs Florentine soup 90
  instant ramen upgrade 168
  Italian wedding soup 75
spring greens
  pot roast chicken with greens & lemon 215
  spring greens with garlic & lemon 126
spring onions
  beef rendang with carrot & cabbage salad 202–204
  braised aubergine with spring 132
  Chinese chicken & sweetcorn soup 76
  congee with sliced belly pork 153
  instant ramen upgrade 168
  Sichuan spicy beef noodles 174
  soto ayam (Indonesian chicken noodle soup) 172
  Vietnamese beef pho 177

Sri Lankan vegetable & coconut soup 101
star anise: bone broth use and method 46
stifado (Greek beef stew) with feta mash 189
stock compared to broth 16
stock cubes 16, 23
stockpots 33
storage of bone broth 50
strainers 34
sultanas: foolproof couscous 137
sumac-spiced tomatoes & green beans 120
swede: Scotch beef & barley broth 109
sweet potatoes: Sri Lankan vegetable & coconut soup 101
sweetcorn: Chinese chicken & sweetcorn soup 76

T
Tabasco: bloody bullshot 67
tagine, classic chicken & apricot 185
tagliolini al tartufo (pasta with white truffle) 167
tea: spiced chai bone broth 66
Thai green chicken curry 199
thyme: bone broth use and method 45
tom yum, hot & sour prawn 72
tomato juice: bloody bullshot 67
tomatoes
  baked rigatoni with aubergine 162
  beef kofta curry 200
  beef tomato soup 94
  bone broth bolognese 194
  bone broth use and method 47
  cheat's bouillabaisse (classic French fish soup) 82
  cheat's ratatouille 122
  foolproof couscous 137
  gazpacho 96
  hot & sour prawn tom yum 72
  light Keralan fish curry with kachumber (Indian salad) 206

Mexican chicken with fresh tomato salsa 187–188
one-pan prawn jambalaya 145
one-pot puttanesca 163
sopa de lima (Mexican lime & chicken soup) 81
sticky short rib birria (Mexican style stew) 218
stifado (Greek beef stew) with feta mash 189
sumac-spiced tomatoes & green beans 120
ultimate chilli 180–181
youvetsi (Greek orzo with lamb) 166
tortellini in brodo 158
tortillas: sopa de lima (Mexican lime & chicken soup) 81
truffle paste: tagliolini al tartufo (pasta with white truffle) 167
tryptophan 14, 27
turmeric
  bone broth use and method 46
  immune-boosting tonic 61
Tuscan ribollita-style minestrone 104

U
umami Marmite tea 65

V
veal: ossobuco alla Milanese (braised veal shanks) 222
Vietnamese beef pho 177
Vietnamese beef stew 205
vodka: bloody bullshot 67

W
waste reduction 19
weight management 27
whisky: hot toddy broth 64
wine
  arroz caldoso (brothy rice with wild mushrooms) 146
  best-ever beef bone broth gravy 207
  best-ever chicken bone broth gravy 209
  bone broth bolognese 194
  boozy beef mushrooms on toast 128

cheat's bouillabaisse (classic French fish soup) 82
comforting chicken & dumplings 201
coq au vin 221
cottage pie with herby lemon mash 192–193
creamed shallots & garlic with pangrattato 121
creamy mustard-glazed fennel 131
leek & mussel chowder in a sourdough bowl 114
linguine alle vongole (pasta with clams) 164
one-pot puttanesca 163
ossobuco alla Milanese (braised veal shanks) 222
red wine, porcini & beef cheek ragu 191
risotto blanco 152
ultimate French onion soup 110
Worcestershire sauce
  beef tomato soup 94
  bloody bullshot 67
  boozy beef mushrooms on toast 128
  cottage pie with herby lemon mash 192–193
  ultimate French onion soup 110

Y
yoghurt
  chicken vindaloo with a cooling raita 196–197
  one-pot butter chicken curry 190
youvetsi (Greek orzo with lamb) 166
yukgaejang (Korean spicy beef soup) 84

Z
zinc 15

ABOUT FREJA

Freja is Britain's leading bone broth brand, founded with a mission to bring back one of the world's oldest and most nourishing foods, and make it fit seamlessly into modern life. The company was born from a belief that the food we eat should be as wholesome as it is delicious, made with simple, natural ingredients you can trust.

Freja was co-founded by Jessica Leather, a full-time working mum of four, who became frustrated with the lack of healthy, real-food options on supermarket shelves. Longing for the slow-simmered broths of her childhood, Jess and her husband Ed began making their own at home using only high-quality ingredients and traditional cooking methods. What started as a family solution quickly evolved into a mission to make naturally protein-packed, collagen-rich bone broth accessible to everyone.

Today, Freja helps thousands of families and home cooks rediscover the joy of cooking with real, nutritious food. Whether used as the base of a comforting soup, the secret depth in a sauce or simply sipped from a mug for a restorative boost, Freja's bone broths are crafted to make wholesome eating both simple and satisfying.

At Freja our vision is to make natural, nourishing food accessible for everyone – celebrating simple ingredients, traditional methods and the belief that good food should help you feel your best.

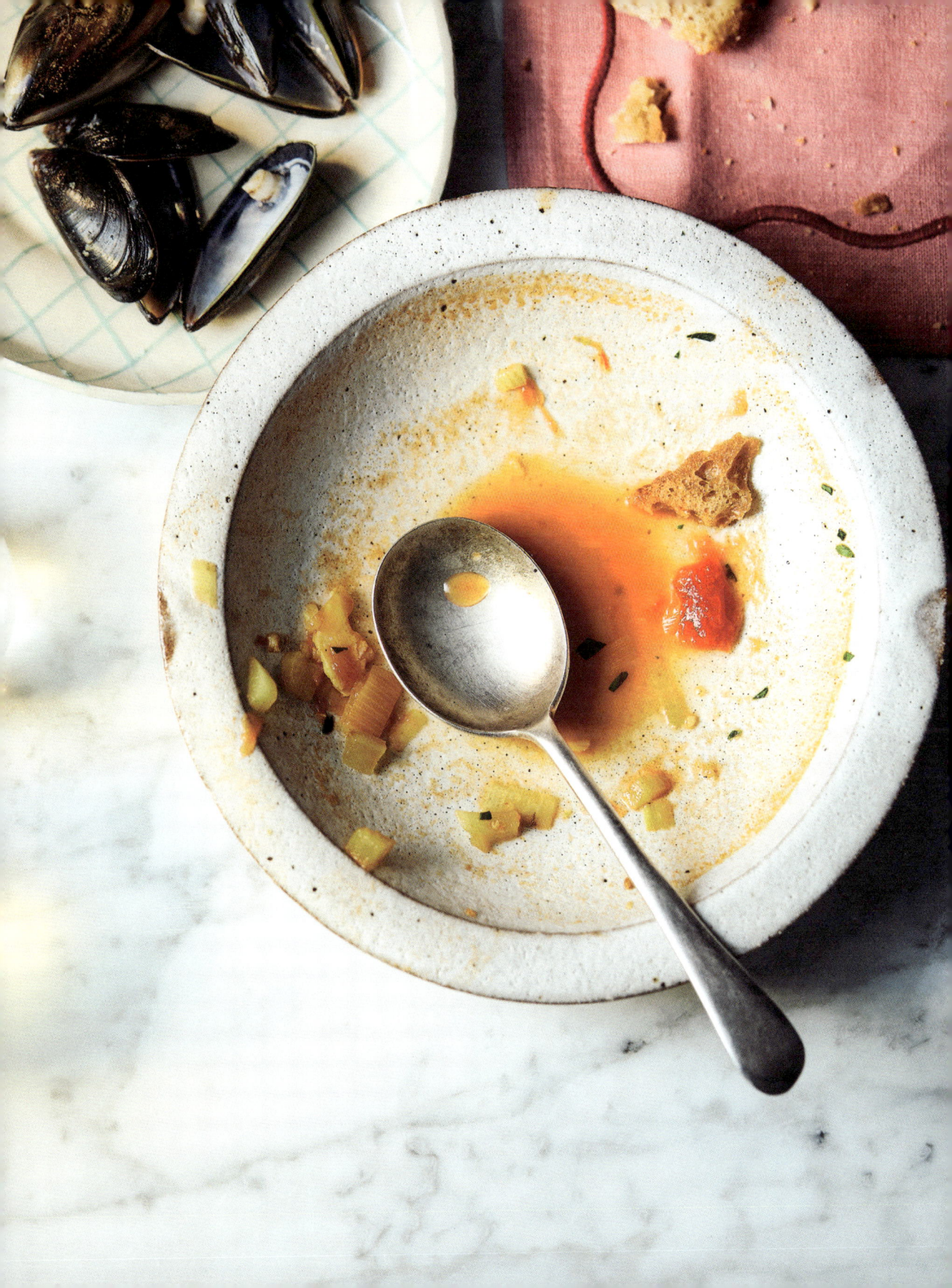

WHEN USING KITCHEN APPLIANCES PLEASE ALWAYS FOLLOW
THE MANUFACTURER'S INSTRUCTIONS

HarperCollins*Publishers*
1 London Bridge Street
London SE1 9GF

www.harpercollins.co.uk

HarperCollins*Publishers*
Macken House, 39/40 Mayor Street Upper
Dublin 1, D01 C9W8, Ireland

First published by HarperCollins*Publishers* 2026

10 9 8 7 6 5 4 3 2 1

Text © Freja 2026
Photography © Andrew Burton 2026

Food styling by Pippa Leon
Prop styling by Faye Wears

Freja assert the moral right to be identified as the author of this work

A catalogue record of this book is available from the British Library

ISBN 978-0-00-879822-2

Printed and bound at GPS

All rights reserved. No part of this publication may be reproduced, stored in a retrieval system, or transmitted, in any form or by any means, electronic, mechanical, photocopying, recording or otherwise, without the prior written permission of the publishers.

Without limiting the exclusive rights of any author, contributor or the publisher of this publication, any unauthorised use of this publication to train generative artificial intelligence (AI) technologies is expressly prohibited. HarperCollins also exercise their rights under Article 4(3) of the Digital Single Market Directive 2019/790 and expressly reserve this publication from the text and data mining exception.

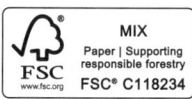